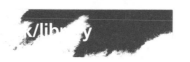

Interventional Pain Control in Cancer Pain Management

Interventional Pain Control in Cancer Pain Management

Edited by

Dr Joan Hester

Consultant in Pain Medicine,
King's College Hospital NHS Foundation Trust,
London
Past President of the British Pain Society

Dr Nigel Sykes

Medical Director and Consultant in Palliative Medicine,
St Christopher's Hospice,
Sydenham,
London

Dr Sue Peat

Consultant in Pain Medicine,
King's College Hospital NHS Foundation Trust,
London

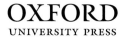

OXFORD
UNIVERSITY PRESS

OXFORD

UNIVERSITY PRESS

Great Clarendon Street, Oxford OX2 6DP

Oxford University Press is a department of the University of Oxford.
It furthers the University's objective of excellence in research, scholarship,
and education by publishing worldwide in

Oxford New York

Auckland Cape Town Dar es Salaam Hong Kong Karachi
Kuala Lumpur Madrid Melbourne Mexico City Nairobi
New Delhi Shanghai Taipei Toronto

With offices in

Argentina Austria Brazil Chile Czech Republic France Greece
Guatemala Hungary Italy Japan Poland Portugal Singapore
South Korea Switzerland Thailand Turkey Ukraine Vietnam

Oxford is a registered trade mark of Oxford University Press
in the UK and in certain other countries

Published in the United States
by Oxford University Press Inc., New York

British Library Cataloguing in Publication Data
Data available

Library of Congress Cataloging in Publication Data
Data available

Typeset in Minion by Cenveo, Bangalore, India
Printed and bound by
CPI Group (UK) Ltd, Croydon, CR0 4YY

ISBN 978–0–19–921908–7

10 9 8 7 6 5 4 3 2 1

Foreword

Professor Irene J. Higginson, BMedSci, BM, BS, PhD, FFPHM, FRCP

I first saw at first hand the importance of interventional pain techniques while working as a junior doctor at St Joseph's Hospice, Hackney, in London, UK, under the leadership of Dr James Hanratty, the medical director. Dr Bob Baxter, the visiting pain specialist, would attend to carry out a variety of interventional pain procedures. The procedures he undertook proved to be a very important component in the care of patients with cancer and non-cancer pain, some of whom had suffered chronic pain for many years. They were helped to live each day well, enjoying time with family and friends.

Pain is one of the most commonly feared symptoms in almost all societies, and one of the first thoughts of patients with cancer is: 'Will I have pain?' These thoughts and fears are quite justified, since 35–96% of patients with cancer will have pain, the incidence and severity being dependent on the type of cancer and the stage of disease. Seventy-five per cent of patients with advanced cancer report pain, which can be overlooked and undertreated by health professionals in many settings. Fortunately, useful assessment measures have been developed for use in palliative care, many of which include pain assessment, e.g. the Edmonton Symptom Assessment System (1) and the Palliative Care Outcome Scale (2).

Managing pain in cancer is becoming more complex, and is liable to become more so as life expectancy is increased, more options become available for the treatment of cancer, and the wide range of co-morbidities experienced by an ageing population become better managed. The World Health Organization (WHO) guidelines on managing cancer pain remain robust and are universally accepted as the core of best practice. This book endorses the principles of the WHO guidance, focusing on those situations where 'adjunct treatments' should be considered. Interventional pain techniques play a valuable role in the management of pain in cancer, and are of significant potential advantage to patients whose pain is not well managed by regular administration of analgesics.

In recent years, as this book shows, there have been considerable developments and improvements in the interventional techniques used, and hence patients can be offered a broader range of strategies. Reversible techniques involving the perineural administration of local anaesthetics and/or opioids administered by constant infusion now largely replace the destructive neurolytic procedures used one or more decades ago. This has reduced some of the fears around interventional techniques, especially the fear of irreversible treatments. Although there is an acknowledged need for greater research into the effectiveness of these approaches, there are numerous case reports demonstrating efficacy, safety, and benefit.

Pain is a multidimensional experience, and the emphasis on listening to the patient's and family's concerns, and individually tailoring treatment, is a core part of this book. Individual specific procedures and their potential place in the management of pain are carefully outlined, offering the reader a detailed overview of the available evidence-based science, illustrated by case reports arising from the authors' extensive practical experience of working in this field. This information will be of advantage to all healthcare professionals involved in the management of patients considering these techniques, explaining what can be expected in terms of procedure, efficacy and potential risk. Neuraxial blocks (epidurals and intrathecals), peripheral nerve and plexus blocks, intrathecal neurolysis, autonomic blockade and cordotomy, as well as wider aspects of management, including nursing care and the use of TENS and acupuncture, are all carefully considered in detail.

This book provides a key guide to interventional pain control for the many specialties concerned with cancer care—palliative care, oncology, surgery, internal medicine, rehabilitation, healthcare of older people—working in all settings: home, hospital, nursing home and hospice. It provides valuable insights into the increasing range of techniques offered by pain specialists, which, when properly integrated into the patients' care, will enable more patients to take advantage of high-quality pain control and improved quality of life.

References

1. Bruera E, Kuehn N, Miller MJ, Selmser P, Macmillan K. (1991) The Edmonton Symptom Assessment System (ESAS): A simple method for the assessment of palliative care patients. *J Palliat Care* 7(2), 6–9.
2. Hearn J, Higginson IJ. (1999) Development and validation of a core outcome measure for palliative care: the palliative care outcome scale. *Qual Health Care* 8(4), 219–27.

Contents

Contributors

Dr Kevin Fai, BSc, MBBS, FRCA
Consultant in Anaesthesia and Pain
Management,
Chronic Pain Unit,
Pembury Hospital,
Maidstone and Tunbridge Wells NHS Trust,
Maidstone,
Kent

**Dr Paul Farquhar-Smith, MA, MB
BChir, FRCA, PhD, FFPMRCA, FFICM**
Consultant in Pain, Anaesthesia and
Intensive Care Medicine,
The Royal Marsden NHS Foundation Trust,
London

Dr Jacqueline Filshie, MBBS, FRCA
Consultant in Anaesthesia and Pain
Management,
Royal Marsden NHS Foundation Trust,
London and Sutton

Ms Margaret Gibbs BSc, MSc, MRPharmS
Specialist Senior Pharmacist,
St Christopher's Hospice,
Sydenham, London

**Dr Richard Griffiths MBBS, FRCA,
FFPMRCA**
Consultant in Anaesthesia and Pain
Management,
Chronic Pain Unit,
Pembury Hospital,
Maidstone and Tunbridge Wells NHS Trust,
Maidstone,
Kent

Ms Rosanna Heal MA, MSc, CQSW
Quality Assurance Adviser,
St Christopher's Hospice,
Sydenham,
London

**Dr Joan Hester, MBBS, FRCA, MSc
(palliative care), FFPMRCA**
Consultant in Pain Medicine,
King's College Hospital NHS
Foundation Trust,
London
Past President of the British Pain Society

**Professor Mark I. Johnson, PhD, BSc,
PGCHE**
Professor of Pain and Analgesia,
Leeds Metropolitan University,
Leeds

**Dr Jon Norman MBBS, FRCA, MRCP,
FFPMRCA**
Consultant in Anaesthesia and Pain
Management,
Chronic Pain Unit,
Pembury Hospital,
Maidstone and Tunbridge Wells NHS Trust,
Maidstone,
Kent

Ms Julie O'Neill, RGN, BSc(Hons)
Ward Manager,
St Christopher's Hospice,
Sydenham,
London

Dr Nicholas Padfield, MBBS, FRCA, FFPMRCA
Consultant in Pain Medicine,
Guys and St Thomas's NHS
Foundation Trust,
London

Dr Sue Peat, BSc, MBBS, FRCA, FFPMRCA
Consultant in Pain Medicine,
King's College Hospital NHS
Foundation Trust,
London

Dr Derek Pounder, MB ChB DA FRCA FFPMRCA
Consultant in Pain Medicine,
St Mary's NHS Trust,
Portsmouth

Nigel Sykes, MA BM BCh FRCP FRCGP
Medical Director and Consultant in
Palliative Medicine,
St Christopher's Hospice,
Sydenham,
London

Professor John W. Thompson, MB, PhD, FRCP, Dip Med Ac
Honorary Consultant in Medical Studies
and Honorary Physician,
St Oswald's Hospice,
Newcastle–upon-Tyne
Formerly Consultant in Charge, Pain
Relief Clinic, Royal Victoria Infirmary,
Newcastle-upon-Tyne

Dr Catherine Elizabeth Urch, FRCP, PhD
Lead Consultant in Palliative Medicine,
Imperial College NHS Trust,
London

Dr Mike Williams, MBBS, FRCA, FFPMRCA, MRCP
Consultant in Anaesthesia and Pain
Management,
St Mary's NHS Trust,
Portsmouth

Chapter 1

Setting the scene

Nigel Sykes

Palliative care as it is known today arose from a desire to relieve the distress of people with cancer. In fact the founding motivation was the distress of one particular man with cancer, a Polish refugee named David Tasma, whose conversations with Cicely Saunders led to the foundation of St Christopher's Hospice and subsequently the worldwide hospice and palliative care movement. The aims of palliative care go far beyond pain control, but the name 'palliative' derives from the Latin 'pallium', meaning 'cloak' and therefore suggests that a prime purpose of the speciality is the cloaking of symptoms arising from a disease that cannot be cured or is not yet cured (but is not necessarily cancer).

The World Health Organization (WHO) places symptom control close to the head of its definition of palliative care, and in their statement the only type of symptom specifically to be identified is pain. No doubt this is because pain is the best known and most feared symptom of cancer, and cancer pain seems widely regarded as being worse than other types of pain. It is, of course, well established that pain is common in cancer, especially in advanced disease. A review of cancer pain prevalence studies found that 74% of 9007 patients reported pain (1) and other estimates range from 38% to 89% depending on the inclusion criteria used. Good pain control for any individual is complicated by the fact that around 80% of people with cancer pain have more than one pain (2), with a median of three pains, each of which might have different mechanisms of causation. Of these pains, between 21% (3) and 49% (4) are reported to be severe, the different estimates again reflecting varying selection criteria and assessment scales.

Pain relief in palliative care was founded on the oral adminstration of morphine. Saunders' work at St Joseph's Hospice at the end of the 1950s marked a rediscovery of the efficacy of morphine when given by mouth. The subsequent demonstration by Twycross that the efficacy of diamorphine, favoured by many doctors in Britain at that time, could be equalled by morphine provided an appropriate dose adjustment was made, and that no more adverse effects resulted, confirmed morphine as the strong opioid of choice for cancer pain relief across the world. In 1986 the WHO issued the first edition of its report *Cancer Pain Relief*, which promoted the regular oral administration of morphine as key to cancer pain management but placed it in the context of a hierarchy of analgesics arranged by potency, often called the 'analgesic ladder' (5). From this point on, cancer pain control rested on the use of drugs 'by the clock and by the ladder', to which the second edition of *Cancer Pain Relief* added 'by mouth', 'for the individual' and 'attention to detail' (6).

The WHO approach to pain control using drugs has been assessed by a number of groups: from the earliest (7) to the latest and largest, which looked at 2118 patients (8). These assessments have found good or satisfactory analgesia to have been achieved in 85–90% of patients.

The effect of the WHO guidance and the organization's accompanying lobbying work to increase morphine availability around the world has been a great increase in the awareness of appropriate use of drugs, especially opioids, to control cancer pain and a new confidence that comfort can be achieved for cancer patients in a wide variety of settings by the use of a relatively simple, standardized approach. A reflection of the effectiveness of the work of the WHO and its Pain and Policy Studies Collaborating Group at the University of Wisconsin is that global morphine consumption has risen from about 3 tonnes in 1985, before the WHO intervention, to almost 40 tonnes now (9). This change in approach to pain management has, in many places, been revolutionary. In particular, the realization that orally administered drugs could provide effective analgesia without unacceptable adverse effects dramatically reduced the reliance that had previously been placed on interventional techniques. In Milan, for instance, the proportion of cancer pain patients receiving nerve blocks fell from 85% to 14% between 1975 and 1987 (10), and similar changes were experienced elsewhere. Such changes in practice were not without repercussions, and some palliative physicians anecdotally experienced a hostile reception when called upon to speak on the WHO approach to pain control in front of audiences that included practitioners of interventional methods.

However, the very success of 'by mouth, by the clock and by the ladder' perhaps brought into sharper relief the minority of patients who remained in an unsatisfactory degree of pain despite the full use of opioids and co-analgesics. Indeed, from the outset, the WHO guidance drew attention to the fact that oral drugs were not necessarily the answer to all types of pain and might need to be combined with or substituted by non-pharmacological interventions such as neurolytic and neurosurgical blocks, as well as other techniques such as radiotherapy (5). The later edition of *Cancer Pain Relief*, which was extensively rewritten, reduced the mention of nerve blocks to inclusion in a table of approaches to pain management and the use of sympathetic blockade as a diagnostic test for sympathetically mediated pain (6). Meanwhile, Swerdlow and Ventafridda had published *Cancer Pain* (11) which, while acknowledging from the evidence then available that drugs could effectively relieve 80–90% of cancer pains, had the express aim of complementing the WHO guidance by 'providing an account of the other modalities—oncological, nerve blocking, neurosurgical' that might help the remaining 10 or 20%. At the same time they placed pain management firmly in the context of rigorous clinical assessment through a multiprofessional approach that took full account of the psychosocial and spiritual as well as the physical dimensions of the pain experience.

There is certainly evidence that the complete mastery of pain that the public image of palliative care sometimes seems to claim is far from the truth. In a series of 111 hospice cancer patients, 50% were pain free or had acceptable relief by the time of the last assessment, but 23% continued to have a quality of pain relief that they felt was unacceptable (12). Most improvement in pain occurred in the first two weeks, after which 97% had at least

50% relief of their pain, but further gains after this time were far less. This is not to imply that all patients necessarily see more complete analgesia as the prime consideration. Another study found that only 39% of palliative care patients with severe pain wanted more treatment. The remainder were too afraid of factors such as the physical and mental side effects of medication, the risks of addiction and were too averse to pills or injections to wish to press for more effective resolution of their pain (13).

Such findings emphasize the more recent WHO document's suggestion that pain control measures must be tailored for the individual: some people are very concerned about swallowing tablets or particular types of medication (perhaps the proliferation of strong opioids in recent years has as much to do with allowing doctor and patient to avoid use of the word 'morphine' as it does with any intrinsic differences in individual response to particular related drugs). Others would rather take any amount of medication than receive a needle prick. At the same time, the analgesic modality of choice depends on the nature of the individual pain as well as that of its owner. A key instance is that of breakthrough pain and, in particular, that subdivision of breakthrough pain termed incident pain, i.e. pain that occurs in response to certain stimuli, most often movement, against a background of otherwise good comfort. Breakthrough pains are common: 218 (89%) of 245 hospice patients with chronic pain also had episodes of breakthrough pain, occurring on average seven times a day but in three-quarters of instances lasting less than 30 minutes (14). The existence of breakthrough pain has a major influence on people's satisfaction with their standard of pain management, 78% of patients without breakthrough pain expressing satisfaction with their analgesia but only 25% of patients with it feeling so positive (14).

A pain that occurs acutely, powerfully but briefly is very hard to control with conventional opioid therapy without giving rise to excessive adverse effects, notably drowsiness, confusion, hallucinations and myoclonus. This is because of the propensity of pain to antagonize such effects of opioids when the dose is proportionate to the pain's intensity. In the case of incident pain, a dose that is high enough to cope with the peak of the pain is excessive in relation to the level of pain that exists most of the time, and hence adverse effects emerge. Here is one situation in which better analgesia may often be achieved by the use of interventional techniques such as nerve blocks, which, by preventing the centrally directed transmission of pain signals, can remove pain from a localized area, whatever its pattern, without the requirement for systemic analgesic drugs.

The purpose of this book is to examine the place and appropriate use of interventional pain techniques in palliative care. Although much diminished compared with what might once have been considered to be the case, the well-directed use of these approaches can achieve good relief in situations where no other analgesic modality could do so. This is not to ignore the importance of other techniques for achieving analgesia, such as the unique effectiveness of radiotherapy for pain arising from metastatic cancer deposits in bone (15), but our focus will be on procedural interventions whose purpose is to interrupt the neural pathways of pain transmission.

The editors' teams, one specializing in pain management and the other a specialist palliative care unit, have worked together for over 30 years. Only about 6% of our palliative care patients receive any form of nerve block (16), but those who do frequently benefit considerably, often when their pain had previously been resistant to all the analgesics used. In a series of 43 patients with ages ranging from 31 to 93 years, neural blockade reduced the median pain score on a 10-point numerical analogue scale from 8 before the procedure to 4 on the day after and 3 one month later. As well as direct benefits to patients there are also considerable educational benefits to palliative care staff from interaction with pain specialist colleagues, and also to pain trainees from the experience they can gain in witnessing analgesic management in a palliative care setting.

However, there is evidence that the possibilities of such a joint approach are not realized in the UK to the extent that they ought to be. A survey of 220 palliative medicine consultants found that although 80% of them had access to a specialist pain service, 55% had made use of it on four or fewer occasions in the last year even though almost all saw over 100 new patients a year. Just 15% had regular weekly sessions with the pain service and trainees in pain management came to only 7% of the palliative care services. On the whole, however, the palliative physicians were satisfied with the availability of pain services, suggesting a lack of appreciation of their possibilities rather than a lack of access (17).

Viewed from the other side, 32% of 106 pain specialists received no more than two referrals relating to patients receiving palliative care. It was notable that, where joint sessions in a palliative care unit existed, referrals were greater, but such arrangements were in place for only 10% of respondents. No less than 63% of pain specialists used hours outside their job plan to accommodate palliative care referrals (18). In addition to an apparent widespread under-use of interventional techniques in palliative care analgesia, there also emerges from these studies a discrepancy in the understanding of the pain specialists' role between the two groups. More than 75% of pain specialists considered they could contribute usefully to advice on drug management of analgesia, whereas less than 25% of palliative physicians viewed them in this light.

It therefore seems that there is a shortfall in the level of mutual understanding and activity between palliative medicine and pain specialists. This must be acting against the best interests of a needy minority of palliative care patients. This situation among doctors may be compounded by a lack of confidence and knowledge elsewhere among the staff of palliative care units, of whom 29%, even of those with full-time consultant medical cover, still felt unable to cope with epidural injections.

It is these issues that this book is intended to address. We aim to explain the place of the techniques available and what is involved in carrying them out and in caring for the patients afterwards. Although interventional approaches to analgesia have a more technical dimension than those generally used in palliative care, requiring specific skills and training for their performance, they still properly belong in the context of a multiprofessional approach to pain control and this book is intended also to reflect that understanding. At the same time, its focus is on encouraging a more appropriate level of use of these procedures in palliative care and so complements rather than repeats the standard accounts of the use of drugs for analgesia in the specialty. It assumes that readers from palliative care will know that material already and hopes that they will recognize that pain specialists know it too!

References

1. Bonica J, Ventafridda V, Twycross RG (1990). Cancer pain. In: Bonica J (ed.). *The Management of Pain* (2nd edn), pp. 400–401. Lea and Febiger, Philadelphia.

2. Twycross RG, Fairfield S (1982). Pain in far-advanced cancer. *Pain* **14**(3), 303–310.

3. Vainio A, Auvinen A (1996). Prevalence of symptoms among patients with advanced cancer: an international collaborative study. *J Pain Symptom Manage* **12**(1), 3–10.

4. Grond S, Zech D, Diefenbach C *et al.* (1994). Prevalence and pattern of symptoms in patients with cancer pain: a prospective evaluation of 1635 patients referred to a pain clinic. *J Pain Symptom Manage* **9**(6), 372–382.

5. WHO (1986). *Cancer Pain Relief.* WHO, Geneva.

6. WHO (1996). *Cancer Pain Relief* (2nd edn). WHO, Geneva.

7. Takeda F (1986). Results of field-testing in Japan of the WHO Draft Interim Guidelines on relief of cancer pain. *Pain Clinic* **1**(2), 83–89.

8. Zech DF, Grond S, Lynch J *et al.* (1995). Validation of the WHO Guidelines for cancer pain relief: a ten year prospective study. *Pain* **63**(1), 65–76.

9. International Narcotics Control Board (2009). Consumption of the principal narcotic drugs. In: International Narcotics Control Board. *Narcotic Drugs 2008*, pp. 248–49. United Nations, New York.

10. Baines M (1989). Pain relief in active patients with cancer: analgesic drugs are the foundation of management. *BMJ* **298**(6665), 36–38.

11. Swerdlow M, Ventafridda V (eds) (1987). *Cancer Pain.* MTP Press, Lancaster.

12. Twycross R, Harcourt J, Bergl S (1996). A survey of pain in patients with advanced cancer. *J Pain Symptom Manage* **12**(5), 273–282.

13. Weiss SC, Emanuel LL, Fairclough DL *et al.* (2001). Understanding the experience of pain in terminally ill patients. *Lancet* **357**(9265), 1311–1315.

14. Zepetella G, O'Doherty C, Collins S (2000). Prevalence and characteristics of breakthrough pain in cancer patients admitted to a hospice. *J Pain Symptom Manage* **20**(2), 87–92.

15. Hoskin PJ (2008). Management of bone pain. In: Sykes N, Bennett MI, Yuan CS (eds). *Cancer Pain* (2nd ed), pp. 256–269. Hodder Arnold, London.

16. Ellershaw JE, Wilkinson P, Durcan T *et al.* (1996). Is there a role for neural blockade in the control of unrelieved pain in hospice inpatients? *Palliative Med* **10**(1), 61.

17. Linklater GT, Leng ME, Tiernan EJ *et al.* (2002). Pain management services in palliative care: a national survey. *Palliative Med* **16**(5), 435–9.

18. Kay S, Husbands E, Antrobus JH *et al.* (2007). Provision for advanced pain management techniques in adult palliative care: a national survey of anaesthetic pain specialists. *Palliative Med* **21**(4), 279–84.

Chapter 2

Difficult pain problems

Sue Peat and Joan Hester

In this chapter we will discuss the use of interventional techniques in situations where they are most helpful: where they can typically offer very significant improvement in pain relief and quality of life. Properly used interventional techniques can provide rapid onset analgesia with few side effects or complications. They are not commonly undertaken, being used in only 3.5% of patients receiving specialist palliative care in one large multi-centre study, and as would be expected, the frequency of use depends to some degree on the expertise of individual teams (1).

Prospective audits have demonstrated effectiveness of interventional techniques in selected patients, where they can produce highly significant reduction in pain scores and improvement in performance status (1, 2) over and above that which would be obtainable without their use. They must be integrated with other analgesic modalities appropriate to the needs of the patient, which may well include continuation of systemic analgesia, radiotherapy and physical methods of pain relief. These can be considered in parallel with interventional techniques and can be used to facilitate them. For example, it is recommended that patients with painful bone metastases should be offered palliative radiotherapy, since an evidence-based approach indicates that they will benefit from this (3). Transport to a radiotherapy centre and positioning for the treatment can be greatly helped by the use of interventional techniques, which also have a place in the patient's ongoing care if the onset of the resulting analgesia from radiotherapy is delayed.

It is vital that the staff looking after patients undergoing these procedures have access to the skills needed to manage them optimally, and that they have clear plans for managing potential side effects and complications. This must include plans for what to do and who to contact in the event of treatment failure. The use of these techniques in a hospital setting has been demonstrated to be highly effective in terms of reduction in pain scores and reduction in the requirement for systemic analgesia in palliative patients (2). Although interventional techniques are much easier to perform in hospital, most of them are transferable to a hospice, or even a home setting.

The issue of consent needs to be carefully considered in patients who are in extreme pain and whose decision making ability is affected by disease and/or drugs. Acting in the best interests of the patient often means that interventional techniques need to be performed in circumstances that would be considered suboptimal outside of a palliative care setting. Pre-intervention investigation (e.g. MRI scanning before insertion of epidural catheters, X-ray to confirm the position of fractures, assessment of coagulation and metabolic status) is often difficult, impossible or inappropriate, particularly in the terminally ill. X-ray screening, routinely used to assist in correct needle placement when managing chronic non cancer pain, will often be completely out of the question. However ultrasound, which is portable and non-invasive, can be of assistance in some situations, particularly when the anatomy is abnormal. Standard 'anaesthetic' monitoring and resuscitation equipment is not available in most hospices. Patient positioning, provision of safe sedation and maintenance of sterility will be difficult, particularly in patients with extremely limited cardiovascular and respiratory reserve, electrolyte disturbances and abnormal states of hydration. Portable monitoring and resuscitation equipment, the immediate availability of emergency drugs, and most of all the presence of skilled assistance, are all vital to the safe and effective use of interventional techniques. This is especially the case when neurolytic, epidural or intrathecal blocks are being undertaken.

We will consider the place of interventional techniques in the following 'difficult' situations:

- fractures
- spinal cord/cauda equina compression
- chest wall pain
- nerve plexus invasion
- visceral upper abdominal pain
- rectal pain
- neural blockade in the opioid toxic patient
- perioperative management of patients dependent on high-dose opioids
- head and neck cancer
- non-cancer pain in palliative care patients.

Fractures

The management of patients with acute fractures presents considerable challenges in palliative care. Conventional assessment and surgical stabilization may be appropriate and should be considered, but is unlikely to be a realistic option in many patients, particularly for those who are terminally ill. Adequate X-ray is vital if the patient is to be assessed for surgical treatment, and in particular the full length of any fractured long bone must be included in the examination. If the patient has experienced prior pain at the site of the fracture, it is probably pathological, but this should not be assumed unless the patient is known to have metastases at the fracture site. The provision of analgesia, particularly if the patient will need to be transported for assessment and further management, is the first priority. Although simple measures to support the affected bone, and the use of a non-steroidal anti-inflammatory drugs combined with opioids may give some pain relief, these will often not provide good analgesia, particularly if the patient moves. Even providing simple nursing care for patient with pelvic, spinal or lower limb fractures may induce severe pain. If the site of the fracture is obvious and surgery is not being contemplated, then simple measures such as the liberal application of EMLA (a eutectic mixture of lidocaine 2.5% and prilocaine 2.5% creams), covered by an occlusive dressing to the fracture site may be very helpful and is free from systemic side effects. There may be skin reactions, which subside when the cream is removed.

Case study

An epidural success?

Saturday morning, 9.30. The phone rang, bringing an unfamiliar and uncertain sounding voice . . .

'Dr Sykes asked me to ring about a patient he feels may need an epidural'.

The patient had fallen during the night; the diagnosis was clear from the end of the bed, she had a mid-shaft femoral fracture. Due to extreme difficulties with pain control she had been very heavily sedated and her leg was in the most unphysiological position imaginable. Even with high-dose opioids, moving her was 'impossible', even with 'stats' on top of the large doses of opioid running via a syringe driver. A quick assessment made it clear that, in anaesthetic/surgical terms, she was 'not fit for a haircut'. Her pulse was just about palpable, and she was clearly very 'dry'. We briefly conferred and agreed that an epidural for pain relief would be in her best interests. The fracture was at the site of a known metastasis. She had been admitted for assessment and terminal care and also suffered with many co-morbidities. Although her relatives were not immediately contactable we made the decision to go ahead with the epidural.

The patient did not flinch when cannulated and intravenous fluids improved her clinical cardiovascular state. A small dose of propofol enabled us to turn her, although once she was in position she developed respiratory obstruction requiring continuous support of her airway.

An epidural was easily inserted, and administration of 10 mL 0.25% bupivicane injected down the catheter meant passive movement of the leg was possible without obvious pain—a nice indication that she was going to get very good pain relief. An ampoule of ephedrine equally divided between her left buttock and the remains of the intravenous fluids staved off the expected acute hypotension.

Her nurses and I were very happy with our performance, everything looked absolutely fine. She was now breathing nicely, had a good palpable pulse and did not react to having her leg moved. I removed her syringe driver and was looking forward to a quick cup of coffee whilst writing up the notes.

'Sue?' Said a familiar voice behind me, 'Now what are you up to?'

The hospice communication had been highly effective; it was one of the senior nurses on duty who had come armed with a pump and bupivicaine. We reviewed the patient's pre-fracture opioid requirements together, and worked out how much diamorphine to put into the infusion.

It felt like a real success story. By midday she had woken up, was pain free and had even had a little to eat. We all know that the patient had very little time to live; she was very cachexic, had multiple bone metastases, and both liver and renal failure. However, she enjoyed a pain free last week of her life. This was acute, multidisciplinary palliative care at its best.

Almost a year later, when the trainee was due to leave St Christopher's for the next bit of her rotation we were discussing the role of anaesthetists in hospices. She described her 'horrendous' first weekend on call. She had been struggling to provide good pain relief for a patient with a metastatic fracture of the femur, and her aim had been to provide a peaceful, pain-free death. Then she was asked by one consultant to ring another consultant and ask them to undertake a highly invasive procedure on this poor dying patient. The anaesthetist she was asked to call came in a rush, failed to communicate with her adequately or take any sort of consent.

Then things got worse—she was asked to assist with a procedure she had never previously seen. The use of propofol, turning a patient with a clearly broken leg and managing respiratory obstruction was all very disturbing. Although it was very clear that both the nurses and the anaesthetist knew each other well, and were perfectly comfortable with the procedure, from her point of view she had been left with a semi-conscious patient receiving an infusion of a drug she had never heard of given via a pump she had never seen. The incomprehensible abbreviations left in the notes were little help. She had no idea how she would answer any questions from the relatives, and exposing her ignorance to anyone or sharing how she felt was completely out of the question; it seemed like everyone but her knew exactly what was going on.

Learning point

Epidural infusions can give excellent pain control for patients with lower limb fractures. Make certain that all who are involved in their care are included in the decision making and are aware of what the procedure involves and what results can be expected, particularly when these are undertaken as an emergency.

Long bone and pelvic fractures

Good analgesia can be provided for lower limb and pelvic fractures using epidural or intrathecal infusions (see Chapters 5 and 6). These techniques are well within the expertise of most anaesthetists and if surgery is to be considered they can be used to provide analgesia for transport and throughout the perioperative period. Turning the patient into the lateral position to insert an epidural or intrathecal catheter can in itself be very painful in the presence of a fracture, and a second anaesthetist will be required to give adequate sedation. However, it is well worth the effort. Usually pain control becomes much less problematic once the fracture has been surgically stabilized, and neuraxial infusions can then be discontinued. If further assessment and surgery are not being considered, the doses required to provide analgesia will be high and will result in bilateral motor weakness, urinary retention and possible haemodynamic instability. However, with adequate planning and care this may well not prevent the patient being hoisted into a wheelchair. If the patient is not experiencing pain above the level of the block then the requirement for systemic analgesia will be markedly reduced.

Brachial plexus, lumbar plexus or appropriate peripheral nerve blocks (e.g. femoral nerve block, which is easily carried out without moving the patient) offer the advantage of unilateral, rather than bilateral, motor block for patients with upper and lower limb fractures, and do not induce urinary retention or haemodynamic instability. More than one injection may be needed to block all nerves to the fracture site, and care needs to be taken in order to avoid local anaesthetic toxicity. Peripheral and plexus blocks are less commonly used than epidural or intrathecal infusions in cancer pain management, in part due to anatomical abnormalities that may be caused by the tumour. They are best undertaken by a specialist with experience of their use, and when correctly placed can give superb analgesia. The use of portable ultrasound for nerve location will make these blocks much safer and more accessible in the future as the quality and use of ultrasound increases. A 'single-shot' block will result in short-term analgesia, which may be useful as a temporary measure, e.g. for transporting a patient or for assessing their suitability for the insertion of a neuraxial catheter. Lumbar and brachial plexus blocks are relatively easy to perform without imaging, and a catheter can be left in situ (see Chapter 8).

Acute rib fractures

Acute rib fractures can considerably interfere with breathing, since each breath is painful, and this can compromise respiratory function. If a rib fractures in two places the patient may develop a 'flail segment' with paradoxical respiration, i.e. sucking in of the chest wall during inspiration. This further compromises respiration and may lead to haemothorax, pneumothorax or infection.

Rib fractures are common in patients with chronic obstructive pulmonary disease who have taken long-term steroids and have osteoporosis, or they may be due to rib metastases or invasion of the rib from an underlying tumour. The diagnosis is principally clinical and can usually be confirmed on palpation of the affected rib(s). X-ray can be used to confirm the clinical diagnosis, but is often not necessary.

Intercostal nerve blocks are easy to undertake and can offer very good pain relief, but often three intercostal nerves need to be blocked to give total pain relief for one rib fracture. Single-shot blocks with bupivacaine will last approximately 6–12 h, allowing the patient a good night's sleep, the opportunity to consider further options and physiotherapy if appropriate. If more than three ribs are affected, consideration should be given to a thoracic epidural, interpleural or paravertebral block (see Chapters 5, 6 and 8).

Spinal cord/cauda equina compression

Typically, this presents with bilateral pain relating to the level(s) of the compression, combined with a sensory and motor neurological deficit. Retention of urine and loss of peri-anal sensation are features of cauda equina syndrome. At the onset the patient will often describe the pain as 'like being sawn in half'. Typically the pain can lessen once compression has become complete. The main aim should be rapid MRI assessment combined with high-dose steroids and evaluation for radiotherapy or surgical decompression (3).

If this is not appropriate, or the patient can not be moved due to pain, then insertion of an epidural well above the level of the lesion will provide good analgesia. It may make transport for MRI and positioning for scanning and radiotherapy possible. If active treatment is being considered, or the diagnosis is uncertain, it should be remembered that any developing motor block that is not responding to a reduction in the concentration and infusion rate of local anaesthetic may reflect progression of compression rather than a side effect of the infusion.

Chest-wall pain

Chest-wall pain can be secondary to direct invasion of the intercostal nerves or irritation of the pleura. Careful assessment with respect to the cause of the pain is vital, as this will significantly affect treatment strategy.

If pain is of sudden onset, unilateral and particularly if it is 'neuropathic' in nature, then it should be remembered that herpes zoster, or shingles, not infrequently occurs in immuno-suppressed patients. Pain can precede the appearance of the rash; it may affect two or three dermatomes, more commonly the thoracic dermatomes, though it can affect the trigeminal nerve, usually the ophthalmic branch, or any other nerve root (see the Appendix). The pain is typically spontaneous, stabbing in quality and associated with extreme allodynia (touch perceived as being painful) of the affected skin. Acute herpes zoster is caused by reactivation of the chicken pox virus in the dorsal root ganglia. Appropriate treatment is the prescription of an antiviral agent. The antineuropathic analgesics (eg amitriptyline, gabapentin, pregabalin) can be effective, as may tramadol. Lidocaine 5% plasters can be applied to the skin once the rash has healed.

If the pain, and particularly neurological deficit, involves the posterior chest wall close to the midline, then the possibility of tumour extension into the epidural space should be considered. This means that all interventions 'downstream' of the lesion (e.g. intercostal nerve block, interpleural infusions) will be ineffective, and placement of an epidural catheter may be difficult. However, an epidural is well worth considering, for both bilateral and unilateral pain. If the pain is unilateral then cordotomy can give highly effective results, particularly in patients with mesothelioma, and the prior placement of an epidural in order to provide temporary analgesia whilst this procedure is considered can be very useful (see Chapter 10).

Nerve plexus invasion

Tumour invasion of the lumbar plexus occurs typically in advanced cervical cancer, although it can be caused by any tumour that spreads into the psoas compartment or paravertebral space at L2, 3 and 4. Tumour invasion of the brachial plexus occurs typically from advanced breast cancer, although a Pancoast tumour of the lung can also be responsible. The pain is typically 'neuropathic' in nature, and will be referred within the distribution of the nerves affected. The configuration of the lumbar plexus is more variable than the brachial plexus, and potential involvement of the sacral plexus should be considered in patients with lower-limb pain secondary to cervical cancer (see Chapter 8).

Case study

A reason for late presentation

'Celia' had a tragic history, and she was admitted to St Christopher's for symptom control under what may have been false pretences. The true story appeared to be that she came from Nigeria and for a while had lived in France, where she had two young children currently living with her estranged partner. She first noticed symptoms of her cervical cancer four or five years previously, but since she was 'an illegal' and was not entitled to treatment in France she had had no option but to just ignore them. She had come to England under a false name, and was living in a room in her 'cousin's' flat when she began to suffer intolerable pain in both legs and intermittent urinary retention. Communication was difficult due both to language barriers and her social history. Her only visible support was from an evangelical church. Her pastor and her 'sisters' visited her regularly.

Her pain appeared to be bilateral, neuropathic in nature, extending to both feet. Examination of her perineum was impossible due to extreme pain when she attempted to abduct her thighs. Even with high dose opioids she was only just comfortable lying on her back at 45 degrees. Examination of the abdomen revealed a large and painful pelvic mass, of uncertain nature. Assessment and management was not going to be helped by her high BMI—she weighed over 120 kg. The minimal investigations she had had left us in no doubt that she had very advanced disease. Attempts at putting in a urinary catheter were clearly going to fail and exacerbate her distress, and her renal function was rapidly deteriorating.

We contacted the urologists who were happy to accept her as an emergency 'day case' and we planned to transfer her to hospital for ultrasound assessment and insertion of an epidural. She could not sit up or lie on her side without extreme pain. She had excessive lumbar lordosis and the spinous processes were not palpable. Giving her a general anaesthetic would have been a significant risk. We inserted an intrathecal catheter with her standing leaning forward on the operating table, and used it to provide spinal anaesthetia for clinical examination, ultrasound assessment and subsequent insertion of a suprapubic catheter.

Her renal function improved significantly over the following three days, and good pain control was provided via the intrathecal catheter with 0.5% bupivicaine running via a syringe driver at 1–2 mL/h. Being pain free very much facilitated her being open to assistance with her social situation, and her children were enabled to visit her before she died.

Learning point

Advanced pelvic cancer can cause very severe neuropathic pain which is not liable to respond well to opioids alone, together with renal failure secondary to obstruction. Consider whether an interventional technique used to facilitate assessment and management could be also be used to provide ongoing pain relief.

Patients with cervical cancer are at risk of bilateral lumbar plexus involvement, and motor weakness in both lower limbs is a common finding. Lumbar plexus blocks are liable to be unreliable due to anatomical considerations and the unpredictable extent of the tumour invasion, but lumbar epidurals will often give superb pain control. Motor block is a particular problem in these patients, since they often already have a significant deficit, and even low doses of bupivicaine may compromise mobility. Under these circumstances ropivicaine may theoretically improve mobility without compromising pain control, although there is little clinical evidence that this agent provides significantly less motor block at equi-analgesic doses when compared with bupivicaine (see Chapter 8).

Pain secondary to brachial plexus invasion at the level of the axilla may well benefit from blockade at a higher level (e.g. supraclavicular or interscalene). A catheter can be inserted at these levels to provide continuous analgesia. Before this is contemplated, a careful assessment of the areas should be undertaken since disease in the nodes at this level may make this approach inadvisable. Before any block is performed it is preferable to have an MRI scan of the plexus, to evaluate the possibility of disease higher in the plexus or at cervical level. This will also differentiate pain secondary to recurrence from that due to radiation-induced fibrosis (see Chapter 8). Ultrasound may be a useful way of identifying the appropriate nerve branches, but if the tumour is closely applied to the nerves, local anaesthesia will not be effective. Neuromodulation techniques (see Chapter 11) may offer a way of providing pain relief; cordotomy (see Chapter 10) or a high cervical epidural (see Chapter 6) could also be considered. Dorsal root entry zone lesions have been successfully used in the treatment of brachial plexopathy (4).

Visceral upper abdominal pain

Upper abdominal pain arising from the liver, pancreas or stomach is particularly responsive to coeliac plexus block, which is one of the few situations where randomized controlled trials of neural blockade versus medical management have been carried out. These demonstrated superiority for coeliac plexus block in terms of pain relief and quality of life; overall opioid consumption was reduced in one study (Stefaniak) (5) but not in the another (Wong) (6). These studies are discussed in more detail in Chapter 9.

It is important to assess the patient carefully and ascertain whether the pain is principally visceral in nature or if there is an added somatic component. Patients with dull, poorly localized epigastic pain, exacerbated by palpation of the epigastrium and/or the tumour mass, and with no evidence of spread to the posterior body wall on imaging, are more likely to respond well to a coeliac plexus block than those with additional 'body-wall' pain in a dermatomal distribution, caused by para-aortic nodes or tumour invasion of the posterior abdominal wall.

During assessment of these patients it is important to appreciate that pain resulting from transection of the intercostal nerves and subsequent neuroma formation following surgery (common after bilateral subcostal incisions) may also be present. This can be associated with allodynia or hyperalgesia of the skin in a dermatomal distribution, and this pain is also exacerbated by palpation. This type of neuropathic pain will not respond to coeliac plexus block, but the patient may well benefit from local injection of steroid (methylprednisolone) into the affected neuroma sites or to local application of 5% lidocaine plasters.

Permanent paraplegia following coeliac plexus block is a rare but significant complication of the procedure, with a reported incidence of 0.15% (4 in 2,730 cases). This data comes from a postal audit carried out in British hospitals between 1986 and 1990, and the information reported was retrospective and anecdotal (7). The techniques and imaging used in the audited patients were variable and often unknown, but this report caused the technique to wane in popularity, almost to the point of extinction, despite the improved pain relief and quality of life that it offers. The safety of the procedure has improved in recent years. Impotence and temporary haemodynamic instability are other potential risks of neurolytic coeliac plexus block. Careful discussion must be undertaken before contemplating this procedure (see Chapter 9).

If the cancer is advanced and in close proximity to the coeliac ganglia, a neurolytic coeliac plexus block may not be effective, since the neurolytic solution cannot reach the ganglia. An up-to-date CT scan should be performed to assess the situation prior to deciding whether a coeliac or splanchnic block is most suitable, and wether this is liable to be feasible (see Chapter 9). If the tumour is invading the posterior abdominal wall, causing somatic pain, or if a neurolytic coeliac plexus block is delayed for any reason, an epidural catheter, sited at mid thoracic level, may be a good option.

Rectal pain

Patients with recurrence in the rectum or rectal stump, following resection of a colonic tumour, can present with both pain and tenesmus, which is sometimes so severe they are unable to sit. This is usually described as a 'burning' pain, and in some patients will respond to topical application of local anaesthetic. If this fails, and particularly if the patient has a permanent colostomy and is already catheterized, then blocking the nerves to the perineum will give effective pain relief with few side effects. This can be done using a 'saddle block', which is performed by injecting 0.5–1 mL of heavy local anaesthetic or phenol into the cerebrospinal fluid with the patient sitting. Urinary retention is a common side effect if the patient is not catheterized, and some patients do not like the resulting area of numbness, which gives the feeling of 'sitting on a ball'. A 'trial block' with local anaesthetic is advisable before phenol is used (see Chapter 8). Ganglion of Impar block or bilateral lumbar sympathetic block are also possibilities for rectal pain and tenesmus (see Chapter 9).

The opioid-toxic patient

Peripheral nerve blocks and epidural or intrathecal techniques are particularly useful in patients whose pain has not responded to opioid escalation and/or are suffering from opioid toxicity. Pain assessment in opioid toxic patients is notoriously difficult, and they often have pain at multiple sites resulting from different pathologies. An assessment of the distribution and dermatomal level of the pain will assist in decision making regarding the appropriateness of peripheral blocks and in evaluating the optimal spinal level for siting epidural catheters. A dermatomal chart is very helpful in this context (see Appendix 1). Somatic pain restricted to small areas supplied by a single nerve root, in the distribution of the brachial or lumbar plexus, or in the distribution of a single peripheral nerve may well benefit from the use of these techniques (see Chapter 8). Any patient whose pain is below T4 and for whom pain control has become 'impossible' may benefit from an epidural or intrathecal local anaesthetic and opioid infusion, whatever the cause or nature of the pain. Such blocks may also be helpful in patients with pain above this level, although high thoracic and cervical techniques are technically challenging and far less commonly used. (see Chapters 5 and 6). Capacity to consent will need to be carefully considered (see Chapter 7).

It has been known for some time that good, long-term results can be obtained in cancer patients with 'refractory' pain using epidural or intrathecal delivery of opioids or opioid and local anaesthetic mixtures (see Chapters 5 and 6). The basic concept lying behind these techniques is the delivery of local anaesthetic directly onto a part of the nervous system responsible for transmitting the pain, and delivery of high concentrations of opioids into the cerebrospinal fluid, from where they gain direct access to the spinal cord and brain. In addition to this a 'synergistc' action between opioids and local anaesthetics can occur.

Exceedingly high levels of drug in the cerebrospinal fluid relative to plasma levels can be achieved using intrathecal and epidural administration, which may well contribute to the improved pain control achieved. The pharmacokinetics of centrally delivered opioids is complex, but may explain their differing efficacy and side effect profile (8, 9). It is also possible that the mechanism by which opioids 'work' is affected by the route of administration—for example in humans intrathecal (but not intravenous) opioids precipitate release of adenosine from the spinal cord (10). Whatever the scientific basis behind its use may be, it is clear that, in selected patients, intrathecal morphine can offer effective and prolonged analgesia when other routes of administration have failed or been associated with unacceptable side effects (11).

The choice between the intrathecal or epidural route will depend on the site of the pain, the patient's anatomy, locally available equipment and, most critically, on the clinical judgement of the operator, particularly if facilities are suboptimal. Anatomical factors, such as scoliosis, previous surgery/radiotherapy and actual or probable malignancy within the spinal canal, can make these blocks exceedingly difficult to perform and render the results less predictable than in patients with normal anatomy, but are no contraindications to their use. There are few data relating to the calculation of an appropriate dose of intrathecal opioid for use in patients previously exposed to high systemic doses, but an oral:intrathecal dose ratio of 100:1 can be used as a good initial working guide if opioids are used in combination with local anaesthetics (12).

Following the instigation of a successful block and reduction of oral and systemic opioids, the patient will need careful and regular assessment of conscious level and opioid requirement. The local anaesthetic component of the epidural infusion will contribute significantly to the patient's analgesia and hence the overall opioid requirement will be greatly reduced. Adequate arrangements must be made for fine and rapid titration of the doses, concentrations and infusion rates used, and bolus injections may be required to give optimum pain control, particularly when these infusions are first initiated. The sudden reduction in pain stimulus may be accompanied by excessive sedation, and an acute reduction of oral and systemic opioids in opioid-dependent patients can lead to withdrawal symptoms, especially vomiting and diarrhoea. However, even small doses of oral or systemic opioids can be effective in preventing or managing withdrawal.

Perioperative management of opioid-dependent patients

Patients dependent on high doses of opioids who are undergoing major surgery require careful peri-operative management. Opioid 'debt' easily occurs if such patients are required to miss even one dose of their usual medication and conventional postoperative analgesic regimes are likely to be totally ineffective. There may also be an understandable reluctance to administer high dose opioids on the part of staff not familiar with their use. This can even be the case when the patient's situation is well understood. It is important that all involved in their care, including the anaesthetist, are aware of the opioids and doses being used, particularly if the pre-operative analgesic regime is likely to be unfamiliar to those caring for them in an acute setting. Careful communication, planning and involvement of the patient in decision making are vital to a smooth peri-operative course. The use of appropriate neural blockade techniques, continued into the postoperative period, combined with continuation of the patient's usual opioid medication (or its equivalent), and adjunct agents such as gabapentin—so-called 'balanced analgesia'—is often the most effective approach.

Pain in head and neck cancers

Major improvements in the multimodal treatment of primary head and neck cancers have recently been reported (13). However, oral cancer pain remains a considerable challenge, and the place of interventional techniques in these patients is limited for multiple reasons, including the nature of the pain, anatomical considerations, localized infection, proximity of vital structures and the position of other nerves adjacent to those it would be desirable to block (14). Mucositis is a common problem during the treatment of many cancers, particularly those involving the oral cavity. Appropriate and effective treatment may well be pivotal in facilitating delivery of effective anticancer therapy. The use of topical analgesia is an essential part of analgesic management (15). There are few published data relating to interventional pain relief for patients with head and neck cancer, but the use of regional anaesthesia for perioperative management of pain during head and neck surgery is very well established. Interventional techniques have been successfully used in the management of intractable head and neck cancer pain when other treatment options fail (16). Commonly used regional techniques, such as mandibular nerve block, can be extended into the palliative setting, using an indwelling catheter to provide long-term relief (17). Blockade of the sphenopalatine ganglion using an endoscopic transnasal approach has given encouraging results in a series of 22 patients with advanced disease who were not responsive to conventional therapy (18).

As with patients with a limited response to morphine for the control of pain in other regions, the use of intrathecal delivery may well have a limited place (19). Of particular interest are reports of benefit from bupivacaine delivered intracisternally, or high in the cervical region, which benefited patients with cancer pain in the mouth, head and neck (20, 21, 22).

Non-cancer pain in palliative care patients

Not all pain experienced by patients with cancer is directly due to the disease, and interventional techniques used for the management of chronic non-cancer pain will be just as useful to cancer patients as they are to those without cancer. Simple measures, first used in a chronic pain setting, may well be very effective for palliative care patients, but careful investigation and appropriate use is required. Neuropathic pain, most notably post-surgical pain, post-herpetic neuralgia and pain secondary to cancer treatments has been apparently effectively treated using lidocaine plasters in a series of 97 patients managed in a cancer centre, where the analgesia was assessed as 'potent' in approximately one-third of patients (23). However, these initial promising results may not be reproduced, as the apparent effectiveness has not been supported by data obtained in well-designed, prospective investigations of specific neuropathic syndromes (24). Despite the development of analgesics, co-analgesics, and physical and psychological techniques now used for management of chronic non cancer pain, neural blockade still has an important place in the management of many patients with co-existing benign disease. These include intra-articular injections for arthritic pain, epidural steroid injections for acute radicular pain, trigger point injections for muscle spasm, peripheral perineural injections for conditions such as occipital neuralgia and chemical sympathectomy for end stage ischemic pain not amenable to surgery. This approach is particularly true for patients with opioid non-responsive pain secondary to coexisting disease who have previously benefited from interventional techniques and are familiar with them.

Conclusion

Despite considerable recent advances in techniques, equipment and pharmacological agents, the management of difficult cancer pain remains a challenge, particularly in patients with acute pain in a palliative care setting. Careful, multidisciplinary individualized assessment, combined with application of techniques not commonly used in the palliative care setting, offers the possibility of progress in the provision of pain relief for these patients. As ever, we have much to learn from carefully reflecting on the patients' own experiences of the use of these techniques, our own practice and that of our colleagues.

Case study

An interpleural option

All attempts at getting an epidural into Gerard were failing. He had a long history of 'arthritis' of the spine, which may well have been ankylosing spondylitis, but the diagnosis was now irrelevant from his point of view. He had lung cancer and a history of recurrent pleural effusions, which had been treated some weeks before with a pleurodesis. This had been successful, in that he no longer suffered recurrent and rapidly accumulating effusions, but he had found the procedure excruciatingly painful, and was now left with constant chest pain, which showed little sign of resolving. He was angry at what had been done to him, and felt that he had not been given sufficient warning of how painful the pleurodesis would be or given enough information about pain control options.

He was understandably very fed up with promises of pain control that turned out not to 'work' for him. He had been promised an epidural for the pleurodesis, which had turned out to be technically impossible, and now he was being asked if he would allow a second attempt. We discussed the options. How about attempting to put a catheter into the pleural space and running bupivacaine into it? His pain was unilateral and the pleurodesis made it unlikely that there was risk of a significant pheumothorax even if the line got disconnected. At least we had a 'plan B' that could be undertaken if inserting an epidural did prove impossible, which, with Gerard heavily sedated and with several attempts having failed, looked like it was the case.

So, using the same kit, the 'epidural' was changed to an interpleural infusion, running bupivacaine 0.25% at 5 mL per hour. This gave him good pain relief, with an occasional 'odd taste' in his mouth, which we could speculate on the cause of.

Learning point

If a patient reports that attempts at an intervention have failed in the past further attempts at undertaking the same procedure are liable to be difficult and unsuccessfull. Under these circumstances it is particularly important to have a 'plan B' and to discuss this with the patient before any procedures are attempted.

References

1. Tei Y, Morita T, Nakaho T *et al.* (2008). Treatment efficacy of neural blockade in specialized palliative care services in Japan: a multicenter audit survey. *J Pain Symptom Manage* **36**(5), 461–7.
2. Boys L, Peat SJ, Hanna MH *et al.* (1993). Audit of neural blockade for palliative care patients in an acute unit. *Palliat Med* **7**(3), 205–11.
3. Dy SM, Asch SM, Naeim A *et al.* (2008). Evidence-based standards for cancer pain management. *J Clin Oncol* **26**(23), 3879–85.
4. Teixeira MJ, Fonoff ET, Montenegro MC (2007). Dorsal root entry zone lesions for treatment of pain-related to radiation-induced plexopathy. *Spine* **32** (10), E316–9.

5. Stefaniak T, Basinski A, Vingerhoets W *et al.* (2005). A comparison of two invasive techniques in the management of intractable pain due to inoperable pancreatic cancer: neurolytic celiac plexus block and videothorascopic splanchnicectomy. *Europ J Surgical Oncol* **31**(7), 768–73.

6. Wong G, Schroeder D, Carns P *et al.* (2004). Effect of neurolytic celiac plexus block on pain relief, quality of life, and survival in patients with unresectable pancreatic cancer. *JAMA* **291**(9), 1092–99.

7. Davies DD (1993). Incidence of major complications of neurolytic coeliac plexus block. *J R Soc Med* **86**(5), 264–6.

8. Bernards CM, Shen DD, Sterling ES *et al.* (2003). Epidural, cerebrospinal fluid, and plasma pharmacokinetics of epidural opioids (part1): differences among opioids. *Anesthesiology* **99**(2), 455–65.

9. Bernards CM (2002). Understanding the physiology and pharmacology of epidural and intrathecal opioids. *Best Pract Res Clin Anaesthesiol* **16**(4), 489–505.

10. Eisenach JC, Hood DD, Curry R *et al.* (2004). Intrathecal but not intravenous opioids release adenosine from the spinal cord. *J Pain* **5**(1), 64–8.

11. Koulousakis A, Kuchta J, Bayarassou A *et al.* (2007). Intrathecal opioids for intractable pain syndromes. *Acta Neurochir Suppl.* **97**(Pt 1), 43–8.

12. Mercadante S, Intravaia G, Villari P *et al.* (2007). Intrathecal treatment in cancer patients unresponsive to multiple trials of systemic opioids. *Clin J Pain* **23**(9), 793–8.

13. Argiris A, Karamouzis MV, Raben D *et al.* (2008). Head and neck cancer. *Lancet* **371**(9625), 1695–709.

14. Epstein JB, Elad S, Eliav E *et al.* (2007). Orofacial pain in cancer: part II—clinical perspectives and management. *J Dent Res* **86**(6), 506–18.

15. Peterson DE, Bensadoun RJ, Roila F (2009). ESMO Guidelines Working Group. Management of oral and gastrointestinal mucositis: ESMO clinical recommendations. *Ann Oncol* **20**(Suppl 4), 174–7.

16. Rosenberg M, Phero JC (2003). Regional anesthesia and invasive techniques to manage head and neck pain. *Otolaryngol Clin North Am* **36**(6), 1201–19.

17. Kohase H, Umino M, Shibaji T *et al.* (2004). Application of a mandibular nerve block using an indwelling catheter for intractable cancer pain. *Acta Anaesthaesthesiol Scand* **48**(3), 382–3.

18. Varghese BT, Koshy RC (2001). Endoscopic transnasal neurolytic sphenopalatine ganglion block for head and neck cancer pain. *J Laryngol Otol* **115**(5), 385–7.

19. Kayahara H, Hamakawa H, Fukuzumi M *et al.* (2000). Indication for epidural morphine for the relief of intractable pain in advanced oral cancer: report of four cases. *Br J Oral Maxillofac Surg* **38**(5), 546–9.

20. Lundborg C, Dahm P, Nitescu P *et al.* (2009). High intrathecal bupivacaine for severe pain in the head and neck. *Acta Anaesthesiol Scand* **53**(7), 908–13.

21. Lambert G, Elam M, Friberg P *et al.* (2006). Acute response to intracisternal bupivacaine in patients with refractory pain of the head and neck. *J Physiol* **570**(2), 421–8.

22. Appelgren L, Janson M, Nitescu P *et al.* (1996). Continuous intracisternal and high cervical intrathecal bupivacaine analgesia in refractory head and neck pain. *Anesthesiology* **84**(2), 256–72.

23. Fleming JA, O'Connor BD (2009). Use of lidocaine patches for neuropathic pain in a comprehensive cancer centre. *Pain Res Manag* **14**(5), 381–8.

24. Cheville AL, Sloan JA, Northfelt DW (2009). Use of a lidocaine patch in the management of postsurgical neuropathic pain in patients with cancer: a phase III double-blind crossover study (N01CB). *Support Care Cancer* **17**(4), 451–60.

Chapter 3

Interventional pain control: Background and current role

Joan Hester

This chapter covers:
Introduction to interventional pain control
Limitations and concerns about opioid therapy
Side effects from opioids
Effects of opioids on immune and endocrine function
Types of pain
Pain assessment
The history of interventional techniques
The place of interventional techniques in cancer pain management
Recommended techniques for specific pain situations
Roles and responsibilities of pain physicians and palliative care physicians

---

Introduction

The prevalence of pain in cancer has been described in Chapter 1 by Dr Sykes, who also mentions the success of the WHO analgesic ladder in the management of cancer pain. However, he also points out the limitations of the oral analgesia approach and the burden of both unrelieved cancer pain and of side effects from opioid analgesics.

There are several other modalities that can be used to improve the management of cancer pain that are outside the scope of this book: the use of adjunct drugs, especially anti-epileptics and antidepressants for the relief of neuropathic pain, topical agents, chemotherapy and radiotherapy, hormones and psychological and physical therapies. These are all an important part of a holistic approach to pain management and are described in a new British Pain Society publication *Cancer Pain Management* (1).

Interventional pain control is an alternative way of approaching pain relief, and involves performing an injection or other invasive procedure, such as neuromodulation or percutaneous cordotomy, primarily to modify nerve transmission from the painful area to the brain. The potential benefit is to provide superior pain relief without the side effects of strong analgesics. There are, of course, difficulties and disadvantages of interventional procedures; each case must be assessed carefully on its own merits and a combination of therapies chosen to offer maximum benefit whilst minimizing the risks. Such is the basic premise of good medical practice. Application of this principle in the management of pain from advanced cancer requires a high level of knowledge and skill.

With the introduction of regular oral opioid administration around the clock in the 1980s and the development of specialist palliative care, the number of cancer patients receiving interventional treatments drastically reduced. Patients were simply not referred any longer to anaesthetists for destructive nerve blocks, and there was a perception of harm rather than benefit.

The number of coeliac plexus blocks, for example, performed for management of pain from pancreatic cancer has reduced markedly since 1985. Serious side effects of neurolytic coeliac plexus block, such as paraplegia, were reported in a UK survey of 2730 neurolytic blocks carried out between 1986 and 1990 (2). The incidence of major complications in this series was one case per 683 blocks or 0.15%. This study made the use of strong oral opioids appear the preferable option, despite inferior pain relief and notwithstanding many side effects, particularly drowsiness. Newer imaging techniques, namely MRI, CT and ultrasound guidance, continue to improve the accuracy of needle placement and safety of injections, and two more recent trials, on 160 patients, did not show any major morbidity or mortality (3, 4).

The training and skills of anaesthetists has developed considerably since the 1980s. It is no longer appropriate to use the term 'anaesthetist', as pain medicine in the UK is now a subspeciality of anaesthesia with its own Faculty of Pain Medicine within the Royal College of Anaesthetists, inaugurated in April 2007.

Pain trainees in the UK undergo an advanced training programme of at least one year, with a detailed curriculum encompassing acute, chronic and cancer pain, with tests of knowledge and skills, including procedural skills and the assessment of the patient with cancer pain. The criteria for entrance to the Faculty of Pain Medicine of the Royal College of Anaesthetists is kept under regular review and is evolving as the speciality develops. The Australian and New Zealand College of Anaesthesists and Faculty of Pain Medicine have a similar training programme, but these are unique in the world, though other countries are developing diplomas and other specialist qualifications in pain medicine. Pain specialists are emerging, both in the UK and internationally, many with a full-time commitment to pain medicine. There are many national and international pain meetings, with a high level of scientific input and contributions from healthcare professionals from many disciplines, including pain, palliative care, neurology, surgery, physiotherapy, psychology, nursing and pharmacy. Training in the management of cancer pain is one of the most demanding parts of the curriculum in both pain medicine and palliative medicine; skills and knowledge are developing rapidly in both disciplines.

Pain specialists have evaluated the effectiveness of interventional techniques for cancer pain.

Banning (1991) assessed pain treatments in 131 patients in Denmark who were referred to a multidisciplinary cancer pain clinic from oncology departments. Multimodal therapies were used, which included analgesic tailoring, non-neurolytic nerve blockades, epidural opioid therapy and combinations of these. In the short term there was moderate to complete pain relief in 72.5% of patients, and in the long term 50%. Pain treatments were supplemented by psychological intervention and social worker assistance in selected cases (5).

Interventional techniques themselves have changed in nature and emphasis, largely moving away from destructive neurolytic techniques to reversible techniques using local anaesthetics and/or opioids by constant infusion, delivered neuraxially (epidurally or intrathecally) or around nerve plexuses, such as the brachial and lumbar plexus. The use of such reversible techniques has been inadequately evaluated for cancer pain, although evidence for remarkable effectiveness of an implantable intrathecal drug delivery system exists with enhanced pain control, a reduction of side effects, particularly sedation, and improved quality of life (6). The same study also showed an improved life expectancy in the group with an implanted pump delivering intrathecal morphine (6). This finding has not yet been reproduced, but morphine is known to suppress immune function, especially natural killer (NK) cell function which appears to be a dose related effect. Using morphine intrathecally instead of orally or subcutaneously reduces the total daily dose dramatically as its potency is approximately 300 times higher by the intrathecal route than by the oral route. Measures to reduce morphine load may become of greater importance in the future.

Several publications support the role of pain management approaches, including interventions, in cancer pain management (7–9). Pain management is based on multidisciplinary care, with detailed assessment of the sources of pain, optimization of pharmacotherapy, combined physical and psychological therapies, and the use of interventional techniques where indicated.

It is widely accepted that interventional techniques are currently underused in cancer pain management. There are complex reasons why this is so, some of which are explored in this chapter.

Limitations and concerns about opioid therapy

It is almost heretical to express concern about opioid therapy, which is rightly used so widely in the management of cancer pain. It should be acknowledged that the WHO ladder was originally produced for the management of cancer pain in developing countries, providing a simple, cheap and effective way of managing cancer pain where there is no access to other methods of pain relief (10).

However, in the UK, and in other developed countries, there are emerging groups of cancer sufferers with complex patterns of pain, such as cancer survivors, who may take opioids long term for persistent pain following cancer treatments or who may be unable to stop opioids that were started during cancer treatment. There are also many patients in whom side effects of opioid medication reduce quality of life.

Side effects from opioids

Eighty per cent of patients taking opioids will experience at least one side effect, and this rises with rapid titration and increasing doses. Analgesics accounted for approximately

17% of admissions to hospital for adverse drug reactions in patients over 60 years of age and opioids were responsible for about 6% of these admissions (11). Glare 2006 (12) studied morphine-related side effects in a cancer population and found the following rates of side effects: dry mouth 70–95%, myoclonus 40–60%, sedation 20–60%, constipation 40–70%, nausea 15–20%, itching 2–10%. Payne *et al.* in 1998 compared pain-related treatment satisfaction and patient-reported side effects in patients receiving either transdermal fentanyl or oral morphine and found self-reported side effects in 54% of the morphine group and 32% of the fentanyl group (13). Satisfaction rates were higher in the fentanyl group, which Payne related to the lower incidence of side effects. Laxatives and anti-emetics are often co-prescribed with opioid analgesics, further adding to the burden of pharmacotherapy. Patients concur with taking analgesic medications and many of them tolerate the side effects without complaint, but if an effective alternative is available many may wish to consider it. Novel opioid analgesics are emerging, such as tapentadol, which has a dual mode of action: central analgesic action and inhibition of noradrenaline re-uptake. Trial data suggest that tapentadol may offer an advantage over convential opioid therapy in terms of a reduced incidence of side effects at equianalgesic doses (14).

It is truly remarkable to see the difference in alertness, function and ability to communicate in a patient who has received successful pain relief from an interventional technique, when oral or systemic opioids have been reduced.

Effects of opioids on immune and endocrine function

The long-term side effects of opioids on the immune and endocrine systems are emerging in importance in non-cancer pain, but the effects are seen in cancer pain patients also.

The effect of morphine in modulating the immune system has been known for over 100 years but it is difficult to quantify how important this effect is in clinical practice. An increased likelihood of infection is associated with opioid abuse, especially HIV infection, and morphine use has been shown to increase susceptibility to *Streptococcus pneumoniae* lung infection (15).

Development of primary cancers and the increased metastatic spread of cancer have been shown to occur more frequently in the presence of opioids.

Opioids alter the function of immunocytes, both directly by inhibiting macrophage function, via interleukins IL-10 and IL-12, and indirectly via the hypothalamic pituitary axis and the sympathetic nervous system. NK cells are particularly sensitive to modulation by morphine (16).

Unrelieved pain also inhibits immune and NK function, and surgery and trauma are also associated with immunosuppression, such that the role of morphine is hard to quantify.

What is known, however, is that some opioids suppress immune function more than others. Morphine has the greatest effect, methadone, codeine and the fentanyl group less so; buprenorphine, oxycodone, hydromorphone and tramadol do not suppress immune function.

Hypogonadal hypogonadism is a dose- and time-related consequence of opioid therapy, mediated indirectly via the hypothalamic pituitary axis and directly via testicular and ovarian receptors. All opioids except buprenorphine and tramadol can cause suppression of testosterone in men, oestradiol in women and dehydroepiandosterone, which is a precursor of adrenal sex hormones. Very low levels of these hormones have been reported leading to fatigue, loss of libido, weakness, small size of the gonads, loss of muscle mass, irregular or absent menses, bone loss and infertility.

In a study of cancer survivors, 20 of whom took opioids and 20 of whom did not, 90% in the opioid group had hypogonadism compared with 40% in the non-opioid group (17).

Other medications

Cancer pain is rarely treated by opioids alone, although these are the mainstay of treatment. Neuropathic pain in cancer is treated with anti-epileptic drugs such as gabapentin, pregabalin and carbamazepine, often in combination with antidepressants such as amitriptyline, nortritriptyline, venlafaxine or duloxetine. All these drugs have their side effects, some major, and any intervention that curtails their use is to be welcomed by the patient. Topical agents such as capsaicin and lidocaine may be applied in creams and skin patches, happily without systemic side effects, although they may cause skin reactions.

A description of these agents is outside the scope of this book, but I would guide the reader to the keynote reviews by Finnerup et al. (18), Dworkin et al. (19) and NICE (20). Ketamine, steroids, hormones, biphosphonates, clonidine and baclofen are also used for treating cancer pain but their use will not be described here.

Under-treatment of pain

One of the main barriers to optimal effective pain relief is inadequate assessment of pain. The initial assessment should be comprehensive and should include a detailed history, psychosocial assessment, physical examination and a diagnostic evaluation for signs and symptoms associated with common cancer pain syndromes.

Inadequate assessment of pain type (nociceptive, neuropathic, visceral) and the precise diagnosis of the location and cause of the pain(s) may mean that treatment is suboptimal. For example, a man with recurrent carcinoma of the bladder may have diffuse suprapubic pain (visceral), back pain (nociceptive) and intense pain with muscle weakness in one leg from lumbar plexus involvement (neuropathic). All the pains are related to his cancer, but each needs a different approach to management.

The importance of diagnosing the type of pain was highlighted by Grond et al., who studied 2266 cancer patients referred to a pain service and assessed the locations, aetiologies and pathophysiological mechanisms of their pain syndromes (21). Pain could be classified as coming from bone in 35%, soft tissues in 45%, viscera in 33% and were neuropathic in 34%. Thirty-nine per cent of patients had two, and 31% three or more distinct pain syndromes. Nine per cent of patients had pain unrelated to cancer.

Types of pain

Pain is categorized according to its physiological origin. Cancer pathophysiology is complex, as described in Chapter 4, and several of these pain types might coexist. The categories of pain are:

- nociceptive (from soft tissue, bone, muscle, joints, ligaments etc.)
- inflammatory pain
- neuropathic pain: "Pain caused by a lesion or disease of the somatosensory nervous system" (22)
- mixed nociceptive and neuropathic
- visceral (from any internal organ; this includes heart, lungs and abdominal organs)
- psychogenic/central (central processing of pain involves many higher centres in the brain, and descending pathways may be inhibitory or facilitatory).

Imaging, such as MRI and CT scanning, is very important to understand which tissues may be invaded by tumour, especially where pain is referred to a more remote location. For example:

- localized chest wall pain in one to two dermatomes from a spinal lesion in the thoracic spine causing radicular pain (e.g. T5,6)
- upper thigh and knee pain from a lesion in the lumbar plexus (L2,3)
- groin and upper thigh pain from a carcinoma in the tail of the pancreas (T12/L1)
- lower abdominal pain from a mesothelioma at T12.

These are examples of neuropathic pain in the distribution of the affected nerves, associated with nociceptive pain at the tumour location.

These types of pain are determined by careful history taking and clinical examination, and use of a dermatomal chart that shows distribution of the nerves, as shown in Appendix 1. Mechanisms of pain are described in Chapter 4.

Nociceptive pain

Nociceptive pain arises from primary or secondary tissue invasion from tumour into fat, ligament, muscle, tendon or bone. Nocicpetive pain may be aching, boring, constant pain, and is often worse on movement if muscle, bone, joint, ligaments or tendons are involved. Recent work from Urch and Dickenson indicates that bone pain from cancer previously assumed to be nociceptive pain, is in fact associated with neuronal changes with both peripheral and central sensitization (23).

Neuropathic pain

Neuropathic pain is often unilateral; it is localized, sharp, spontaneous, severe pain associated with burning, numbness, itching and sometimes hypersensitivity of the skin to non-noxious stimuli (allodynia). Clinical examination may reveal sensory or motor changes in the location of the nerve and, in the case of a spinal tumour, possibly an upper motor neurone lesion in the legs.

Different means of diagnosing neuropathic pain have been described in the literature. One example is the LANSS (Leeds Assessment of Neuropathic Signs and Symptoms) scale (24). In this example the patient completes a questionnaire, as shown below, and the doctor tests the affected area for mechanical allodynia and/or pinprick alteration. If the combined score is more than 12, neuropathic pain is very likely.

- Question 1: pricking, tingling, pins and needles (0–5)
- Question 2: skin mottled, red, pink (0–5)
- Question 3: abnormally sensitive to touch (0–3)
- Question 4: electric shocks, jumping, bursting (0–2)
- Question 5: hot, burning (0–2)
- Sensory testing: Mechanical allodynia (0–5)
- Pinprick alteration (0–5)

There are other neuropathic pain scales available such as Douleur Neuropathique (DN4) (25) and PainDETECT (26).

It is important to diagnose neuropathic pain, as the treatment(s) will be different from nociceptive pain; a course of steroids, palliative radiotherapy or chemotherapy may be indicated or an anti-epileptic drug such as pregabalin and/or tricyclic antidepressant such as amitriptyline may be a first choice of medication. Opioids tend to be less effective for neuropathic pain. Some severe neuropathic pains, especially plexopathies, respond well to interventional techniques.

Visceral pain

Visceral pain is diffuse, hard to localize and difficult to describe in words. It may be referred to a distant location, for example from the liver and spleen via the diaphragm, innervated by C3, 4 and 5, to the shoulder, or from lower abdominal organs to the groin and leg. Tenesmus is an example of visceral pain. There is often an associated area of segmental hyperalgesia on the skin of the abdomen and/or back that can be detected by bedside testing with a pin. Visceral afferents travel through the sympathetic and parasympathetic nervous systems to the spinal cord, but in advanced cancer there is usually also a somatic component to the pain. Neurotransmitters and central projections are different in somatic and visceral pain, as described in Chapter 4.

Psychogenic/central pain

The concept of total body pain was first described by the late Dame Cicely Saunders, founder of St Christopher's Hospice, in her writings through the 1950s and 1960s. She described the complex interaction between physical pain, emotional pain, the social setting, family relationships and spirituality. Her work is nicely encapsulated in an article by David Clark, in 1999 (27).

Scientific advances, especially through imaging of the brain, are beginning to explain the complexity of some of these interactions. Pain within the context of suffering and imminent death has a different dimension from non-cancer pain, and the palliative care movement continues to explore these relationships; the hospice movement provides a level of holistic care that was unimaginable 50 years ago.

Complex regional pain syndrome

Complex regional pain syndrome has previously had many names, reflex sympathetic dystrophy or causalgia, for example. It was renamed complex regional pain syndrome (CRPS) by the International Association for the Study of Pain (IASP) taskforce in 1996 but the name is still not used consistently (28). Diagnostic criteria and causality continue to be discussed at international meetings and by consensus groups. Harden has recently commented on the diagnostic criteria (29).

Basically CRPS is a syndrome of persistent pain in a limb, of diffuse distribution, which is out of proportion to the inciting event and associated with two or more symptoms or signs from the following categories:

- sensory abnormality in the form of allodynia or hyperalgesia
- inappropriate temperature and/or colour changes
- sweating, swelling and/or trophic changes
- weakness, dystonia and/or motor neglect.

It is now considered by some authorities to be a form of neuropathic pain with predominantly central changes. Treatment of CRPS is out of the scope of this book, but the IASP has some excellent resources at www.iasp-pain.org. CRPS can coexist with other types of pain or could follow fracture, radiotherapy and central nervous system lesions.

Pain assessment

When assessing a patient with cancer pain it is important to decide from the history, clinical examination, investigation results and knowledge of the spread of the tumour where the pain is coming from and, particularly, which nerve roots, plexuses or peripheral nerves may be is a useful aide memoire (Appendix 1) as is pictorial documentation of the site and nature of the pain (Fig. 3.1).

Simple pain scales can be used to monitor severity of the pain, psychological distress and quality of life. There are many of these, but some of the simplest and most useful in clinical practice are:

- a verbal rating scale: none, mild, moderate, severe
- a numerical rating scale: an 11 point scale of 0–10 is used most often, 0 being no pain and 10 being the worst pain imaginable
- a visual analogue scale: a 10-cm line with 'no pain' at one end and 'worst pain imaginable' at the other end of the line
- the Brief Pain Inventory (30) (see Fig. 3.2)
- the Hospital Anxiety and Depression Scale (31)
- Euroqol EQ-5D (see http://euroqol.org).

There is a wealth of literature about the merits and validity of pain measurement scales, which is outside the scope of this book. The authors recommend that pain is measured regularly, at least daily, using a simple verbal or numerical rating scale, with pain at rest and pain on movement recorded. Preferably the patient will give his/her own rating when asked.

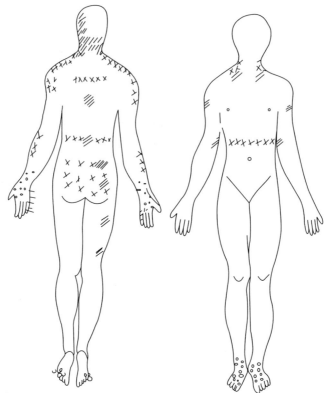

Fig. 3.1 Pain drawing, indicating sites of pain. A body outline for the patient to mark the location of the pain can be helpful.

A pain diary may be kept when the patient is at home. Changing pain levels are then registered and an assessment of the effects of treatment can be made more accurately than by the usual questioning.

History of interventional techniques

The WHO guidance about its analgesic ladder (10) states:

> *"Surgical intervention on appropriate nerves may provide further pain relief if the drugs are not wholly effective"*

It is simplistic to assume that cutting a nerve to a painful area will relieve the pain. This approach causes numbness in the distribution of the nerve, motor weakness if the nerve has a motor component or paralysis if it is a major nerve, and pain returns as the nerve attempts to regenerate. Animal experiments on transected or ligated sciatic nerves show that the animal will shake and chew the affected paw and autotomy may occur. This phenomenon is related to central sensitization. Human models include amputation of a limb, during which the sciatic and femoral nerves or their branches are transected. There are immediate phantom sensations, which are painful in 80–90% of amputees initially, subsiding in the majority of people in months or years. The stump may become sensitized

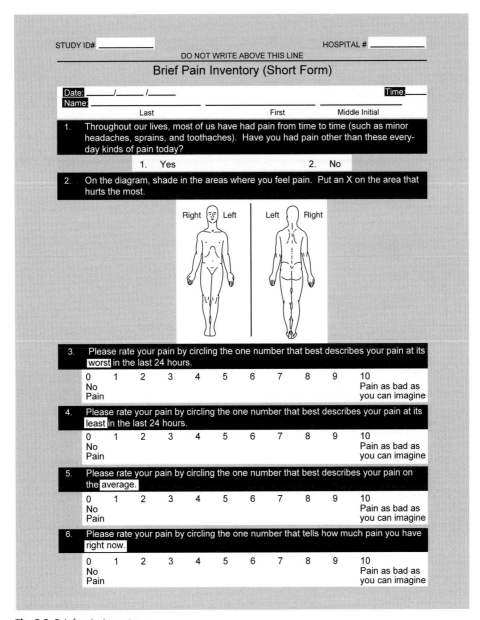

Fig. 3.2 Brief pain inventory.

and allodynic. As explained in Chapter 4, there is alteration of neurotransmitters in the spinal cord. In addition, brain representation, or mapping, of the amputated limb takes many years to readjust.

Another example of nerve destruction causing an increase in pain is that of transection, or alcohol injection, of a trigeminal nerve for trigeminal neuralgia. This leads to numbness on the affected side of the face, loss of corneal sensation, some facial muscle weakness and intense burning pain, called anaesthesia dolorosa, which is often more intolerable than the original neuralgia, and is constant and untreatable.

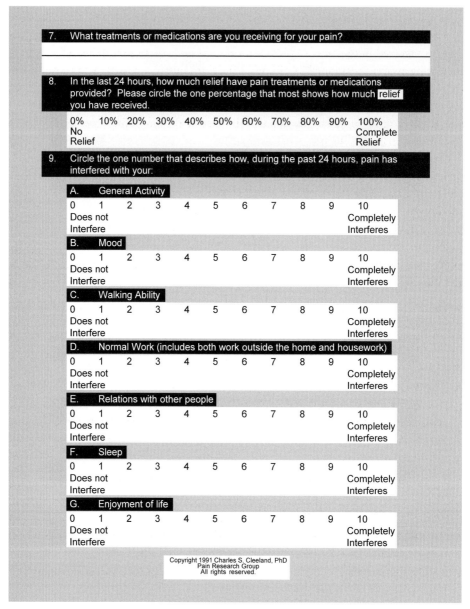

7. What treatments or medications are you receiving for your pain?

8. In the last 24 hours, how much relief have pain treatments or medications provided? Please circle the one percentage that most shows how much relief you have received.

0% 10% 20% 30% 40% 50% 60% 70% 80% 90% 100%
No   Complete
Relief   Relief

9. Circle the one number that describes how, during the past 24 hours, pain has interfered with your:

A. General Activity

0 1 2 3 4 5 6 7 8 9 10
Does not   Completely
Interfere   Interferes

B. Mood

0 1 2 3 4 5 6 7 8 9 10
Does not Completely
Interfere Interferes

C. Walking Ability

0 1 2 3 4 5 6 7 8 9 10
Does not Completely
Interfere Interferes

D. Normal Work (includes both work outside the home and housework)

0 1 2 3 4 5 6 7 8 9 10
Does not Completely
Interfere Interferes

E. Relations with other people

0 1 2 3 4 5 6 7 8 9 10
Does not Completely
Interfere Interferes

F. Sleep

0 1 2 3 4 5 6 7 8 9 10
Does not Completely
Interfere Interferes

G. Enjoyment of life

0 1 2 3 4 5 6 7 8 9 10
Does not Completely
Interfere Interferes

Fig. 3.2 (Continued)

Despite these and other examples, the belief that pain transmission runs through the nervous system like a 'hard wired telephone cable' and that cutting a nerve will therefore relieve pain persists in the minds of lay people, and this view is even held by some professionals.

Techniques have been pursued that involved partly destroying a nerve, with the intention of disrupting the pain pathways while leaving sensory and motor parts intact. The foremost pioneer of modern pain therapy was John Bonica (1917–1994) of the USA, who wrote the seminal book *The Management of Pain* in response to the enormous challenge of the millions wounded during the Second World War. This book became a bible for doctors involved in the relief of pain. John Bonica went on to found the IASP in 1973. Increasing awareness amongst clinicians of the gate control theory of pain transmission (32)—a breakthrough in understanding prompted by the discovery that pain impulses are modulated in the spinal cord—and the discovery of endogenous opioids led to a new era in pain therapy. Modulation of pain became the aim rather than temporary or permanent nerve destruction.

There are undoubtedly some destructive procedures that work extremely well in skilled hands, with minimal complications, notably percutaneous cordotomy for painful, unilateral mesothelioma, neurolytic coeliac plexus block for upper abdominal cancer, and intrathecal neurolysis for selected pelvic and perineal cancers.

As the understanding of the science of pain transmission has advanced, interventional techniques have moved away from the destruction of nerves to the use of drugs applied directly to part of the nervous system in a low-dose infusion, particularly via the epidural and intrathecal routes. There are several reasons for this:

- Destructive procedures may destroy the sensory or motor part of the nerve, causing numbness (anaesthesia dolorosa) and/or motor weakness or, when applied to the spinal cord, permanent loss of bladder or bowel control.
- The effect of neurodestructive procedures is unpredictable and irreversible.
- Technological advances have improved the equipment used to perform reversible invasive techniques, such as non-kinkable epidural catheters, special intrathecal catheters, accurate implantable pumps, high-quality, 'user-friendly' external pumps, nerve-locating devices, and availability of good X-ray, CT scanning and ultrasound machines to aid placement of the needle.
- Healthcare professionals have become more educated about the possibilities offered by interventional techniques, are aware of the limitations of medical management in some cases, and seek to diminish opioid toxicity and side effects.
- Patients are wary of the potential complications of a destructive procedure and may refuse consent.
- The ability to programme an electrical device is a more familiar skill than it was 20 years ago.
- Apprehension about an invasive procedure is easier to allay if the process is reversible.
- Electrical stimulation techniques such as peripheral nerve stimulation and spinal cord stimulation are becoming more accessible as technology improves.

These techniques are described in greater detail elsewhere in this book.

The place of interventional techniques in cancer pain control

The most challenging decisions are when to offer interventional pain control, which procedure to offer and where and how to manage the patient after the procedure. There is little guidance in the literature, apart from case series and an occasional randomized controlled trial on a specific procedure, but these may not help the decision-making process.

A request for an interventional procedure is usually initiated by a palliative care physician or oncologist who has already been treating the patient, often for a considerable time. Requests are less often initiated by a general practitioner. The request for consideration of a procedure is often not made until all other possible means of pain relief have been tried, or the patient is opioid toxic, or pain control is still inadequate despite the application of varying drug regimes. Such requests may be made in a very advanced stage of illness and can reflect desperation on the part of the referring team, patient or relatives.

A better way to make earlier and more considered referrals to a pain specialist is to establish weekly regular joint discussion about a variety of patients with difficult cancer pain problems, thereby each discipline learns from the others, with the outcome of earlier and more timely intervention and an ability to put into place the support needed for aftercare.

Liaison between pain specialists and palliative care remains sporadic in many places and there are very few centres that provide joint working with the oncology team, although this would be optimal.

The pain specialist needs to have an understanding of the natural history of the illness and current treatments that can be provided for cancer patients, and a working knowledge of symptom control in palliative care. Pain specialists need to have realistic expectations of what can be achieved with an intervention and the ability to explain this clearly to the patient, relatives and healthcare professionals involved in the patient's management. Selecting the right intervention depends on a detailed assessment of the cause(s) of pain at the time of referral.

Interventional techniques that may be used for cancer pain

Local anaesthetic may be combined with a steroid as a 'single-shot' procedure, or with opioids such as morphine, diamorphine and fentanyl, or with other drugs such as clonidine or baclofen. A novel agent for intrathecal use only is ziconotide.

Table 1 Reversible techniques: Local anaesthetic nerve block (± opioids), with or without infusion

Peripheral nerve block (e.g. intercostal nerve block, femoral nerve block)
Plexus block (lumbar plexus block, brachial plexus block)
Paravertebral block
Spinal cord and nerve roots, via the epidural and intrathecal routes
Brain via the intracerebroventricular route (opioids only)
Autonomic nervous system
Stellate ganglion block
Coeliac plexus block
Lumbar sympathetic block
Superior hypogastric block
Ganglion of Impar block

Reversible techniques are described in Chapters 5, 6, 8 and 9.

Table 2 Destructive techniques
Neurolytic blocks
Peripheral nerve (rarely used)
Epidural
Intrathecal
Coeliac plexus
Other sympathetic nerve blocks
Percutaneous cordotomy
Radiofrequency lesioning

Destructive techniques are described in Chapters 6, 8, 9 and 10.

Table 3 Stimulation techniques
TENS
Acupuncture
Peripheral nerve stimulation
Spinal cord stimulation (percutaneous)
Deep brain stimulation

Stimulation techniques are described in Chapters 11 and 12.

Table 4 Neurosurgical techniques
Surgical Cordotomy
Midline myelotomy

Neurosurgical techniques are not described in this book.

Table 5 Examples of difficult cancer pain that may respond to an interventional technique:	
Cancer pain syndrome	**Interventional technique to consider**
Brachial plexus involvement	Brachial plexus block, high thoracic or cervical epidural, cordotomy (if unilateral)
Lumbar plexus involvement	Lumbar plexus block, paravertebral block, epidural or intrathecal infusion
Central nervous system involvement (brain, spinal cord, meninges)	Intrathecal or epidural infusions
Rib pain/secondary/intercostal neuralgia	Intercostal nerve block
Unilateral chest wall pain from mesothelioma	Interpleural block/cordotomy
Visceral pain	
Upper abdominal	Coeliac plexus block
Lower abdominal, tenesmus	Lumbar sympathetic block
Pelvic organs, tenesmus	Superior hypogastric plexus block
Lower rectum, tenesmus	Ganglion of Impar block
	(continued)

Table 5 (Continued)

Mixed somatic and visceral pain	
Bilateral generalized chest/upper abdominal pain from advanced cancer	Epidural or intrathecal infusion
Bilateral lower abdominal, hip or leg pain	Epidural or intrathecal infusion
Pathological fractures	Plexus block, paravertebral block, epidural or intrathecal infusion
Widespread body pain with bony metastases	Intrathecal infusion
Localized perineal pain from somatic nerve involvement	Intrathecal phenol saddle block
Unilateral hip pain	Lumbar plexus block
Unilateral shoulder pain	Suprascapular nerve block

Who is responsible for treating cancer pain?

This depends on the stage of the cancer, the severity and complexity of the illness, geographical location of the patient and availability of services. The NHS cancer plan has done much in recent years to provide timely and expert diagnosis and treatment of cancer throughout the UK(7). However, liaison between cancer services and specialist pain services is not clearly defined, and there is inconsistent partnership between the specialities of pain medicine and palliative care. This inconsistent pattern is reproduced in other countries to a greater or lesser extent.

Surveys of working between pain management and palliative care

A national survey of pain management services in palliative care was conducted in 2002 by Linklater *et al.*, who sent a postal questionnaire to all consultant members of the Association of Palliative Medicine asking if they had contact with a pain management specialist (33). Most respondents had access to 'as required' anaesthetic pain consultations, 72% feeling that the frequency of consultations was adequate, but 20% desiring more frequent input. Fifteen per cent had access to regular weekly sessions. Trainee anaesthetists featured in only 7% of sessions. Half the respondents used pain management services fewer than four times per year. All respondents felt that the anaesthetist's input involved advice on performing practical procedures, but only 25% felt that a joint consultation about analgesic therapy would be beneficial. The authors advocated the establishment of a regular weekly session with a pain specialist, and their experience showed that this increased the number of referrals to 11% of inpatients, with procedures performed on 8% and advice given on 3%.

A survey of anaesthetists in UK pain clinics was conducted in 2007 by Kay *et al.* by postal questionnaire and they found that referral rates from palliative medicine to pain clinics were low: only 31% respondents received more than 112 referrals per year (approximately 2/week) (34). Only 25% of pain anaesthetists' job plans had time allocated for palliative medicine referrals and joint consultations were rare.

A 2007 survey of hospices and palliative care units in England has shown that, while 92% palliative care units have access to specialist pain management advice, only 16% have regular sessions (35). The situation has not changed over the past 5 years, despite the increasing complexity of illness. Only 41% of pain services provided a comprehensive range of pain treatments, including non-invasive therapies such as TENS or minimally invasive techniques such as acupuncture and trigger point injections. In about 50% of palliative care units neuraxial infusions are not available. There are distinct barriers to sending patients home with invasive therapies, related to multiple factors, but particularly to a lack of training and experience of the home care team and drug supply issues.

The barriers to interdisciplinary team working in complex cancer care are summarized in Box 1. Both pain medicine and palliative medicine have much to contribute to symptom control, teaching and training, and the contributions each discipline can make are summarized in Boxes 2 and 3.

Palliative medicine has been a recognized speciality since 1987, when speciality training programmes were established by the Royal College of Physicians. Funding of the speciality was further enhanced as a result of the Calman–Hine report in 1995, when palliative care was integrated with cancer services. Pain medicine is not yet a recognized speciality, although a Faculty of Pain Medicine of the Royal College of Anaesthetists was established in April 2007 to set and uphold standards of training of doctors practising pain medicine in the future. Cancer pain management is an essential part of this training. Interventional pain control is also a vital part of the training of palliative medicine doctors, thus providing hope for enhanced future collaboration, to the benefit of patients with pain from advanced cancer.

Box 1 Barriers to links between specialist pain management and palliative medicine

These can be summarized as follows:

- funding of the service
- time on the part of the pain specialist for regular assessment and discussion (allocated and funded sessions)
- facilities for performing interventions may not be easily accessible
- complexity/lack of in-depth understanding
- staff training in the management of pumps and catheters
- pharmacy issues, procurement of solutions/availability of preservative-free opioids/ lack of sterile facilities for making up infusions
- cost of implanted devices
- palliative care doctor may be unaware of potential benefits/unsure how to access expertise
- pain doctor may not be adequately trained in the management of cancer pain/ selection of an appropriate technique.

Box 2 What can specialist pain medicine offer in palliative care?

- Assessment of complex cases
- Detailed knowledge of the neurophysiology of pain
- Specialist knowledge of treating different types of pain, e.g. neuropathic pain, complex regional pain syndrome
- Interventional techniques
- TENS, acupuncture
- Psychological aspects of pain management
- Provision of sedation
- Management of non-cancer pain
- Recognition and advice about the management of addiction
- Tapering and withdrawal from opioids

Box 3 What can palliative medicine offer to specialist pain medicine?

- Detailed knowledge and experience of using opioids
- Management of opioid toxicity
- Understanding of cancer pain and all cancer treatments
- Good communication skills
- Team working
- Family therapy
- Holistic medicine
- Home care
- Complementary therapies
- End-of-life care

Concluding remarks

Treating complex cancer pain is challenging for patients, carers, and clinicians and will become more so as cancer treatments advance and survival rates improve. The development of interventional pain techniques over the past 50 years, a better understanding of the science of pain, improvement in technology, enhanced education and skills of healthcare professionals make the practice of complex interventions a realistic goal in advanced cancer. It is a goal that requires work and perseverance, never losing sight of the desire not only to do no harm, but also to enhance the quality of life for many sufferers.

Case study 1

Lumbar plexopathy

A 70-year-old man presented with pain in the anterior right thigh radiating from hip to knee. It was intense and unremitting, present at rest and made worse by walking. It also woke him several times at night. He complained of numbness in the thigh and burning pain, and found it difficult to walk upstairs.

Three years previously he had a total cystectomy and ileal conduit for transitional cell carcinoma of the bladder, and considered himself cured. Recent review from the urologist had been satisfactory and his ileal conduit was functioning well. An orthopaedic surgeon had screened his hip and knee and found no joint pathology to account for his pain. He was known to have degenerative disease of the spine, which was presumed to be the cause of his pain, and he was referred to a pain specialist for a possible lumbar epidural steroid injection, although no nerve root compression showed on MRI.

On examination there was 3/5 weakness of right hip flexors and reduced pin-prick perception in the L2/3 distribution. In view of the history and spine MRI findings a CT scan of the abdomen and pelvis was performed, which confirmed recurrent tumour invading the anterior sacrum, enlarged para-aortic glands and invasion of the right psoas muscle compressing the right L2 and 3 nerve roots.

His pain was difficult to control with opioids, tricyclic antidepressants and anti-epileptic drugs. He received palliative radiotherapy, which did not help. A tunnelled epidural catheter was inserted in the upper lumbar region, connected to an external pump and an infusion of bupivacaine and diamorphine started. He spent his last 12 weeks of life with the epidural *in situ*, giving him excellent pain control. The majority of this time was spent at home. He needed one replacement of the epidural catheter because of migration and pain on injection, but there were no signs of infection.

Learning point

Pelvic tumours often recur in the posterior abdomen and pelvis, invading the lumbar plexus and causing neuropathic pain in the leg. CT scanning of the abdomen and pelvis is essential to confirm the diagnosis. MRI of the spine will not identify nerve involvement within the psoas muscle. Management may include medication for neuropathic pain, steroids, palliative radiotherapy, palliative chemotherapy and neuraxial local anaesthetics and opioids.

Case study 2

The importance of careful clinical assessment

A lady of 55 years was referred with unilateral chest wall pain in a T5/6 distribution. She was known to have carcinoma of the breast, with widespread bony metastases that had been static for some months. The pain was thought to be coming from a rib secondary and she was referred for an intercostal nerve block.

However, after a careful history and examination it was found that she had difficulty in walking with weakness of her legs, the pain was worse when she was standing, when she became quickly short of breath, with pain on both sides of the chest wall. Neurological examination revealed upgoing plantar reflexes with leg spasticity, hyper-reflexia and weakness. There was no localized chest-wall tenderness. Urgent MRI scanning revealed a secondary in the vertebral bodies of T5 and T6, eroding the pedicles, with incipient spinal cord compression and narrowing of the T5 and T6 neural foraminae.

She was admitted urgently to the hospice, given high dose dexamethasone, and, as no further radiotherapy could be performed, she was referred for consideration of urgent decompressive neurosurgery.

Learning point

Incipient spinal cord compression can present as pain. Although this is usually bilateral it can be worse on one side and should be considered if there is no clear cause for dermatonally distributed pain.

References

1. The British Pain Society with the Association for Palliative Medicine (2009). *Cancer Pain Management*. Available from: http://www.britishpainsociety.org/pub_professional.htm#cancerpain (Accessed 11 February 2011).

2. Davies DD (1993). Incidence of major complications of neurolytic coeliac plexus block. *J Royal Soc Med* **86**(5), 264–66.

3. Stefaniak T, Basinski A, Vingerhoets W *et al.* (2005). A comparison of two invasive techniques in the management of intractable pain due to inoperable pancreatic cancer: neurolytic celiac plexus block and videothorascopic splanchnicectomy. *Eur J Surgical Oncol* **31**(7), 768–73.

4. Wong G, Darrell R, Schroeder P *et al.* (2004). Effect of neurolytic celiac plexus block on pain relief, quality of life, and survival in patients with unresectable pancreatic cancer: a randomized controlled trial. *JAMA* **291**(9), 1092–99.

5. Banning A, Sjøgren P, Henriksen H (1991). Treatment outcome in a multidisciplinary cancer pain clinic. *Pain* **47**(2), 129–34.

6. Smith T, Staats P, Deer T *et al.* (2002). Randomized clinical trial of an implantable drug delivery system compared with comprehensive medical management for refractory cancer pain: impact on pain, drug-related toxicity and survival. *J Clinical Oncology* **20**(19), 4040–49.

7. *NHS cancer plan: a plan for investment, a plan for reform*. September 2000. Available from: www.dh.gov.uk.

8. Control of pain in adults with cancer. A national clinical guideline no.106. Scottish Intercollegiate Guidelines, November 2008. Available from: www.sign.ac.uk.

9. *Supportive and palliative care; the Manual*. March 2004. Available from: www.nice.org.uk.

10. World Health Organization. WHO's pain relief ladder. http://www.who.int/cancer/palliative/painladder/en/.

11. Zhang M, Holman C, Price S *et al.* (2009). Comorbidity and repeat admission to hospital for adverse drug reactions in older adults: retrospective cohort study. *BMJ* **338**, a2752 doi:10.1136/bmj.a2752.

12. Glare P, Walsh D, Sheehan D (2006). The adverse effects of morphine: a prospective survey of common symptoms during repeated dosing for chronic cancer pain. *Am J Hosp Palliat Care* **23**(3), 229–35.

13. Payne R, Mathias S, Pasta D *et al.* (1998). Quality of life and cancer pain: satisfaction and side effects with transdermal fentanyl versus oral morphine. *J Clin Oncology* **16**(4), 1588–93.

14. Candiotti KA, Gitlin MC (2010). Review of the effect of opioid-related side effects on the undertreatment of moderate to severe chronic non-cancer pain: tapentadol, a step toward a solution? *Curr Med Res Opin* **26**(7), 1677–1684.

15. Wang J, Barke RA, Charboneau R *et al.* (2005). Morphine impairs host innate immune response and increases susceptibility to *Streptococcus pneumoniae* lung infection. *J Immunol* **174**(1), 426–34.

16. Saurer TB, Ijames SG, Lysle DT (2006). Neuropeptide YY_1 receptors mediate morphine-induced reductions of natural killer cell activity. *J Neuroimmunol* **177**(1–2), 18–26.

17. Rajagopal A, Vassilopoulou-Sellin R, Palmer JL *et al.* (2004). Symptomatic hypogonadism in male survivors of cancer with chronic exposure to opioids. *Cancer* **100**(4), 851–58.

18. Finnerup NB, Otto M, McQuay HJ, Jensen TS *et al.* (2005). Algorithm for neuropathic pain treatment: an evidence based proposal. *Pain* **118**(3), 289–305.

19. Dworkin RH, O'Connor AB, Backonja M *et al.* (2007). Pharmacologic management of neuropathic pain: evidence-based recommendations. *Pain* **132**(3), 237–51.

20. Neuropathic pain: the pharmacological management of neuropathic pain in adults in non-specialist settings. Nice Guidance CG96. Available from: http://guidance.nice.org.uk/CG96.

21. Grond S, Zech D, Diefenbach C *et al.* (1996). Assessment of cancer pain: a prospective evaluation in 2266 cancer patients referred to a pain service. *Pain* **64**(1), 107–114.

22. Classification of Chronic Pain, IASP Taskforce on Taxonomy 2nd edition (1994). *Part III: pain terms, a current list with definitions and notes on usage* pp209–214, eds H Merskey amd N Bogduk, IASP Press, Seattle

23. Urch CE, Dickenson AH (2008). Neuropathic pain in cancer. *Eur J Cancer* **44**(8), 1091–96.

24. Bennett M (2001). The LANSS pain scale: the Leeds assessment of neuropathic symptoms and signs. *Pain* **92**(1–2), 147–57.

25. Bouhassira D, Attal N, Alchaar H *et al.* (2005). Comparison of pain syndromes associated with nervous or somatic lesions and development of a new neuropathic pain diagnostic questionnaire (DN4). *Pain* **114**(1–2), 29–36.

26. Freynhagen R, Baron R, Gockel U *et al.* (2006). PainDETECT: a new screening questionnaire to identify neuropathic components in patients with back pain. *Curr Med Res Opin* **22**(10), 1911–20.

27. Clark D.(1999). 'Total Pain', disciplinary power and the body in the work of Cicely Saunders 1958–1967. *Soc Sci Med* **49**(6), 727–36.

28. Janig W, Stanton-Hicks M (1996). *Reflex Sympathetic Dystrophy: a Reappraisal.* IASP Press, Seattle.

29. Harden RN, Bruehl SP (2006). Diagnosis of complex regional pain syndrome: signs, symptoms and new empirically derived diagnostic criteria. *Clin J Pain* **22**(5), 415–419.

30. Cleland CS (1991). Pain assessment in cancer. In: Osoba D (ed.). *Effect of Cancer on Quality of Life.* CRC Press, Boca Raton.

31. Zigmond AS, Snaith RP (1983). The hospital anxiety and depression scale. *Acta Psychiatr Scand* **67**(6), 361–70.

32. Melzack R, Wall P (1965). Pain mechanisms: a new theory. *Science* **150**(699), 971–979.

33. Linklater GT, Leng MEF, Tiernan EJ *et al.* (2002). Pain management services in palliative care; a national survey. *Pain Reviews* **9**(3–4), 135–40.

34. Kay S, Husbands E, Antrobus JH *et al.* (2007). Provision for advanced pain management techniques in adult palliative care: a national survey of anaesthetic pain specialists. *Palliative Med* **21**(4), 279–84.

35. Petrovic Z, Hester JB (2007). *A national survey of pain management services in palliative care.* (Personal communication).

Chapter 4

Mechanisms of cancer pain

Catherine Elizabeth Urch

Introduction

Pain is one of the most common symptoms that occur in patients with cancer, alongside fatigue, anxiety and cachexia. Incidence and prevalence varies between tumour types and stage of disease, and thus over 70% of patients with advanced head and neck cancer experience pain, whilst pain is a less common feature of lymphoma (1). With the advent of improved surgery, chemotherapy and radiotherapy regimes for solid tumours, life expectancy has increased. Patients are now living, often for many years, with increased symptoms and pain either from the cancer or its treatment (2).

In order to understand the many unique features of cancer pain it is important to revise our knowledge of the mechanisms of pain pathways in 'normal' acute pains, and some of the more common pathophysiological changes in chronic pain states (such as neuropathy).

Cancer pain cannot be considered as a single entity; it comprises several separate pathological entities:

- direct cancer invasion resulting in combinations of neuropathic, visceral, ischaemic and bone pain
- inflammatory syndromes
- pathologies relating to its presence, e.g. bowel obstruction or raised intracranial pressure
- pathologies caused by cancer treatments, such as chemotherapy or radiation-induced neuropathy

A common debate in recent times has been whether cancer pain represents a different pain state from the accepted mechanisms of neuropathy and inflammation, or whether it is a cause of neuropathy in the same manner that herpes zoster is a trigger. The former camp will cite the many fascinating advances in the understanding of cancer pain pathophysiology, such as unique dorsal horn signalling patterns, the different mode of damage to neurons in chemotherapy-induced neuropathy or the relative resistance to conventional analgesics (3). The latter camp will suggest that cancer pain is not a unique state, but produces multiple concurrent and different triggers onto well understood pain pathways, such as inflammatory, neuropathic and ischaemic pathways, with a rapidly changing time frame of pain development (4).

Acute pain transmission

Acute pain transmission of peripheral noxious stimuli to higher brain centres is often considered the 'normal' pattern from which the protective pain pathway has evolved. The body, in order to protect itself, needs to be rapidly aware of noxious stimuli that may produce actual or potential tissue damage and thus pain pathways have evolved as a protective mechanism for survival, incorporating reflex withdrawal of the sensing limb, rapid coding of 'aversion' and 'threat to self' (affective) pathways, through to higher conscious awareness, attention and localization. These mechanisms in turn enable withdrawal of the affected part, protection (of self and others) and learning or memory (5). The system has elegant thresholds: to filter unnecessary stimuli (tonic inhibition), to feed forward excitatory loops, to ensure rapid magnification of noxious stimuli and counter-balancing negative feedback loops, and to ensure restoration of the conscious pain-free state.

The system is complex, with some aspects hard-wired, for example $A\delta$ and C fibre afferents, whilst others are 'plastic', dynamic and allow differential coding, attention and response (6). An infinite number of interactions with the environment, immune system and higher brain centres create a highly sensitive and reactive system, capable of identifying, reacting to and learning from noxious stimuli.

Afferent fibres

Stimuli below a threshold of actual or potential tissue damage are termed non-noxious and are transmitted to Lamina III of the dorsal horn via $A\beta$ fibres. Noxious stimuli, however, are transmitted via lightly myelinated $A\delta$ or virtually unmeyelinated C fibres to Lamina I and II, respectively, in the dorsal horn (6).

C fibres can be divided into two types. The first type is peptidergic and consists of neuropeptidergic-expressing calcitonin gene-related peptide (CGRP), the vallinoid receptor (TRVP1) and others, and peptide-releasing neurotransmitters such as substance P. The second type consists of non-peptidergic fibres releasing only amino acids (glutamate, aspartate, etc.).

Both $A\delta$ and C fibres have thresholds that must be exceeded before depolarization and transmission of the input. C fibre thresholds vary to the extent that a proportion remain silent in all but the most persistent noxious stimuli (7). Even when the thresholds have been exceeded, the pattern of firing of the $A\delta$ and C fibres varies according to the type, intensity and duration of the stimuli. Stimuli are transduced into electrical conduction via the triggering of specific receptors, i.e. heat, chemical and pressure (Fig. 4.1). Local rapid depolarization is achieved after receptor stimulation, which in ion channels allows positive ion influx. Multiple or persistent local depolarizations are required to trigger wider activation (depolarization of the neuron) and onward transmission. Sequential depolarizations via sodium and voltage gated calcium channels (VDCC) allow the depolarization to be propagated along the neuron to the dorsal root ganglia (DRG) and to the termination areas within the superficial dorsal horn (8). The speed of primary afferent transmission varies in proportion to the depth of the myelin sheath produced by

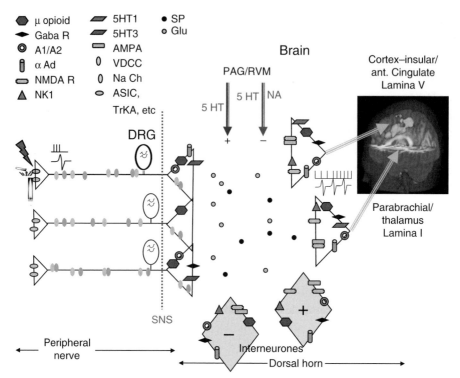

Fig. 4.1 The diagram simplistically summarizes normal acute noxious input from the periphery, through the dorsal horn to the brain. From the left, noxious stimuli, such as heat, chemical or mechanical injury, are transduced via specific receptors, namely temperature coding receptors, acid sensing ion channels (ASIC), TrkA (inflammation) or pressure receptors. Transduction allows a flow of positive ions into the cell, which causes depolarization and action potentials. This is transmitted along the neurone via sodium (NaCh) and calcium (VDCC) channels to the dorsal root ganglion (DRG) and the dorsal horn. The sympathetic nervous system (SNS) lies close to the DRGs but is unaffected in acute noxious transmission. In the dorsal horn extensive modulation of the input can occur. Neurotransmitters such as substance P (SP) or glutamate (Glu) amongst others are released from the primary afferent and diffuse across the synapse. An array of receptors can be triggered, including N-methyl D-aspartate (NMDA), α-amino-3-hydroxy-5-methylisoxazole-4-propionic acid (AMPA), neu-rokinin 1 (NK1) and adenosine (A1/A2). Other inhibitory neurotransmitters are also released either locally, (such as enkephalins [μ opioid receptor] and gamma-aminobutyric acid (GABA)) or as a result of descending inhibition (noradrenalin [α Ad receptor] and serotonin). The overall modulated signal (either increased as shown or decreased) is transmitted to the brain via ascending pathways, predominately the spinothalamic from Lamina V, which terminates in the cortex, and the parabrachial from Lamina I, which terminates in the thalamic areas. Descending pathways arise from the brain and pass through the peri-aquaductal grey (PAG) and rostro-ventral medulla (RVM) areas before terminating in the dorsal horn. Also appears in colour in the colour plate section, Plate 1.

Schwann cells. Aβ fibres are large, thickly myelinated fibres, with the fastest transmission at around 50 m/s, compared with Aδ, more thinly myelinated, at 10 m/s and the unmy-elinated C fibres at 2 m/s. The myelin sheath allows the depolarization to jump to subse-quent nodes of Ranvier (areas of thinning or lack of myelin). The neuronal cell body in turn may alter receptor and neurotransmitter production and transportation, which become increasingly important in pathological pain states.

Dorsal root ganglia

The DRG are situated laterally to the spinal cord, surrounded by the vertebral column. The sympathetic chain lies anterolateral to vertebral column and maintains a close relationship with the spinal cord. The DRG hold the DNA and protein synthesis capacity of the cell, and are thus responsible for all neurotransmitter, receptor and scaffolding protein production together with continuous anterograde and retrograde translocation (9). DRG mechanisms are sensitive and influenced by alterations in internal calcium levels, secondary messenger systems and depolarizations. Altering protein synthesis within neurons produces longer-term changes, which may result in increased or decreased activation threshold, increased or decreased excitation and neurotransmitter release (10).

Dorsal horn

Passing through the dorsal horn entry zone the primary afferents terminate in a specific topographic manner. The dorsal horn is divided into laminae, based originally on the appearance obtained from a light microscope, which fortunately correspond to functional groupings of neurons, such as afferent or motor, primary termination or ascending pathways. Thus Aδ fibres terminate within lamina I, whilst peptidergic and non-peptidergic C fibres terminate in lamina II, inner and outer, respectively (5). Synapses are closely held junctions between two or more neurons or glia. These highly specialized junctions allow communication between neurons and modulation of the original input. Communication occurs via the release of neurotransmitters, which can be excitatory (such as glutamate, glycine or substance P) or inhibitory (such as enkepahlins or GABA) (11), or extra-neuronal signalling such as chemokines and nitric oxide (12, 13). Neurotransmitters diffuse across the synapse to bind to receptors, which may or may not trigger onward depolarization. Each synaptic junction allows for modulation, with excitation or inhibition of the previous input. Modulation can occur at any point in the pathway. Modulation at the receptor level: the receptor may be held in an inhibited or activated state. Modulation at the neuronal level: there may be alteration of neuroreceptor expression, secondary messenger system expression, and synaptic strength allowing different summation from inputs. Modulation throughout CNS involves alteration in descending controls, release of diffusable neurotransmitters (nitric oxide), extra-synaptic transmission and activation, and glial activation. (14, 15).

  The dorsal horn is held in a state of tonic inhibition through the release and effect of the endorphin and cannabinoid systems from inhibitory interneurones (16, 17). Endorphins bind to μ receptors and are part of a wider inhibitory opioid family, including enkephalins, dynorphin and orphanin, which bind respectively to κ, δ and orphanin receptors (18). These are tonically released through out the central nervous system (CNS) and are a central part of preventing overexcitation and death of neurons. In addition to tonic release, endorphins are released following excitation of descending inhibitory pathways and within the dorsal horn and the higher CNS. In the dorsal horn opioids primarily act on presynaptic terminals inducing a hyper-polarization of the primary afferents and in inflammation-activated receptors allow peripheral inhibition (19). Endogenous cannabinoids are equally ubiquitous and act via cannabinoid receptors but also via direct transmembrane diffusion (20). Opioid and cannabinoid systems are both part of the immune–neuron interactions (21).

The overall response that is transmitted to higher centres as a result of an initial primary afferent stimulation is dependent on the intensity and duration of the stimulation, modulation of Aδ and C fibres and further complex modulation within the dorsal horn. This allows a commonly experienced phenomenon to be explained (for example pain following a skin incision: one of sudden severe pain initially (with rapid transmission of noxious input and excitation within primary afferents and dorsal horn), followed by a reduction in pain sensation (with peripheral and central inhibition) then persistent hyperalgesia during tissue healing, reduced sensation (overshoot of tonic inhibition) and gradual restoration of normal sensation. In addition there is a fast reflex arc, which connects the dorsal and ventral horn and which allows very rapid, 'unconscious' withdrawal from pain stimuli.

Glia

More recently the role of glia cells in the generation and maintenance of pain pathways has been demonstrated. Far from being merely bystander cells, whose role was only to support neurones, it has now been acknowledged that astrocytes and the immune-derived microglia play an intrinsic role in pain pathways as do neurones (22, 23). These roles have been demonstrated in numerous pain states such as neuropathy and inflammation, where hypertophy of glia, with activation morphology (with the formation of numerous stellate processes), and an increased number of glia have been shown. Microglia activation is in part due to intrinsic glia division, but also reflects invasion and capture of circulating immune cells. Thus centrally and peripherally there is an intrinsic and dynamic interaction between the fixed neuronal system and the mobile immune system. Neuronal-glia interaction is fundamental to the excitation state of neurons, maintenance of synaptic homeostasis and tonic inhibition (24, 25). For example, glia are responsible for the scavenging of glutamate, which is a potent excitatory neurotransmitter amino acid, via the GALT receptor family, thus terminating synaptic and extra-synaptic activation. The chemokine–receptor interaction responsible for glia leads neuronal excitation (26, 27). Attenuation of behavioural hyperalgesic response to a noxious stimulus has been achieved through application of glia inhibitors alone (28, 29).

Connections with higher centres

The dorsal horn is intimately connected to the brain via several pathways (Fig. 4.1). The spinothalamic tract carries information via the thalamus, ultimately to the cortical areas of the brain. The pre-frontal cortex corresponds to conscious awareness of pain, topographic location and intensity rating of the given noxious stimulus, whilst other cortical and cingulated areas correspond to the attentive, evaluative and discriminatory aspects of pain (30).

Another important ascending pathway is the parabrachial or hypothalamic pathway, which ultimately projects onto limbic and amygdala regions of the brain (affective coding areas), hippocampal region (memory coding area) and the brain stem (physiological response) (31). These are non-topographical and lack intensity thresholds, but are responsible for the unpleasantness and aversive qualities of the pain experience, and affect core homeostatic functions such as mood, sleep, appetite, blood pressure, etc. and trigger memory recall and learning. The mid-insular region preferentially codes for visceral/autonomic stimuli, and links viscero-visceral loops and autonomic responses (32).

The brain

Recent functional MRI (fMRI) research has demonstrated a pattern of central neuronal response of closely connected and interdependent areas termed the pain matrix or pain networks. Thus experiments have elegantly demonstrated that the anterior cingulated cortex is required for attention to a task or input, whilst altered mood pre-excites the limbic and the amygdala systems, which centrally sensitizes the pain matrix (33). Thus a larger response is seen to a fixed stimulus in depressed as opposed to non-depressed people (34). Empathy to pain and mirror pain can be demonstrated by activation of the brain pain matrix in response to a loved one receiving a painful stimulus (35). This has gone some way to explain the clinical and human experience of feeling 'pain' in intense emotional states such as bereavement, or in response to witnessing pain in a loved one. The response of the central pain matrix is just as dynamic as, and can be modulated to an even greater degree than, the dorsal horn response. Thus CNS activation can be altered by anticipating pain, by anticipating analgesia (as in placebo) and during distraction from the stimulus, or indeed suppressed where inflicted pain is a retribution or punishment.

It is important that the brain can both consciously and unconsciously modulate the dorsal horn response. The numerous descending pathways converge in the peri-aquaductal grey and rostroventral medulla. These complex areas receive inputs from other central areas, and further modulate the descending output (36). A dynamic of excitation, inhibition and disinhibition, and neutral firing of neurons results in two major descending pathways to the dorsal horn. One is inhibitory (noradrenergic and serotonin-releasing), terminating on primary interneurons and projection neurons. The effect of excitation of this pathway is to inhibit or reduce excitation of the dorsal horn. A more recently described descending pathway is excitatory (serotonin) (37), which terminates on primary afferents. Thus potential feed-forward or inhibition loops can be generated entirely centrally.

Neuropathic pain

Neuropathic pain arises from damage to a nerve, usually peripherally (e.g. post-herpetic neuralgia from herpes zoster, or trauma to a peripheral nerve) but can also be centrally induced (i.e. post-stroke pain). The damage to the nerve allows a train of pathological events to be initiated and then maintained, resulting in classical symptoms and signs of allodynia, hyperalgesia, dysaesthesia and sensory loss. Fig. 4.2 gives a brief summary of the changes that occur (38).

Altered transmission

Normal transmission relies on ordered sequential functioning of sodium and calcium channels, allowing depolorization to occur in a specific place and time. In damaged neurones (such as transection, as may occur following surgery or amputation) the severed neurone responds to the loss of its distal portion by trying to re-grow (sprouting), forming neuroma (whorls of neuronal tissue with or without myelin), and developing abnormal accumulations of sodium and calcium channels (4). These channels are not only abnormal, having increased density, but also undergo a change in character and activation properties. In other neuropathic models there is an overall reduction of sodium channels in damaged neurones and an increase in neighbouring, otherwise undamaged, neurones (39). This results in previously normal neurones becoming 'abnormal' and contributes to the clinical phenomenon of primary hyperaglesia.

At present nine different sodium channels have been identified, which possess different characteristics with respect to the voltage at which they open, how long they stay open, how quickly they close (inactivate) and the refractory time before re-opening. The distribution of sodium channels alters with development (during foetal and early childhood), type of neurone and in response to damage. It has been shown that a foetal sodium channel, $Na_v1.3$, is upregulated following neuropathy. $Na_v1.8$ is located on small diameter primary afferents (Aδ and C fibres), whilst $Na_v1.7$ is on all sizes of fibre (40). Work suggests that the differential expression and accumulation of sodium channels is responsible for spontaneous discharges in damaged neurones, which may be perceived as spontaneous pain. Likewise, the calcium channels belong to a large family and are differentially located depending on neuronal type and damage (41). All calcium channels contain a sub-unit α2δ, which is an important therapeutic target for gabapentin (42). Remodelling of other membrane channels, such as potassium channels, is important, if not as well characterized.

The chaotic depolarization and transmission affects events within the neurone (such as altered retrograde translation of nerve growth factor) and the dorsal root ganglion (with activation of *c-fos* and other genes), and results in altered receptor and secondary messenger translation, both between neurones and within the dorsal horn. In the periphery, the abnormal neuronal sprouting can lead to an enlargement of the receptive field (area of body) that feeds the abnormal pain transmission (43). These nerve endings also 'cross-talk' to other non-damaged nerves, in turn altering the normal nerves to become abnormal and chaotic (44). Likewise the damaged neurone itself engages in 'epiphatic' cross-talk to non-damaged neurones within its bundle. This cross-talk causes a synchronous depolarization and perpetuates the pathological characteristics onto otherwise normal non-damaged neurones (43).

Alterations within the dorsal horn

This area, as noted above, is a central point of modulation of normal pain signals, and is also vital to the onward transmission of the abnormal and chaotic inputs from damaged (and adjacent) non-damaged neurones. The Aδ and C fibres terminate predominately in the superficial layers (Lamina I and II) of the dorsal horn, also Aδ in Lamina V, and the

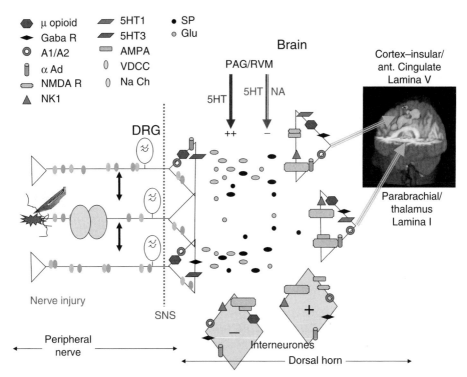

Fig. 4.2 The same simplified diagram is used to summarize the changes that occur in the peripheral and central neuronal pathways following a peripheral nerve injury (nerve transection shown), resulting in chronic neuropathy. In the periphery, the nerve distal and the injury dies and regenerates in an abnormal manner. The sodium (NaCh) and calcium (VDCC) channels alter in expression (to be more responsive) and number (increase particularly around the area of damage). Aberrant transmission in the damaged nerve leads to spontaneous discharge and epiphatic cross-talk between damaged and undamaged neurones, and between DRG and SNS. This results in an increase in the receptive field size and spontaneous and lower threshold discharge of neurones, and can lead to the aberrant excitation of the sympathetic nervous system. Within the dorsal horn, glutamate (Glu) and substance P (SP) are released in increased and irregular amounts (not necessarily in response to a threshold stimuli), although there may be reduced or absent release in the damaged neurone termination. Increased excitatory amino acid release results in an overall excitation of the inter-neurones and increased transmission to the brain. This is further enhanced by the overall reduction in inhibition, by the loss of GABAergic neurones, the relative inactivation of μ opioid receptors and facilitation of descending serotonin–5HT3 excitation pathways. Also appears in colour in the colour plate section, Plate 2.

non-noxious Aβ fibres terminate in Lamina III (45). Work some years ago suggested that there was abnormal re-sprouting of Aβ fibres into Lamina II following axotomy, thus allowing non-painful thresholds to be translated in the dorsal horn as pain. This would have accounted nicely for the symptom of allodynia. This theory, whilst widely quoted and beguiling in its neatness, has largely been disproved and dorsal horn neuronal reorganization should be viewed as contentious. It appears that C fibres take on characteristics of and express receptors that are normally confined to low-threshold Aβ fibres (45).

Within the dorsal horn, the abnormal primary afferent inputs result in areas of 'silence' (with no input) and areas of chaotic overactivity. The increased release of neurotransmitters allows the prolonged depolarization of the post-synaptic neurones, and the activation of the important N-methyl-D-aspartate (NMDA) receptor (7, 46). This receptor is important, as it usually remains held closed by magnesium ion block until the cell is depolarized and there continues to be glutamate (and glycine) binding to the receptor. Once these multiple events occur, the receptor opens and allows a flood of calcium (and sodium) into the cell (47). The effect is one of massive excitation within the neurone—the phenomenon of wind-up, a greatly increased response to a given stimuli. An increase in calcium within the cell not only depolarizes/activates it, but also sets in train a series of events that modify receptors (either more open or more closed), activates secondary messenger pathways, alters gene expression, increases the production of excitatory gases such as nitric oxide and also has other effects. The overall effect is one of neuronal excitation.

In addition it appears that there is an overall reduction in the inhibition within the dorsal horn, either by loss or downregulation of GABAergic neurones, or loss of active intrinsic opioid receptors and/or reduction in descending inhibitory pathways (45) (Fig. 4.2).

Central alterations in neuropathic pain states

Peripheral and dorsal horn alterations have been investigated extensively for decades in animal models. The areas are readily accessible and much has been elucidated about the pathophysiological state, which has been confirmed in human studies (where possible). The more central areas within the brain have remained a black box for some time, but over the last decade sophisticated animal work within the rostro-ventral medulla (RVM) and peri-aquaductal grey (PAG) have revealed a complex web of interconnecting neurones, with specific ON, OFF and neutral cells that are central in controlling descending pathways back to the dorsal horn (48). These areas in turn have projections to and from other areas such as the sensory cortex and hypothalamus (Fig. 4.2). The recent refinement of fMRI and positron emission tomography imaging has allowed a more clinical-based approach to understanding the complex interconnections and plasticity within the brain following neuropathic injury (49).

Extensive modulation, excitation and abnormal changes that occur in primary afferents and dorsal horn continue throughout the higher pain centres, in particular the RVM, PAG, thalamus, primary somatosensory cortex (S1 and S2) and anterior cingulate cortex (50). Recent fMRI work has suggested that distinct regions of the brain are activated with noxious stimuli, pain, anticipation, recall and emotion, and are altered in states of chronic pain. Also fMRI has allowed the study of clinical pain states and has shown extensive plasticity, re-mapping and excitation, which alter pre- and post-pain control (51). For example, in complex regional pain syndrome the areas that map body location in the cortex showed a reduction in the space between them; this reverted to normal spacing when the pain had been controlled (52). Thus a long-term pathological state of central sensitization can be maintained via central feed-forward loops, with or without continued peripheral input.

Descending controls

Serotonergic pathways appear to be central in the descending facilitatory pathway. From spinal cord lamina I, the parabrachial pathway ascends to the brainstem (hypothalamus). The signals are modulated and transmitted to the PAG and RVM, from where the descending system commences and terminates back within the spinal cord (53). In animal neuropathy it has been shown that this 5HT pathway is facilitated. In humans it has been shown that the attention/distraction centre of the PAG is altered in humans with chronic pain, leading to a reduction in descending inhibition (54). It must be remembered that, whilst the ascending spinothalamic pathways retain a strict location mapping, the parabrachial and descending systems are diffuse and lack location mapping (Fig. 4.2).

Inflammatory pain

A state of central hyperalgesia is produced in inflammatory pain secondary to sensitization of the primary afferents, in response to inflammatory mediators, such as bradykinin, histamine, nerve growth factor (NGF), interleukins, cytokines and ATP (from dying cells), etc. (6). The neuronal response establishes a feed-forward loop, with release of neurokinins (e.g. substance P), which in turn triggers depolarization of the primary afferent. The overall effect is one of reduced threshold for primary afferent depolarization and increased input to the dorsal horn (12). Within the dorsal horn activation of the non-neuronal cells, glia and astrocytes are now understood to be essential in the initiation and maintenance of central neuronal activation. Neuronal–non-neuronal communication is intricate and frequently relies on chemokines and interleukin production. In inflammatory pain states there is increased COX-II activity, both peripherally and centrally (55). Inflammatory pain has inbuilt inhibitory loops with the co-activation of peripheral and central opioid receptors, allowing for effective termination if the inflammatory stimulus is removed. Peripheral opioid receptors, whilst expressed, are only coupled to G-proteins and activated following inflammatory stimuli (56). This has a dual effect of allowing immune modulation of the neuronal pathway and a peripheral inhibition to be activated. The dorsal horn response to inflammatory stimuli includes increased expression of cholecystokinin which in turn facilitates opioid receptor activation, thus rendering inflammatory pain more sensitive to the modulating effects of opioid agonists (57). Whilst inflammatory states can be chronic and trigger central sensitization and CNS activation, they require ongoing inflammatory stimulus and input sufficient to overcome the innate inhibitory pathways. This is in contrast to neuropathic damage, where there is an overall reduction in innate inhibition.

Cancer-induced pain

The main problem encountered when establishing an animal model of any cancer-induced pain is the well-being of the animals. Systemic cancer or chemotherapy regimes often induce unacceptable side effects, and the pain behaviours are hard to interpret. In the last 20 years, models of confined tumour growth (either within a bone, around a nerve or within viscera) have allowed detailed pathophysiology to be investigated in otherwise well animals (58–60). It is acknowledged that animal models have limitations: in time (most models run over days or weeks, not months and years as in humans), in higher-centre perceptions of suffering, and also in the presence of co-morbidities. However, animal models have allowed the exploration and interpretation of the mechanisms of pain patho-physiology and exploitation of new therapeutics. In cancer pain they are allowing a deeper understanding of this complex pain state. In therapeutic terms, animal models do appear to have face validity, with broad equivalence demonstrated in clinical trials, albeit at a lower level of efficacy (61).

Cancer-induced bone pain

During the past decade there have been numerous models of cancer-induced bone pain (CIBP) reported. The initial work inoculated mouse osteosarcoma cells into a femur, which led to an evolving state of pain behaviours, bone destruction–remodelling and pathological fracture (58). The model appeared to closely parallel the clinical pattern, with radiologically obvious bone destruction and pathological fracture, and increasing pain behaviours of limping, limb guarding and tenderness (Fig. 4.3). Until recently primary afferents were thought to be present only in the periosteum, but with different bone preparation it has been found that bones are densely innervated. The majority of primary afferents are A-delta and peptidergic C fibres as well as contributions from the sympathetic nervous system. This rich primary afferent network could be triggered by alterations within the bone or marrow without periosteal damage.

As cancer invades and grows within the marrow it induces a profound inflammatory response, as well as intrinsic activation of the osteoclast/osteoblast axis (primarily via the receptor activator of NF-kappa B (RANK–Ligand pathway). The result is progressive bone destruction, aberrant bone remodelling, cell death, inflammation and primary afferent deafferentation (62). Depolarization of primary afferents arises from a combination of inflammatory and neuropathic stimuli occurring simultaneously. The dorsal horn also undergoes unique alterations. In a rat model of breast cancer the dorsal horn excitation paralleled the evolution of pain behaviours, but the pattern of neuronal, glial and receptor excitation was different from pure neuropathy or inflammation (3). Superficial Lamina I neurons became hyperexcitable with an expansion of wide-dynamic range (WDR) neurons (i.e. neurons that depolarize to a wide range of stimuli) from 25 to 50% of the population and a relative reduction of nociceptive specific neurons occurs (63) (Fig. 4.3). The expansion leads to overall dorsal horn pro-excitation, however it is as yet unclear whether this represents an alteration of nociceptive specific neurons or an activation of a previously silent WDR population. Immunocytochemistry also suggests a unique combination of neuroreceptor activity, with activated glia, raised dynorphin, but a notable lack of the changes expected in neuropathic (i.e. raised neuropeptide Y, galanin, etc.) or inflammatory pain states (raised CGRP, etc.) (58, 64).

In addition, in CIBP the significant astrocyte and microglia activation implies a central role for glia-neuronal interactions (65). Experimental CIBP has been shown to increase spinal levels of a non-histone chromosomal protein, high mobility group: box 1 (HMGB1)

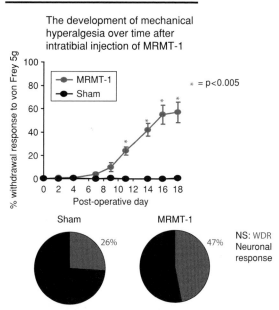

Fig. 4.3 Results of intra-tibial injection of MRMT-1 breast cancer cells in rat model of cancer-induced bone pain (CIBP). Left, two scanning electron microscope pictures of a normal rat tibia (top) and the pathological fracture (bottom) after day20. Note abnormal bone resorption (osteoclast action) and abnormal bone formation (osteoblast action). Right, the top panel demonstrates the withdrawal response to von Frey 5g filament over day0-day18 post MRMT1 injection (red) and sham injection (blue). Note the significant withdrawal from day11 showing that hyperalgesia occures in this model of cancer induced bone pain. The bottom panel demonstrates the ratio of nociceptive specific (NS) to wide-dynamic range (WDR) in normal (or sham) and in CIBP (from day15 onwards). It can be seen that the percentage of WDR neurones increases from 25% to almost 50%. Also appears in colour in the colour plate section, Plate 3.

and interleukin 1 (IL-1); both activate microglia and upregulate the superfamily of TOLL receptors (which, in turn, also upregulate IL-1 and tumour necrosis factor (TNF)). HMGB-1 or IL-1 antagonists can attenuate experimental CIBP, and increased opioid sensitivity can be induced via antagonism of TOLL-4 receptors (66). In an rodent model of CIBP (breast cancer cells infused into a rat tibia on D0), the development of CIBP behaviours (usually manifest by day9) could be delayed by systemic administration of minocycline (a potent inhibitor of microglia but not astrocytes) during day0-day9. But not when the minocycline administration start was delayed. This observation indicates a role for microglia in the induction and generation of neuronal excitation and activation of the pain pathway, but less of a role in maintenance.

Attenuation of CIBP has been demonstrated using conventional analgesics such as opioids, albeit at doses more akin to neuropathy models, as well as neuropathic agents such as gabapentin (67). In addition, novel targets of inhibition of bone turnover (i.e. osteoprogetergin), blocking of peripheral NGF (inflammatory) via Trk A receptor sequestering or antagonism of the endothelin-A receptor (a key factor in cancer cell spread and a primary afferent receptor) have all been demonstrated to significantly reduce pain behaviours in animal models and in some cases clinical studies (68, 69). Other drugs such as bisphosphonates may attenuate pain indirectly by altering and inhibiting osteoclast activation, and thus reducing the acid microenvironment, bone destruction and de-afferentation.

Cancer and chemotherapy-induced neuropathy

Neuropathic pain in cancer patients may arise as a result of physical compression of the nerve by the growing tumour or through direct infiltration into the nerve. Pain can also be secondary to a change in tissue pH (acidosis) or to the release of chemical algogens by the tumour, either in areas surrounding the nerve or directly in the nerve itself following tumour infiltration. Paradoxically, neuropathy can also arise as a consequence of cancer-directed therapy, from chemotherapy, radiotherapy or surgery. Drugs such as paclitaxel, vincristine and cisplatin have been widely reported to produce sensory neuropathies, evoking tingling sensations, paresthesiae or numbness in the distal extremities consistent with a glove-and-stocking distribution (70).

Despite the existence of a wide range of rodent neuropathy models, there exist only a limited number of animal models involving cancer-related nerve damage. Of these, the most widely studied models involve the use of chemotherapy agents (e.g. taxol, platins) or the inoculation of tumour cells adjacent to peripheral nerves (e.g. sarcoma, mammary carcinoma). However, in all models animals are often generally unwell (71, 72). Although the originating source of pain may differ between malignant (e.g. tumour compression) and non-malignant neuropathic pain (e.g. diabetic neuropathy), the mechanisms and neural pathways involved in the generation of the pain state are essentially similar and, as such, much of the underlying pathology can be inferred from mechanisms operating in non-malignant neuropathic pain. For example, inoculation of Meth-A sarcoma cells in the vicinity of the mouse sciatic nerve results in the growth of a tumour mass embedding the nerve (72). Pain behaviours reach a maximum by three weeks post-inoculation, at a time when clear histological signs of nerve damage can be identified. Further immunohistochemical analysis reveals enhanced spinal expression of c-fos (a marker of neuronal activation) and neuropeptides (e.g. substance P, CGRP, dynorphin A), indicating enhanced pain transmission within nociceptive circuits, consistent with behavioural findings (73).

However, there is a gradual decline of pain behaviours and subsequent appearance of hyposensitivity, which may in part correspond to progressive motor paralysis in the animals. Evidence for nerve damage and neural infiltration of immune and malignant cells (with mild oedema) would suggest the involvement of neuropathic, as well as inflammatory, processes in cancer-induced pain, highlighting the complex pathology of this condition.

Models of chemotherapy-induced neuropathy are more common and indicate novel mechanisms for neuropathic pain, but have difficulty in reproducing the hypoaesthesia alongside the hyperalgesia seen in humans. In a rat model of taxol-induced neuropathy the rat sciatic nerves revealed evidence of marked microtubular aggregation within axons, which appear to be the primary site of target of this drug (74). This interferes with microtubule dynamics, arresting cellular division and engaging apoptosis. Taxol has been shown to accumulate in peripheral nerves and DRGs (75). In addition, neuroimmune reactions are evoked with pro-inflammatory cytokine release (e.g. TNF-α., IL–6), which may underlie the flu-like symptoms experienced by patients and may contribute to the development of sensory neuropathy.

Visceral pain

Over the last five years there has been an increase in the understanding of visceral neurons and central processing of visceral pain. However, clinical management remains difficult and has been unchanged for years (76). The innervation of viscera is complex, with contributions from both the autonomic system (e.g. the vagus) and C fibers (77). Visceral pain is diffuse in nature and may be referred and difficult to locate, in contrast to somatic pain. Visceral afferents represent 10% of all spinal afferent input and are found throughout the spinal cord and synapse, with second order neurones over several segments, which in turn receive input from several visceral and non-visceral afferents. The majority (80%) of visceral afferents are 'silent', being recruited only after pre-sensitization or after dorsal horn excitation (78). Both events may occur via non-visceral stimuli, for example anxiety may produce both descending facilitation and increased gut motility, which in turn can be interpreted consciously as discomfort and 'pain'. Higher CNS input differs from somatic nociception in that visceral inputs are transmitted in greater number to the hypothalamus pathway and to the cingulate, but localization to the pre-frontal cortex is sparse. This typically leads to unconscious perception, feelings of aversion and threat to self, attention to and attempted escape from the discomfort, but poor pain location and poor intensity rating (79).

Two neural pathways, typically parasympathetic via the vagus and sympathetic via the sympathetic chain or hypogastric plexuses in the pelvis, innervate each organ. Only high-threshold mechano-sensitization produces aversive sensation in viscera, in contrast to skin afferents, where low-threshold mechanoreceptors also sensitize, providing a significant increase in spinal cord input in certain conditions (such as inflammation). Chemosensitivity is complex. For example, proton exposure can lead to adverse or painful response but typically nutrient proton exposure does not (80). From animal knock-out work it appears that the acid sensing ion channel 3 (ASIC3) is critical to mechanosensitivity in the colon, whereas ASIC2 contributes an inhibitory or facilitatory function depending on the class of neurones (81).

Cancer-induced visceral pain is complex and difficult to reproduce in murine models. Many are painless despite considerable tumour load, such as the murine adenomatous polyposis model (genetic mutation in APC gene), which develops multiple colonic polyps allowing evaluation of pharmacological agents. However, pain/hypersensitivity has not been described (82). Mantyh *et al.* have recently reported a pancreatic cancer model in transgenic mice. Cancer was present with invasion, increased angiogenesis and immune infiltration by week 6. But pain was a late feature, occurring up to 16 weeks post-innoculation and characterized by sudden onset writhing and hypersensitivity. Opioids were effective analgesics, but importantly, mu opioid receptor antagonist (naloxone), given intrathecally prior to week 16, precipitated pain behaviours (83). This suggests that one reason for the sudden onset of cancer pain is not due to the expansion of the cancer or new destruction; rather it is secondary to the loss of tonic inhibition provided by endogenous opioids.

Conclusion

It is clear from the above discussion that cancer pain, whilst employing the same basic mechanisms of pain transmission as non-cancer pain, i.e. mechanisms involving transduction, neurotransmitters and receptors, is a highly complex pain situation. The diverse nature of the multiplicity of inducers means that cancer pain is rarely a pure neuropathic, inflammatory or visceral pain. Rather, cancer pains are perhaps unique in being a combination of interactions, modulations and interplay from each mechanism and type. In addition, the ever-changing stimuli as the tumour progresses or regresses lead to a complex re-emergence of pain and an alteration in the balance of pain (for example from visceral to neuropathic) and, consequently, complex polypharmacy and non-drug interventions are required to treat pain. It is clear that extrapolation from non-cancer pain physiology is possible, but further work is needed to elucidate what aspects of cancer-induced pain are indeed unique.

References

1. van den Beuken-van Everdingen MH, de Rijke JM, Kessels AG *et al.* (2007). Prevalence of pain in patients with cancer: a systematic review of the past 40 years. *Ann Oncol* **18**(9), 1437–49.
2. van den Beuken-van Everdingen MH, de Rijke JM, Kessels AG *et al.* (2007). High prevalence of pain in patients with cancer in a large population-based study in The Netherlands. *Pain* **132**(3), 312–20.
3. Urch C (2004). The pathophysiology of cancer-induced bone pain: current understanding. *Palliat Med* **18**(4), 267–74.
4. Hansson PT, Dickenson AH (2005). Pharmacological treatment of peripheral neuropathic pain conditions based on shared commonalities despite multiple etiologies. *Pain* **113**(3), 251–4.
5. D'Mello R, Dickenson AH (2008). Spinal cord mechanisms of pain. *Br J Anaesth* **101**(1), 8–16.
6. Besson JM (1999). The neurobiology of pain. *Lancet* **353**(9164), 1610–5.
7. Herrero JF, Laird JM, Lopez-Garcia JA (2000). Wind-up of spinal cord neurones and pain sensation: much ado about something? *Prog Neurobiol* **61**(2), 169–203.
8. Treede RD (1995). Peripheral acute pain mechanisms. *Ann Med* **27**(2), 213–6.
9. Woolf CJ, Costigan M (1999). Transcriptional and posttranslational plasticity and the generation of inflammatory pain. *Proc Natl Acad Sci USA* **96**(14), 7723–30.
10. Luo ZD, Chaplan SR, Higuera ES *et al.* (2001). Upregulation of dorsal root ganglion (alpha)2(delta) calcium channel subunit and its correlation with allodynia in spinal nerve-injured rats. *J Neurosci* **21**(6), 1868–75.
11. Carpenter KJ, Dickenson AH (2002). Molecular aspects of pain research. *Pharmacogenomics J* **2**(2), 87–95.
12. Dickenson AH (1995). Spinal cord pharmacology of pain. *Br J Anaesth* **75**(2), 193–200.
13. Mannion RJ, Woolf CJ (2000). Pain mechanisms and management: a central perspective. *Clin J Pain* **16**(3 Suppl), S144–56.
14. Woolf CJ (2000). Pain. *Neurobiol Dis* **7**(5), 504–10.
15. Ji RR, Woolf CJ (2001). Neuronal plasticity and signal transduction in nociceptive neurons: implications for the initiation and maintenance of pathological pain. *Neurobiol Dis* **8**(1), 1–10.

16. Melzack R (1999). From the gate to the neuromatrix. *Pain* 82(Suppl 1), S121–6.

17. McCormack K, Prather P, Chapleo C (1998). Some new insights into the effects of opioids in phasic and tonic nociceptive tests. *Pain* **78**(2), 79–98.

18. Milligan G (2005). Opioid receptors and their interacting proteins. *Neuromolecular Med* **7**(1–2), 51–9.

19. Stein C, Zollner C (2009). Opioids and sensory nerves. *Handb Exp Pharmacol* **194**, 495–518.

20. Anand P, Whiteside G, Fowler CJ *et al.* (2009). Targeting CB2 receptors and the endocannabinoid system for the treatment of pain. *Brain Res Rev* **60**(1), 255–66.

21. Vigano D, Rubino T, Parolaro D (2005). Molecular and cellular basis of cannabinoid and opioid interactions. *Pharmacol Biochem Behav* **81**(2), 360–8.

22. Haydon PG (2000). Neuroglial networks: neurons and glia talk to each other. *Curr Biol* **10**(19), R712–4.

23. Watkins LR, Milligan ED, Maier SF (2001). Spinal cord glia: new players in pain. *Pain* **93**(3), 201–5.

24. Aldskogius H, Liu L, Svensson M (1999). Glial responses to synaptic damage and plasticity. *J Neurosci Res* **58**(1), 33–41.

25. Watkins LR, Hutchinson MR, Milligan ED *et al.* (2007). 'Listening' and 'talking' to neurons: implications of immune activation for pain control and increasing the efficacy of opioids. *Brain Res Rev* **56**(1), 148–69.

26. Gegelashvili G, Dehnes Y, Danbolt NC *et al.* (2000). The high-affinity glutamate transporters GLT1, GLAST, and EAAT4 are regulated via different signalling mechanisms. *Neurochem Int* **37**(2–3), 163–70.

27. Lindia JA, McGowan E, Jochnowitz N *et al.* (2005). Induction of CX3CL1 expression in astrocytes and CX3CR1 in microglia in the spinal cord of a rat model of neuropathic pain. *J Pain* **6**(7), 434–8.

28. Raghavendra V, Tanga F, Rutkowski MD *et al.* (2003). Anti-hyperalgesic and morphine-sparing actions of propentofylline following peripheral nerve injury in rats: mechanistic implications of spinal glia and proinflammatory cytokines. *Pain* **104**(3), 655–64.

29. Ledeboer A, Sloane EM, Milligan ED *et al.* (2005). Minocycline attenuates mechanical allodynia and proinflammatory cytokine expression in rat models of pain facilitation. *Pain* **115**(1–2), 71–83.

30. Hudson AJ (2000). Pain perception and response: central nervous system mechanisms. *Can J Neurol Sci* **27**(1), 2–16.

31. Gauriau C, Bernard JF (2002). Pain pathways and parabrachial circuits in the rat. *Exp Physiol* **87**(2), 251–8.

32. Apkarian AV, Bushnell MC, Treede RD *et al.* (2005). Human brain mechanisms of pain perception and regulation in health and disease. *Eur J Pain* **9**(4), 463–84.

33. Ploghaus A, Tracey I, Gati JS *et al.* (1999). Dissociating pain from its anticipation in the human brain. *Science* **284**(5422), 1979–81.

34. Ploghaus A, Narain C, Beckmann CF *et al.* (2001). Exacerbation of pain by anxiety is associated with activity in a hippocampal network. *J Neurosci* **21**(24), 9896–903.

35. Cheng Y, Chen C, Lin CP *et al.* (2010). Love hurts: an fMRI study. *Neuroimage* **51**(2), 923–9.

36. Gebhart GF (2004). Descending modulation of pain. *Neurosci Biobehav Rev* **27**, 729–37.

37. Suzuki R, Rahman W, Hunt SP *et al.* (2004). Descending facilitatory control of mechanically evoked responses is enhanced in deep dorsal horn neurones following peripheral nerve injury. *Brain Res* **1019**(1–2), 68–76.

38. Suzuki R, Dickenson AH (2000). Neuropathic pain: nerves bursting with excitement. *Neuroreport* **11**(12), R17–21.

39. Djouhri L, Koutsikou S, Fang X *et al.* (2006). Spontaneous pain, both neuropathic and inflammatory, is related to frequency of spontaneous firing in intact C-fiber nociceptors. *J Neurosci* **26**(4), 1281–92.

40. Devor M (2006). Sodium channels and mechanisms of neuropathic pain. *J Pain* **7**(1 Suppl 1), S3–S12.

41. Matthews EA, Dickenson AH (2001). Effects of spinally delivered N- and P-type voltage-dependent calcium channel antagonists on dorsal horn neuronal responses in a rat model of neuropathy. *Pain* **92**(1–2), 235–46.

42. Gilron I, Flatters SJ, Bennett GJ (2006). Gabapentin and pregabalin for the treatment of neuropathic pain: A review of laboratory and clinical evidence studies of peripheral sensory nerves in paclitaxel-induced painful peripheral neuropathy: evidence for mitochondrial dysfunction Ethosuximide reverses paclitaxel- and vincristine-induced painful peripheral neuropathy. *Pain Res Manag* **11**, (Suppl A 3), 16A–29A.

43. Koltzenburg M, Scadding J (2001). Neuropathic pain. *Curr Opin Neurol* **14**(5), 641–7.

44. Campbell JN (2001). Nerve lesions and the generation of pain. *Muscle Nerve* **24**(10), 1261–73.

45. Costigan M, Scholz J, Woolf CJ (2009). Neuropathic pain: a maladaptive response of the nervous system to damage. *Annu Rev Neurosci* **32**, 1–32.

46. Woolf CJ, Thompson SW (1991). The induction and maintenance of central sensitization is dependent on N-methyl-D-aspartic acid receptor activation; implications for the treatment of post-injury pain hypersensitivity states. *Pain* **44**(3), 293–9.

47. Dickenson AH, Chapman V, Green GM (1997). The pharmacology of excitatory and inhibitory amino acid-mediated events in the transmission and modulation of pain in the spinal cord. *Gen Pharmacol* **28**(5), 633–8.

48. Heinricher MM, Tavares I, Leith JL *et al.* (2009). Descending control of nociception: Specificity, recruitment and plasticity. *Brain Res Rev* **60**(1), 214–25.

49. Bridges D, Thompson SW, Rice AS (2001). Mechanisms of neuropathic pain. *Br J Anaesth* **87**(1), 12–26.

50. Tracey I (2005). Functional connectivity and pain: how effectively connected is your brain? *Pain* **116**(3), 173–4.

51. Borsook D, Becerra LR (2006). Breaking down the barriers: fMRI applications in pain, analgesia and analgesics. *Mol Pain* **2**, 30.

52. Becerra L, Schwartzman RJ, Kiefer RT *et al.* (2009). CNS measures of pain responses pre- and post-anesthetic ketamine in a patient with complex regional pain syndrome. *Pain Med epub ahead of print* www.ncbi.nlm.nih.gov/pubmed/19254342.

53. Suzuki R, Rygh LJ, Dickenson AH (2004). Bad news from the brain: descending 5-HT pathways that control spinal pain processing. *Trends Pharmacol Sci* **25**(12), 613–7.

54. Fairhurst M, Wiech K, Dunckley P *et al.* (2007). Anticipatory brainstem activity predicts neural processing of pain in humans. *Pain* **128**(1–2), 101–10.

55. Scheuren N, Neupert W, Ionac M *et al.* (1997). Peripheral noxious stimulation releases spinal PGE2 during the first phase in the formalin assay of the rat. *Life Sci* **60**(21), 295–300.

56. Stein C, Lang LJ (2009). Peripheral mechanisms of opioid analgesia. *Curr Opin Pharmacol* **9**(1), 3–8.

57. Stanfa L, Dickenson A (1995). Spinal opioid systems in inflammation. *Inflamm Res* **44**(6), 231–41.

58. Honore P, Schwei J, Rogers SD *et al.* (2000). Cellular and neurochemical remodeling of the spinal cord in bone cancer pain. *Prog Brain Res* **129**, 389–97.

59. Urch CE, Dickenson AH (2003). In vivo single unit extracellular recordings from spinal cord neurones of rats. *Brain Res Brain Res Protoc* **12**(1), 26–34.

60. Asai H, Ozaki N, Shinoda M *et al.* (2005). Heat and mechanical hyperalgesia in mice model of cancer pain. *Pain* **117**(1–2), 19–29.

61. Kontinen VA, Meert TF (2003). Predictive validity of neuropathic pain models in pharmacological studies with a behavioural outcome in the rat: a systematic review. In: Dotrovsky JO, Carr DB, Koltzenburg M, (eds). *Proceedings of the 10th World Congress on Pain*. IASP, Seattle; pp. 489–98.

62. Fine PG (2002). Analgesia issues in palliative care: bone pain, controlled release opioids, managing opioid-induced constipation and nifedipine as an analgesic. *J Pain Palliat Care Pharmacother* **16**(1), 93–7.

63. Urch CE, Donovan-Rodriguez T, Dickenson AH (2003). Alterations in dorsal horn neurones in a rat model of cancer-induced bone pain. *Pain* **106**(3), 347–56.

64. Cao F, Gao F, Xu AJ *et al.* (2010). Regulation of spinal neuroimmune responses by prolonged morphine treatment in a rat model of cancer induced bone pain. *Brain Res* **1326**, 162–73.

65. Hald A, Nedergaard S, Hansen RR *et al.* (2009). Differential activation of spinal cord glial cells in murine models of neuropathic and cancer pain. *Eur J Pain* **13**(2), 138–45.

66. Watkins LR, Hutchinson MR, Rice KC *et al.* (2009). The 'toll' of opioid-induced glial activation: improving the clinical efficacy of opioids by targeting glia. *Trends Pharmacol Sci* **30**(11), 581–91.

67. Donovan-Rodriguez T, Dickenson AH, Urch CE (2005). Gabapentin normalizes spinal neuronal responses that correlate with behavior in a rat model of cancer-induced bone pain. *Anesthesiology* **102**(1), 132–40.

68. Lassiter LK, Carducci MA (2003). Endothelin receptor antagonists in the treatment of prostate cancer. *Semin Oncol* **30**(5):678–88.

69. Sevcik MA, Ghilardi JR, Peters CM *et al.* (2005). Anti-NGF therapy profoundly reduces bone cancer pain and the accompanying increase in markers of peripheral and central sensitization. *Pain* **115**(1–2), 128–41.

70. Malik B, Stillman M (2008). Chemotherapy-induced peripheral neuropathy. *Curr Neurol Neurosci Rep* **8**(1), 56–65.

71. Nozaki-Taguchi N, Chaplan SR, Higuera ES *et al.* (2001). Vincristine-induced allodynia in the rat. *Pain* **93**(1), 69–76.

72. Shimoyama M, Tanaka K, Hasue F *et al.* (2002). A mouse model of neuropathic cancer pain. *Pain* **99**(1–2), 167–74.

73. Shimoyama M, Tatsuoka H, Ohtori S *et al.* (2005). Change of dorsal horn neurochemistry in a mouse model of neuropathic cancer pain. *Pain* **114**(1–2), 221–30.

74. Flatters SJ, Bennett GJ (2006). Studies of peripheral sensory nerves in paclitaxel-induced painful peripheral neuropathy: evidence for mitochondrial dysfunction. *Pain* **122**(3), 245–57.

75. Cavaletti G, Cavalletti E, Oggioni N *et al.* (2000). Distribution of paclitaxel within the nervous system of the rat after repeated intravenous administration. *Neurotoxicology* **21**(3), 389–93.

76. Bielefeldt K, Gebhart GF (2005) *Textbook of Pain*, 5th edn. Churchill-Livingstone, Edinburgh.

77. Lindsay TH, Halvorson KG, Peters CM *et al.* (2006). A quantitative analysis of the sensory and sympathetic innervation of the mouse pancreas. *Neuroscience* **137**(4), 1417–26.

78. Cervero F (1991). Mechanisms of acute visceral pain. *Br Med Bull* **47**(3), 549–60.

79. Dunckley P, Wise RG, Aziz Q *et al.* (2005). Cortical processing of visceral and somatic stimulation: differentiating pain intensity from unpleasantness. *Neuroscience* **133**(2), 533–42.

80. Bueno L, Fioramonti J (2002). Visceral perception: inflammatory and non-inflammatory mediators. *Gut* **51**(Suppl 1), 19–23.

81. Cervero F, Laird JM (2004). Understanding the signaling and transmission of visceral nociceptive events. *J Neurobiol* **61**(1), 45–54.

82. Oshima M, Dinchuk JE, Kargman SL *et al.* (1996). Suppression of intestinal polyposis in Apc delta716 knockout mice by inhibition of cyclooxygenase 2 (COX-2). *Cell* **87**(5), 803–9.

83. Lindsay TH, Jonas BM, Sevcik MA *et al.* (2005). Pancreatic cancer pain and its correlation with changes in tumor vasculature, macrophage infiltration, neuronal innervation, body weight and disease progression. *Pain* **119**(1–3), 233–46.

Chapter 5

Neuraxial (epidural and intrathecal) infusions I: Anatomy and commonly used drugs: mode of action, pharmacokinetics, side effects, and evidence base for effectiveness

Paul Farquhar-Smith

Introduction

Neuraxial (epidural and intrathecal) infusions of local anaesthetic, with or without opioid, are the most important interventional procedures that are currently used for the management of severe cancer pain. Chapters 5, 6 and 7 examine neuraxial infusions in detail, and explain to the reader the rationale for the technique, precisely how it is done, what drugs are used, the benefits, risks, how to select patients and the practical nursing management.

Many patients with severe cancer pain can be relieved by the appropriate use of neuraxial infusions, and it is sad that they are not always available. It is hoped that these chapters will increase understanding of the technique and help to ensure that they will be used with more confidence in the future.

This chapter describes:

◆ the anatomy of the spine in relation to neuraxial infusions

◆ the therapeutic agents used

◆ the evidence for their effectiveness.

Anatomy

It is important to clarify the difference between an epidural and an intrathecal injection or infusion. Sometimes the word 'spinal' is used in this context, but the word can mean either epidural or intrathecal and should be avoided. The following definitions apply:

◆ **epidural**—into the epidural space, outside the dura mater

◆ **intrathecal**—into the cerebrospinal fluid (CSF) between the pia and arachnoid maters.

There are very important differences between the two routes in terms of potency and spread of drugs, and a clear understanding of the anatomical differences is essential.

The spinal cord starts at the foramen magnum at the base of the skull and is enclosed within the vertebral column. At birth it extends the length of the spinal canal, but during growth the vertebral column grows longer than the spinal cord, which normally ends in adults at the level of L1 or L2. Below this level the spinal canal contains the lumbar and sacral nerve roots, known as the cauda equina.

The spinal cord is covered directly by the pia mater, which is a thin but vascular membrane. The spinal cord, invested in the pia mater, is surrounded by CSF. The second of the three membranes that are considered here is the arachnoid mater, which is a fine non-vascular membrane closely adherent to the dura mater. The intrathecal space lies between the pia and arachnoid maters and is filled with CSF. Blood vessels to the spinal cord are also present, passing through this space.

There is a potential space between the arachnoid and dura maters called the subdural space. The dura mater is a tough and fibrous membrane, continuous with the brain dura mater and descending normally to S2. The epidural space is a virtual space that runs external to the dura mater, from the foramen magnum to the sacro-coccygeal hiatus. The anatomy of the spinal canal is shown in cross-section in Fig. 5.1.

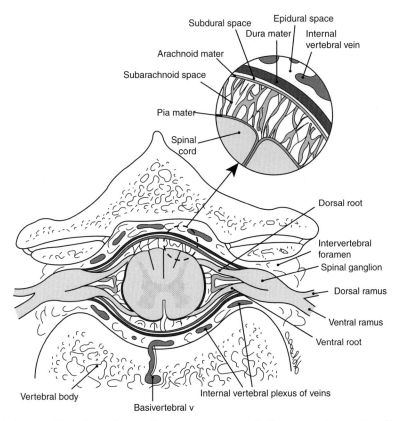

Fig. 5.1 Cross section of spinal cord. Also appears in colour in the colour plate section, Plate 4.

CSF is produced by the choroid plexuses in the lateral cerebral ventricles and by brain ependymal cells. CSF flows through the ventricles and foramina to the spinal cord. It is thought that the total amount of CSF present in the CNS is 70–120 mL and that it is normally produced at the rate of approximately 0.35 mL/min.

Anatomical relations of the epidural space

The epidural space exists between the dura mater and the periosteum of the vertebral canal. The vertebral canal is enclosed by a ring of structures; posteriorly by the laminae and arch of the vertebrae and the ligamentum flavum (yellow ligament). The ligamentum flavum connects adjacent laminae and consists of inelastic connective tissue, which affords the high resistance experienced whilst undertaking an epidural using the loss of resistance technique for performing an epidural. Injection of saline or air into the ligamentum flavum is difficult due to this high resistance. The epidural space is identified as the resistance suddenly decreases at the point of needle exit into the epidural space. Injection into the epidural space has little or no resistance. A midline interlaminar (also known as translaminar) epidurally sited needle enters the posterior epidural space. However, in the thoracic and cervical regions there may be a gap between the lateral parts of the ligmamentum flavum, potentially causing variable loss of resistance using the midline approach (1). The vertebral bodies and intervertebral discs lie anteriorly and are covered by the posterior longitudinal ligament along the whole length of the vertebral canal. Laterally are the intervertebral foraminae (which communicate with the paravertebral space) and the periosteum of the vertebral pedicles. Indeed, fluid injected into the epidural space might preferentially flow through the intervertebral foraminae rather than within the epidural space itself (2). The spinal nerve roots are covered with a thinning sleeve of dura and pass through the epidural space laterally. The anatomical relations of the epidural space are shown in Figs 5.2, 5.3 and 5.4.

Contents and size of the epidural space

The epidural space contains fat, a valveless plexus of veins (especially in the anterior epidural space), sparse lymphatics and spinal arteries. The anterior spinal artery, which takes its origin from the vertebral artery, carries 75% of the blood supply to the spinal cord. The epidural space is not regular or uniform, differing in shape, extent and contents along the course of the spine. The posterior space in the lumbar region is approximately 5 mm (from front to back), decreasing in the thoracic region and often less in the cervical region. Continuing cephalad, there is diminishing fat in the posterior epidural space, which may allow easier and more consistent spread of injectate in thoracic and cervical epidural blockade. Excess epidural fat has been linked to failure of epidural analgesia (3). Interestingly, the depth of ligamentum flavum from skin in the lumbar region is similar to the cervical region but the volume of the cervical epidural space is less. Indeed, some MRI studies have showed little or no posterior epidural space above C7 (4). The adult caudal epidural space is approximately 34 mL in volume but can vary widely with sacral anatomy. It contains the termination of the dural sac, the cauda equina, fat and sacral epidural veins. It is usually accessed through the sacral hiatus.

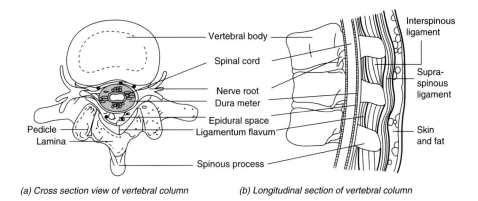

(a) Cross section view of vertebral column

(b) Longitudinal section of vertebral column

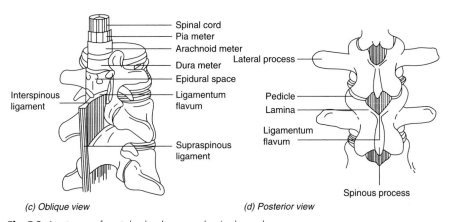

(c) Oblique view

(d) Posterior view

Fig. 5.2 Anatomy of vertebral column and spinal canal.

It is unclear how the epidural space changes with age, but epidural injection consistently demonstrates, for a given volume, increased segmental (up and down, cephalad to caudad) spread in older patients. A transverse section of the spinal canal demonstrating the relations of the epidural and intrathecal compartments is shown in Fig. 5.5.

Compartments of the epidural space: reality or artefact?

It is known that drugs placed in the epidural space may not spread evenly, giving an inconsistent or patchy (only some areas becoming analgesic) block. The anatomical reasons for this are discussed below.

The understanding of the anatomy has been confounded by the methods of examination (such as epiduroscopy or injection of contrast for imaging), which can differ from the *in vitro* anatomy. Early cadaveric studies often displayed post-mortem artefacts. The technique of cryomicrotome sectioning has previously been generally accepted as being the least disruptive, and allows examination without tissue movement artefact. However, the increasing resolution of MRI gives a direct comparator in elucidating the true anatomy.

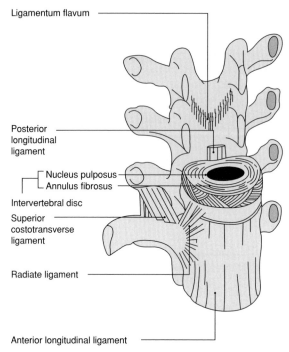

Ligamentum flavum

Posterior
longitudinal
ligament

Nucleus pulposus
Annulus fibrosus

Intervertebral disc

Superior
costotransverse
ligament

Radiate ligament

Anterior longitudinal ligament

Fig. 5.3 Anterior view of thoracic vertebrae. Bodies have been removed from upper two. Also appears in colour in the colour plate section, Plate 5.

At certain places the dura contacts the periosteum directly, which compartmentalizes the epidural space. Some authors suggest that there are areas anteriorly where the dura adheres to the posterior longitudinal ligament and limit the extent of the anterior epidural space. However, others state there are no such connections and that they are artefactual (5). Nevertheless, even the places of contact could potentially disrupt the free

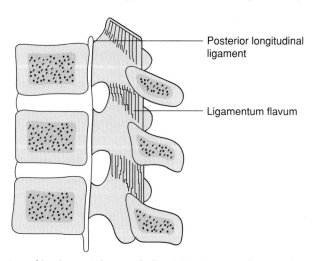

Posterior longitudinal
ligament

Ligamentum flavum

Fig. 5.4 Lateral view of lumbar vertebrae excluding interspinous and supraspinous ligaments. Also appears in colour in the colour plate section, Plate 6.

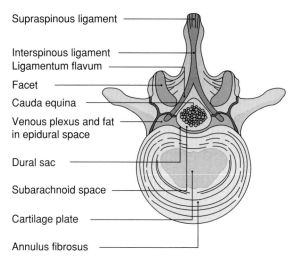

Supraspinous ligament

Interspinous ligament
Ligamentum flavum

Facet

Cauda equina

Venous plexus and fat
in epidural space

Dural sac

Subarachnoid space

Cartilage plate

Annulus fibrosus

Fig. 5.5 Transverse section of an intervertebral disc, showing the subarachnoid space. Also appears in colour in the colour plate section, Plate 7.

flow of liquid in the epidural space. Another anatomical band, the existence of which has been debated, is the plica mediana dorsalis. This is thought to be a fold of dura that divides the posterior epidural space into two lateral halves and has been cited as the cause of unilateral block. Although it has been identified under epidurography (6), others suggest it is an artefact and that anterior, lateral or transforaminal (injecting into the lateral intervertebral foramen, rather than the midline) catheter position is the likely cause of unilateral block (7). However, even a transforaminal placement infrequently leads to unilateral block since injectate appears to still distribute into the spinal canal (5). Acquired changes to spinal anatomy may also have an impact on the placement and use of neuraxial blockade, including spinal stenosis and scoliosis.

The route to the epidural space

The needle route for a midline interlaminar approach will initially pass through the supraspinous ligament that joins the tips of spinous processes. Deeper to this is the interspinous ligament that connects the rest of the spinous processes. This is in continuation with the ligamentum flavum, which unites adjacent laminae. The midline approach is suitable for the lumbar and cervical regions. The average depth of the lumbar epidural space is 4.5–5.5 cm but may range from 3 to 9 cm depending on interspace and the angle of the needle, and is often influenced by the body mass index of the patient (5). The anatomy of the interlaminar approach is demonstrated in Fig. 5.6.

The paramedian approach (needle insertion approximately 2 cm lateral to the midline) is often used in the mid-thoracic region, where there may be overlap of spinous processes hindering a midline approach. The lateral part of the ligamentum flavum is reached directly, usually after walking the needle off the vertebral laminae.

The sacral epidural space is accessed at the sacral hiatus via the sacro-coccygeal membrane. This hiatus is between S4 and S5, posteriorly, on the sacrum.

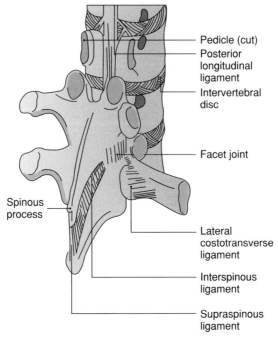

Pedicle (cut)

Posterior
longitudinal
ligament

Intervertebral
disc

Facet joint

Spinous
process

Lateral
costotransverse
ligament

Interspinous
ligament

Supraspinous
ligament

Fig. 5.6 Dorsolateral view of the thoracic vertebrae and ligaments. The vertebral arch of the upper vertebra has been removed. Also appears in colour in the colour plate section, Plate 8.

Most epidurals inserted for the management of cancer pain are sited at lumbar or low thoracic level.

The epidural space in cancer

The epidural space is a site of metastasis and local spread of several cancers including breast, lung, melanoma, prostate, kidney and myeloma. In a series of 124 myelograms done in 100 patients with breast cancer who presented with radiculopathy or myopathy, 53% indicated epidural disease (8). Pain is often a presenting complaint and in these patients may be associated with signs of radiculopathy or nerve root irritation secondary to infiltration by cancer (9). These symptoms may require further investigation in order to establish the diagnosis and epidural steroid injection may be considered (10). Epidural disease is also being increasingly recognized as a cause of malignant spinal cord compression (11). Risk of bleeding by direct injury from the epidural needle may be increased in these patients. Furthermore, distortion of the anatomy by the epidural disease may lead to compromised spread and lack of efficacy of both single injection of steroid and continuous infusions via a catheter. The presence of epidural disease has also been associated with the presence of intractable pain (12). Of 57 patients with 'refractory pain' (refractory to opioids and, in 29%, refractory to epidural local anaesthetic and opioids), 70% had evidence of epidural metastatic disease when investigated with imaging. Spinal canal stenosis in these patients was associated with a higher incidence of complications, including paraplegia, and also required higher dosage of intrathecal drugs (12). An MRI scan can provide useful information before neuraxial blockade, although this may not be possible for practical reasons (13).

Intrathecal and subdural space

The intrathecal space is contained by the dura mater. The arachnoid mater is closely applied to the inside of the dura. However, between the dura and the arachnoid is the potential subdural space, which is only really of relevance in misplaced epidurals. Being of lower volume, injection here can cause excessive spread or a patchy block compared to true epidural placement. In the intrathecal space, CSF surrounds the spinal cord, which itself is covered with a vascular membrane called the pia mater. Denticulate ligaments extend from the pia mater from the lateral sides of the spinal cord to the dura and may impede free flow of injectate. All arteries supplying the spinal cord pass through the intrathecal space.

The intrathecal space in cancer

Metastases in the epidural space are unlikely to spread into the intrathecal space due to the presence of the dura. The presence of tumour in the epidural space is unlikely to significantly affect the intrathecal spread of injectate. A potential problem would be the necessity of passing through tumour mass to enter the intrathecal space. The presence of epidural metastatic disease may increase neurological complications of intrathecal blockade, such as unexpected paraplegia, thought to be caused by medullary coning (12).

Neuraxial therapy
'Single shot' steroid neuraxial injections

Epidural steroid injections are one of the most commonly utilized interventions for back pain due to degenerative disc disease and radicular pain emanating from a 'trapped nerve' or nerve root irritation, most commonly from disc prolapse into the lateral recesses of the spinal canal. Knowledge of the anatomical distribution of the nerves is essential in diagnosing radicular pain. This presents as pain with pins and needles or numbness and sometimes also weakness in the distribution of the affected nerve; to the leg if coming from the lumbar spine (sciatica) or to the arm if coming from the cervical spine.

Thoracic disc prolapse is relatively rare in non-cancer pain, but this causes pain to radiate around the chest wall in the distribution of the thoracic nerve roots.

Mode of action

Although several mechanisms of action have been proposed, the precise means of how analgesia is achieved with epidural steroid has not been elucidated. Conceivably it would be expected to reduce pro-inflammatory processes contributing to the development of central sensitization. Epidural steroids have been shown to reduce the pain behaviours seen in animal models of radicular pain (14, 15). Activation of phospholipase A2 (PLA2), which has been demonstrated in radicular pain models, releases arachidonic acid, which is the substrate for cyclooxygenase and lipoxygenase pathways. These pathways produce many key pro-inflammatory moieties, including prostaglandin E_2, leukotriene B_4 and several hydroperoxyeicosatetraenoic acids (HPETEs) (16). HPETEs are endogenous agonists at the capsaicin TRPV1 receptor and contribute to pain (17). Inhibition of activated PLA2 by epidural steroids has been shown to be a mechanism that reduces radicular pain (15). It is more difficult to understand any putative effect of epidural steroid in cases of chronic pain where there is little evidence of inflammation.

Evidence for effectiveness

A large meta-analysis of epidural steroids for chronic spinal pain concluded that there was strong evidence of a short term benefit following interlaminal lumbar epidural steroid for lumbar radicular pain. However, evidence for a long term effect was described as limited for interlaminal injection and moderate for the transforaminal approach. The use of caudal epidural steroid injections for alleviation of lumbar radicular pain was also supported by strong evidence in the short term and moderate evidence in the long term. However, although not excluded a priori, there have been no studies involving cancer radicular pain. Moreover, there is insufficient evidence to verify a role for epidural steroid in non-malignant spinal stenosis (18).

Cancer can cause radicular pain by either direct root involvement by local tumour (e.g. epidural disease) or by spinal metastatic disease altering vertebral architecture, resulting in nerve impingement. Malignant spinal cord stenosis can also cause pain by direct contact. These mechanisms would be expected to have a significant inflammatory component and therefore implicate epidural steroid as an effective treatment. However, there are few data for the efficacy of epidural steroids in malignant back pain or radicular pain. Nevertheless, although the cancer aetiology is different, the inflammatory pain mechanisms are comparable and amenable to epidural steroid injection. Epidural steroid injection should therefore be used for the same indications as in non-cancer spinal pain, i.e. radicular pain where the pathology is at the spinal level. Several steroid preparations are used, most commonly triamcinolone. Methylprednisolone (Depomedrone) has been implicated in causing adverse neurological sequelae secondary to adhesive arachnoiditis, probably after inadvertent intrathecal injection, although it appears to have been used safely in millions of epidural injections globally. There has also been some concern that cervical epidural injection of steroid preparation with larger particulate size could increase the risk of anterior spinal artery syndrome, resulting in cord ischaemia and paralysis (4). It is recommended that dexamethasone be used for cervical steroid injection due to its small particulate size.

Duration of effect is variable and the epidural steroid injection may need to be repeated. Theoretically, steroid inhibition of the hypothalamic-pituitary axis may prevent repetition any more frequent than monthly.

Similarly, there are few studies looking at epidural steroids for cancer-induced cord compression. Studies have investigated the use of high-dose systemic steroids in respect of their effect on the neurological consequences of cord compression but also their effect on pain (19). It is unclear whether targeted epidural steroid would have the same beneficial effect.

Drugs commonly used for neuraxial infusions
Opioids

Opioids are chemicals that bind to opioid receptors. Opiates are naturally occurring opioids. Opioid receptors are present throughout the body but are present predominately in the central nervous system and gastrointestinal tract. The body produces endogenous opioids that act on these receptors. Opioid receptors that are involved in pain transmission and modulation are found in key areas in the brain, spinal cord and periphery. Although the analgesic properties of opioids have been known for thousands of years, opioid receptors were only discovered in the spinal cord of mammals in the 1960s. These receptors are located in the superficial dorsal horn, which is integral to spinal pain processing.

Epidural opioids penetrate the dura, gaining entry into the CSF and act directly on the spinal cord. Intrathecal opioids are injected directly into the CSF. The theoretical advantage of neuraxial delivery of opioid in proximity to the spinal site of action is to allow a significant reduction in effective dose compared to systemic administration, potentially reducing the incidence of side effects (20–23).

Mode of action

At a molecular level, opioids act by activation of predominantly pre-synaptic opioid receptors in the superficial dorsal horn of the spinal cord, reducing transmitter release by inhibiting calcium channels. Part of the anti-nociceptive action occurs post-synaptically by induction of hyperpolarization secondary to activation of G-protein coupled inwardly rectifying potassium channels (GIRKs) (24).

Pharmacokinetics

Opioids display large variations in pharmacodynamics. Minimum effective analgesic blood concentration may vary by up to a factor of four between patients. Clinically effective analgesic dosages may vary widely between patients and thus require individual titration to effect. For neuraxial administration, as well as drug half-life, opioid lipid solubility (lipophilicity) and relative water solubility (hydrophilicity) influence analgesia and side effects. High lipid solubility allows membrane absorption and rapid uptake by neural tissue, while high water solubility increases dissolution into the CSF. Lipid soluble opioids (e.g. fentanyl) have a rapid onset of action but also a more rapid systemic absorption and potentially more systemic side effects. Less lipid- and more water-soluble agents (e.g. morphine) are absorbed more slowly and have a slower onset time but a longer duration of action. Higher concentrations of morphine would theoretically be able to diffuse up to the brain and cause delayed side effects such as respiratory depression. However, this complication is extremely rare even in previously opioid naïve patients. The pharmacokinetics of some commonly used neuraxial opioids are shown in Table 5.1.

Table 5.1 Pharmacokinetics of some neuraxial opioids

	Lipid solubility	Speed of onset	Duration of action	CSF solubility (possible higher spread)
Morphine	+	Slow	Long	High
Fentanyl	++++	Rapid	Short	Low
Methadone	+++	Fast intermediate	Short	Low
Hydromorphone	++	Intermediate	Intermediate	Intermediate

Tolerance (more opioid required to achieve the same effect) is often observed with any route of administration. This is also possible for neuraxial administration and often increasing doses are required for continuing analgesia (25).

Practically, the choice of neuraxial opioid is governed more by operator choice and staff experience rather than pharmacokinetics.

Side effects

Many of the serious side effects of opioids result from activation of central receptors located in the brain. These include respiratory inhibition, drowsiness, nausea and vomiting. Dysphoria, hallucination and delirium have also been associated with opioids as well as myloclonus, which is seen at 'toxic' opioid levels. The action of opioids on gut opioid receptors decreases intestinal motility, increases transit time and results in constipation or opioid-induced bowel disorder. This effect is less apparent when neuraxial opioids are used. Rarely, neuraxial opioids may cause urinary retention, although this is more common with the use of concomitant local anaesthetics (LAs). Opioid-induced itch can be severe enough to cause dose limitation and it may be more prevalent with neuraxial administration. Other long-term effects include interference with the immune system and decreased testosterone levels in men, although the lower doses associated with neuraxial infusion reduce the risk of this.

There is increasing evidence that chronic long-term and high-dose opioid use may cause hyperalgesia and worsening of pain (26); this is associated with 'central sensitization' of pain pathways similar to that found in neuropathic pain states (see Chapter 4). Other less common side effects have also been observed with neuraxial opioids, including dry mouth, oedema, headache, muscle rigidity and withdrawal.

Neuraxial administration of opioids aims to reduce dose and thus reduce all these side effects, but they may still occur.

Local anaesthetics
Types
Chemically, LAs are divided into amide and ester types. The most commonly neuraxially used agents are amides such as bupivacaine, lidocaine and ropivacaine. Lidocaine is commonly used for local anaesthesia of short duration for many indications, but is not often used neuraxially for chronic pain. Bupivacaine is a mixture of two stereoisomers (each have a chemical structure that is the mirror image of the other), known as the D- and L-isomers. The D-isomer form is more likely to cause cardiac arrhythmias (especially after intravenous injection), and these are potentially fatal. The L-isomer is available as levobupivacaine and is theoretically and practically less likely to cause these side effects.

Ropivacaine is less lipid soluble, has been shown to have less motor blockade at equianalgesic doses with epidural use and may also have fewer cardiotoxic side effects (27).

Liposomal technology has been used with bupivacaine to attempt to increase the duration of neuraxial LA (28), but is not widely available at present.

Mode of action

LAs act by impairing the membrane permeability of sodium ions that are necessary for nerve conduction. Thus electrical transmission is reduced or blocked. The degree to which this occurs varies with concentration of the LA and with the diameter of the nerve exposed to LA. Small unmyelinated nerves are blocked more easily than larger myelinated ones. This potentially allows LAs to have a differential action on motor and sensory nerves, allowing analgesia without inducing muscle weakness. Moreover, C and Aδ fibres (small unmyelinated and lightly myelinated) mediating pain transmission are more easily blocked than Aβ fibres (myelinated) that transmit touch sensation and proprioception (positional awareness). Therefore pain can theoretically be reduced without numbness.

Pharmacokinetics

Intrathecal administration delivers LA directly into the CSF and into the superficial spinal cord. Epidural LA diffuses through the dura into the CSF, explaining the slower onset of action.

Several properties influence the action of LAs, including lipid solubility, protein binding and degree of ionization at body pH (also known as the pKa). Most of the nerve cell membrane is lipid, and increased lipid solubility is associated with increased potency. Increased protein binding is related to longer duration of action. The less the LA is ionized at body pH, the faster onset and more effective the block. High lipid solubility of many LAs also promotes uptake into the spinal cord at the point of injection, thereby reducing potential cephalic spread and risk of respiratory depression.

The metabolic clearance of LA from the body is predominantly by the liver. However, the wearing off of the effect of LA is by diffusion into the vascular compartment.

Side effects

Neuraxial LA can block sensory nerves other than those mediating pain, resulting in numbness. Furthermore, motor nerves may also be affected, causing muscle weakness. Alteration of infusion rate and concentration of LA may reduce these effects without compromising analgesia. However, other serious CNS and cardiovascular side effects can result from excessive systemic absorption or inadvertent intravascular injection of LA. Both epidural and intrathecal administration can lead to rapid systemic absorption and it is thus recommended that safe total LA doses should be adhered to (e.g. 2 mg/kg for bupivacaine without adrenaline). Increasing systemic levels of LA initially cause light headedness, dizziness, tinnitus, circumoral numbness and decreased consciousness. Further increases to toxic levels can lead to tonic-clonic convulsions, coma and even death. Cardiac toxicity resulting in arrhythmia and myocardial inhibition are often the cause of death. However, at the doses normally used, LA toxicity is not usually a problem. If it does occur, prompt intravenous intralipid treatment can effectively treat the sequelae of LA toxicity.

Table 5.2 summarizes the physiology of LA actions, side effects and toxicity.

Table 5.2 Physiology of local anaesthetic effect, side effects and toxicity

Usage	Nerve fibres/ function blocked	Effect
With normal use	C	Analgesia
With normal use	Aβ	Numbness
With normal use	Aα	Weakness
With normal use	Aδ	Lack of positional awareness (propiroception)
With normal use	Sympathetic	Hypotension
		Bradycardia (high block)
After high serum levels from rapid absorption/inadvertent intravascular injection	CNS	CNS symptoms leading to convulsion and coma
After high serum levels/inadvertent intravascular injection	Myocardium and cardiac conduction	Cardiotoxic effects: intractable arrhythmias, decreased contractility

Evidence for effectiveness of commonly used neuraxial drugs
Evidence for epidural opioids

Theoretically a tenfold reduction in epidural opioid dose compared to systemic has been suggested (23), but clinical empirical ratios may be less opioid sparing (29). Equal pain relief but a clinical reduction in side effects was demonstrated by the epidural administration of morphine compared to oral morphine (30). Kalso compared epidural and subcutaneous routes of patient-controlled administration of morphine in ten patients with severe cancer-related pain. Analgesic efficacy was similar but the epidural group used a median dose of 106 mg compared to the subcutaneous group's usage of 372 mg. Efficacy and side effects improved in both groups compared to prior to the study, when the patients were taking oral morphine (29). Other studies have also shown not only good pain relief for epidural morphine (31) but also reduction of systemic opioid requirements (32).

In an uncontrolled retrospective trial, 105 patients (90% with pain from malignancy) were treated with boluses of epidural opioids (86% morphine), with 67% reporting 'satisfactory' pain relief (33). Two other studies examined cancer pain relief and complications from long-term epidural catheters (34, 35). All of the 40 patients receiving 10 mg/day of epidural morphine experienced initial significant or complete pain relief but required a trebling of average dose within the first three weeks (34). However, nearly all of the 32 patients required replacement of catheter, chiefly due to mechanical leakage (34). A comparable increase in epidural morphine requirement with time (tolerance) was demonstrated in 146 patients who had external catheters inserted for cancer pain (35). The initial mean epidural dose of morphine was 18 mg/day (compared to a mean oral dose of 164 mg) and the mean epidural morphine dose increased to 69 mg at the end of treatment. Ineffectiveness of therapy led to 19% stopping epidural morphine, an observation which was more common in people with neuropathic, visceral or incident pain (35).

These studies and others were included in a Cochrane review looking at the efficacy of epidural, subarachnoid and intracerebroventricular opioids in cancer pain. An exhaustive search of 18 databases failed to find any controlled studies, meaning the 1343 patients studied were from 31 uncontrolled trials. Morphine was the opioid used in nearly all of these studies. This review concluded that 87% of patients reported excellent or good pain relief from epidural opioids for cancer pain. Of the 656 patients from 19 out of 31 of the studies who reported side effects, 194 (30%) complained of transient or protracted side effects, with nausea and vomiting (10%), pruritis (8%) and urinary retention (5%) most common. In non-implanted or reservoir systems there was a 39% incidence of catheter-related problems such as misplacement/dislodgement (12%), blockage (9%), leakage (6%), superficial infection (6%) and pain on injection (5%). Less than 1% (6 out of 757) reported a spinal infection. Where an implantable reservoir was used, overall system problems occurred in 28%, with relatively more blockages (15%) (36).

Very little has been published concerning the use of other epidural opioids in cancer pain, but there are some data on the use of epidural methadone. Of the 70 cancer patients that received epidural methadone (up to 8 mg four times a day) good pain control was reported by 56 (80%) (37). Fourteen (20%) required rotation to epidural morphine due to inadequate analgesia and of these only four had a good response (37).

Table 5.3 summarizes selected evidence for epidural opioid alone in cancer pain.

Table 5.3 Selected evidence for epidural opioid alone in cancer pain

Study	Type of study, n	Opioid	Outcome
Kalso et al. (29)	Randomised controlled trial 10	Morphine	Equi-analgesic to s.c. Lower dose
Vainio and Tigerstedt (30)	Prospective uncontrolled	Morphine	Equi-analgesic to oral Fewer side effects
Crawford et al. (33)	Prospective uncontrolled, 105	Mostly morphine (some buphrenorphine)	67% satisfactory pain relief No serious side effects
Driessen et al. (34)	Prospective uncontrolled, 32	Morphine	All significant pain relief 3× increase morphine in first 3 weeks
Samuelsson et al. (35)	Prospective uncontrolled, 146	Morphine	83% some analgesic response 19% stopped because of increasing pain
Shir et al. (36)	Prospective uncontrolled, 70	Methadone	80% good pain control No serious side effects
Hassenbusch et al. (32)	Prospective uncontrolled, 69	Morphine	Decrease in systemic morphine by 80%
Waterman et al. (31)	Prospective uncontrolled, 33	Morphine	80% excellent/good pain relief

Evidence for intrathecal opioids

Historically, the intrathecal techniques have been used less than the epidural route for acute, chronic and cancer pains. However, despite previous anxiety about the potential for increased infection risk (meningitis), there is an increasing body of evidence for the efficacy and safety of long-term intrathecal catheters for chronic pain, including cancer pain (38–50). Furthermore, advances in implantable technology have facilitated safe and effective administration of intrathecal opioids. Similarly to epidural administration, intrathecal opioids act on opioid receptors in the substantia gelatinosa of the superficial dorsal horn, resulting in inhibition of transmitter release and post-synaptic hyperpolarization and, by virtue of closer spinal proximity, require a lower effective dose than epidural opioids.

Most of the data on intrathecal opioids in cancer pain has been gathered from small retrospective trials using morphine. Indeed, as for the epidural opioids, the same Cochrane review found only uncontrolled trials to assess (37). Of the 28 trials (722 patients) analgesic efficacy data was only extractable from 19, comprising 404 patients. Nonetheless, 84% of these achieved good or excellent analgesia (37). However, 50% experienced transient or prolonged side effects, including pruritis (18%), nausea and vomiting (17%), and urinary retention (10%) (37). Overall there was a 2% incidence of protracted headache, possibly indicative of dural puncture headache (37). Catheter or system-related problems were less than for epidural administration (22% vs 39%) (37). Spinal infections were also rare using external systems (37). There were 12 out of 229 (5%) spinal infections with implantable reservoir systems, which was significantly higher than the proportion for external epidural catheters, but none were reported for the 138 patients with totally implantable pumps (37). These data are taken from uncontrolled trials and therefore it is difficult to state categorically that intrathecal catheters are more likely to result in significant infection. There is also no definitive evidence that external or non-implanted intrathecal catheters are more likely to suffer complications such as infection. The incidence of complications in 200 consecutive patients with external intrathecal catheters was found to be equivalent to the figure for those with implanted intrathecal catheters taken from published literature (51).

Similarly to epidural opioids, intrathecal administration is associated with some tolerance and often an increasing dose is required over time. In 53 patients with pain from metastatic cancer, intrathecal morphine requirement had increased by 250% 16 weeks after starting the infusion (25). Table 5.4 summarizes selective evidence for intrathecal morphine in cancer pain.

Two other major reviews examined intrathecal delivery of pain medication (52, 40). An expert panel identified 52 studies of intrathecal analgesia for cancer pain, all either case series or retrospective uncontrolled trials (52). Four years later the evidence was updated, but of the 25 additional studies, only 4 involved cancer pain (40). The authors highlighted the paucity of randomized controlled trials, but based on these data produced consensus guidelines for intrathecal drug delivery for cancer and non-malignant pain (40). This algorithm is shown in Fig. 5.7.

The evidence supports morphine as the first-line intrathecal opioid.

Table 5.4 Selected evidence for intrathecal morphine in cancer pain

Study	Study type, n	Outcome
Rauck et al. (41)	Prospective uncontrolled, 119	91% >50% reduction in pain at 4 months Fewer opioid side effects
Onofrio and Yaksh (25)	Prospective uncontrolled, 53	64% excellent/good pain relief 2.5× increase spinal dose at 16 weeks
Gestin et al. (42)	Retrospective, uncontrolled, 50	50% good pain relief, 50% fair
Sallerin-Caute et al. (43)	Retrospective uncontrolled, 159	80% excellent/good pain relief 2–3× increase in dose at 3 months
Penn and Paice (44)[44]	Retrospective uncontrolled, 35	80% good/excellent pain relief
Paice et al. (45)	Multicentre survey, 133	95% excellent/good pain relief 2× increase dose at 3 months
Devulder et al. (46)	Retrospective uncontrolled, 33	80% good pain relief
Schultheiss et al. (47)	Prospective uncontrolled, 79	96% excellent or good pain relief
Follett et al. (48)	Retrospective uncontrolled, 35	77% good pain relief
Madrid et al. (49)	Retrospective uncontrolled 35	78% excellent/good pain relief
Brazenor (50)	Retrospective uncontrolled, 26	88% excellent/good pain relief

Intrathecal delivery of morphine using a patient-controlled analgesia system, whereby the patient delivers boluses as required has also been shown to provide good, long-term analgesia (41, 42).

Intrathecal morphine has also been shown not only to improve analgesia in intractable cancer pain, but also may have an impact on survival. Implantable morphine intrathecal infusions were added to the comprehensive medical management (CMM) of patients with pain scores greater than 5/10 and who were receiving more than than 200 mg oral morphine per day (or equivalent) (53). Intrathecal morphine resulted in improvement in pain, reduction in total morphine and reduction in opioid-induced side effects. Moreover, at six months, over 50% of the intrathecal morphine group were still alive compared to 32% in the CMM group (53). Opioids have been implicated in the inhibition of immune-mediated tumour surveillance. Reduction in total opioid requirement may allow re-establishment of this surveillance and reduce cancer spread and subsequent mortality.

Other opioids have been used intrathecally, including fentanyl, hydromorphone, fentanyl and sufentanil (40). There are no controlled trials and no cancer pain studies, but two

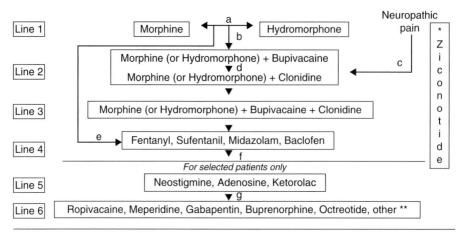

Fig. 5.7 Algorithm for the management of pain by intrathecal drug delivery; report of an expert panel, Polyanalgesic Consensus Panel, 2003. Reproduced from (40) with permission from Elsevier.

retrospective studies have looked at intrathecal hydromorphone in non-cancer pain (54, 55). Twenty-four patients who had received intrathecal hydromorphone were reviewed at time periods after insertion of the implantable system (54). Pain scores were significantly improved, but only 13 out of 24 patients could be analysed at one month and just 7 out of 24 at 12 months (54). In another trial, intrathecal morphine was switched to hydromorphone in 37 patients, mostly due to side effects or lack of analgesic efficacy (55). Side effects were improved and some of those who had switched due to lack of pain relief displayed improved pain scores (55). This evidence was considered strong enough to suggest hydromorphone as a first-line intrathecal agent or first change from morphine if intolerable side effects were occurring (40). Animal studies have also implied that hydromorphone is less likely to be associated with catheter tip grannulomata (56). Whether or not these are less common clinically is unclear and, indeed, inflammatory masses have been described clinically (57) (see Chapter 6).

There are very few studies into the effect of intrathecal methadone and none in cancer pain. Intrathecal methadone for acute post-operative pain demonstrated efficacy comparable to morphine, with shorter duration and a higher incidence of side effects (58).

Evidence for the co-administration of local anaesthetics and opioids

Epidural

Epidural opioids are more routinely administered with LAs. The synergistic direct inhibition of nerve conduction by LA potentially reduces the opioid requirements and may improve the quality of analgesia (59). Smitt retrospectively reviewed 91 patients with chronic cancer pain, who had 137 epidural catheters inserted over a three-year period. Adequate pain relief (>50% decrease in opioids and as described by patient and physician) was attained in 75% of patients receiving a mixture of LA and opioid (60).

Intrathecal

Animal studies have demonstrated the possibility of a synergistic analgesic effect of intrathecal opioids with LAs (61). This has also been shown in clinical studies for acute (62) and chronic pain (63). In acute pain, these reductions in opioid requirements did not necessarily result in fewer opioid-induced side effects (62). Sjöberg demonstrated efficacy of a morphine–bupivacaine mixture in an uncontrolled trial of 53 patients with intractable pain or unacceptable opioid-induced side effects (64). All the patients described good pain relief (visual analogue scale (VAS) < 4), but there was a significant increase in LA-mediated side effects such as urinary retention, leg weakness and hypotensive episodes (64).

In another non-randomized study, 44 out of 52 patients with severe (VAS > 6) complicated cancer pain (often due to difficult-to-treat types of pain, e.g. visceral or ischaemic) reported pain scores of 0–2 after intrathecal morphine and bupivicaine. Over half of these patients (26/44) achieved this analgesia at a bupivacaine dose of less than 30 mg/day and did not experience any LA-mediated adverse effects. Intrathecal therapy reduced total morphine dose and improved other quality of life measures such as sleep and activities of daily living (65). However, these were non-comparative trials and only demonstrate the efficacy of intrathecal administration of opioid and LA in refractory cancer pain. They do not support intrathecal synergism.

In a randomized trial of 20 patients with cancer pain, van Dongen demonstrated a reduction in intrathecal morphine escalation when intrathecal bupivacaine was co-administered (66). The clinical utility of LA/opioid intrathecal mixture has been reinforced by the Tyneside Spinal Group, who instigated a new and considered intrathecal policy, and have demonstrated the safety of 100 external (non-implanted) intrathecal delivery systems, achieving analgesic effectiveness in two-thirds of patients using a diamorphine/bupivacaine mixture (67).

The addition of intrathecal LA to intrathecal opioid can therefore reduce overall opioid requirements, may reduce opioid-induced side effects and, for moderate dosage of LA, is not associated with additional LA-induced side effects.

Direct comparison of intrathecal and epidural administration

Both intrathecal and epidural analgesic techniques have been shown to be effective in refractory cancer pain, yet there are few data on direct comparison of these routes of opioid and LA administration. Rates of complications appear to be comparable. One retrospective review compared intrathecal and epidural pain relief for chronic non-cancer pain and found an overall intrathecal advantage in terms of improved analgesia, lower failure rate, fewer replacement catheters and fewer complications (68). In another study, 25 patients with continuing severe pain despite epidural morphine and bupivacaine were changed to receive intrathecal morphine and bupivacaine. Total opioid requirements were reduced and pain scores improved significantly (69). Nevertheless, in cancer pain data are scarce, which makes it difficult to state a clear preference for either route. The analgesic requirements of each patient should be assessed individually and an appropriate technique utilized. Often this will be more influenced by local practice than other factors.

Other neuraxial drugs α_2 receptor agonists: clonidine

Mode of action

Adrenergic α_2 receptors are found in the superficial dorsal horn of the spinal cord and are thought to be activated by descending inhibitory pathways and by local release of endogenous agonists. Adrenergic α_2 agonists are thought to be analgesic at a spinal level, acting via inhibitory G proteins and by potassium channel activation.

Evidence for effectiveness: epidural

There is a wealth of preclinical evidence supporting a spinal analgesic action of clonidine (70). Clinically, evidence has mostly been for acute post-operative or obstetric pain (63). However, in a randomized double-blind controlled trial of 85 patients with severe cancer pain, 30 µg/h of epidural clonidine or placebo was administered over 14 days and epidural morphine used as rescue analgesia (71). Using decrease in morphine dose or reduction in pain score as a positive outcome, 45% of the clonidine group improved compared to 21% in the placebo group, and this benefit was even more likely in patients with neuropathic pain (56% compared to 5%) (71). Hypotension was regarded as serious in two of the clonidine patients and in one placebo but clonidine was associated with slightly less nausea (71). Addition of epidural clonidine to other agents may therefore be beneficial in refractory cancer pain.

Addition of low-dose adrenalin to epidural LA/opioid mixtures in post-operative patients has also been shown to improve pain relief significantly, putatively by its α_2 action (72). However, there is no clear evidence for the use of adrenaline in cancer pain neuraxial blockade.

Evidence for effectiveness: intrathecal

The evidence base for intrathecal clonidine is even more limited and is mostly at the level of case reports (73, 74). It may be a useful addition to other intrathecal medication.

Ketamine

Mode of action

The N-methyl-D-aspartate (NMDA) receptor is pivotal to the multiple mechanisms of central sensitization. Normally relatively quiescent in the resting state, the spinal post-synaptic NMDA receptor is activated by increased noxious afferent barrage from the periphery (or from viscera in visceral pain) and contributes greatly to the activation and sensitization of pain pathways. Recent animal evidence has suggested a role for the spinal NMDA receptor subunit NR2B in cancer bone pain, and development of targeted therapies may herald future analgesic opportunities (75).

Evidence for effectiveness: epidural

The NMDA antagonist ketamine has been used epidurally for post-operative pain with mixed results (63). Epidural ketamine-induced analgesia seems to be better in combination with other agents (76). Lauretti *et al.* looked at a number of non-opioid epidural drugs, including ketamine (77). After reducing VAS pain scores to less than or equal to 4/10 with epidural morphine given at a dose of 2 mg twice daily 48 patients with chronic cancer pain were randomized to receive a daily dose of either 2 mg morphine (control) or 0.2 mg/kg epidural ketamine, 100 µg neostigmine or 500 µg midazolam if pain scores increased to over 4 (77). Only the ketamine group achieved significantly improved pain scores compared to the morphine control group.

Evidence for effectiveness: intrathecal

There is little evidence for the intrathecal used of ketamine in cancer pain. Case reports have described apparently safe, effective analgesia but also have reported significant spinal cord pathology after long-term intrathecal $S(+)$-ketamine infusion (78, 79). Intrathecal ketamine should therefore be used with caution.

Ziconotide

Ziconotide is a compound based on the neurotoxin produced by *Conus magus* (cone snail). The ω-conotoxin acts by blockage of the N-type voltage-sensitive calcium channel. This calcium channel is important in mediating excitatory transmitter release (e.g. glutamate) at the level of the spinal cord (80). In a trial of 111 patients with cancer or HIV-related pain (VAS >50/100), intrathecal ziconotide reduced mean pain scores by 53% compared to 18% in the placebo group (81). However, 97% of the ziconotide group complained of an adverse event (such as confusion and dizziness), which was described as serious in 30% (81). Combination of ziconotide with a stable dose of intrathecal morphine in 26 patients with refractory chronic pain improved VAS by 14.5% (82). Ziconotide may have a role in cancer pain refractory to neuraxial treatment and there is no evidence for tolerance with long-term usage. However, evidence is limited, side effects are common and there have been no direct comparisons with intrathecal opioids.

Conclusions

Neuraxial administration of opioids, when combined with LA or otherwise, is an effective method of analgesia for cancer pain. Opioids delivered by both routes can show tolerance and may need escalation of dose with time. Epidural administration of opioids can reduce the dose requirement, the epidural/systemic ration for dose equivalence being in the region of 1/3. This may be further reduced by using epidural opioids in combination with local anaesthetics but the data related to this is limited. Published side effects and complication rates are variable and often not reported, but even at the lower doses there can be significant opioid-induced problems associated with epidural and intrathecal administration. However, intrathecal administration of opioids generally requires an even lower dose than epidural without analgesic compromise. The incidence of intrathecal adverse effects is comparable to those seen with epidural administration and may be less with long-term use. Most of the literature suggests that serious neuraxial catheter-related infections are rare, but investigation where the focus has been on complications suggests this is clinically still a potentially serious problem. Although there is little evidence of effectiveness, consideration should be given to administration of prophylactic antibiotics. Mechanical issues such as displacement, leakage and blockage may necessitate catheter replacement, but tunnelling catheters or the use of implantable ports may reduce these problems.

There are limited data to support the use of agents other than opioids or LAs, but these may be used in refractory cases.

The evidence does not clearly indicate the best choice of neuraxial technique for any one situation. The decision will require a careful assessment of each patient and often be more influenced by the expertise and experience of the team involved in the management of the neuraxial infusion than by available objective evidence.

References

1. Hogan QH (1996). Epidural anatomy examined by cryomicrotome section. Influence of age, vertebral level, and disease. *Reg Anesth* **21**(5), 395–406.
2. Hogan Q (2002). Distribution of solution in the epidural space: examination by cryomicrotome section. *Reg Anesth Pain Med* **27**(2), 150–6.
3. Lang SA, Korzeniewski P, Buie D *et al.* (2002). Repeated failure of epidural analgesia: an association with epidural fat? *Reg Anesth Pain Med* **27**(5), 494–500.
4. Huston CW (2009). Cervical epidural steroid injections in the management of cervical radiculitis: interlaminar versus transforaminal. A review. *Curr Rev Musculoskelet Med* **2**(1), 30–42.
5. Hogan QH (1998). Epidural anatomy: new observations. *Can J Anaesth* **45**(5 Pt 2), R40–48.
6. Stevens DS, Balkany AD (2006). Appearance of plica mediana dorsalis during epidurography. *Pain Physician* **9**(3), 268–70.
7. Asato F, Goto F (1996). Radiographic findings of unilateral epidural block. *Anesth Analg* **83**(3), 519–22.
8. Boogerd W, van der Sande JJ, Kroger R (1992). Early diagnosis and treatment of spinal epidural metastasis in breast cancer: a prospective study. *J Neurol Neurosurg Psychiatry* **55**(12), 1188–93.
9. Weissman DE (2006). Early diagnosis of epidural metastases #62. *J Palliat Med* **9**(2), 480–81.
10. Boswell MV, Shah RV, Everett CR *et al.* (2005). Interventional techniques in the management of chronic spinal pain: evidence-based practice guidelines. *Pain Physician* **8**(1), 1–47.
11. Cole JS, Patchell RA (2008). Metastatic epidural spinal cord compression. *Lancet Neurol* **7**(5), 459–66.
12. Appelgren L, Nordborg C, Sjoberg M *et al.* (1997). Spinal epidural metastasis: implications for spinal analgesia to treat 'refractory' cancer pain. *J Pain Symptom Manage* **13**(1), 25–42.
13. Rathmell JP, Roland T, DuPen SL (2000). Management of pain associated with metastatic epidural spinal cord compression: use of imaging studies in planning epidural therapy. *Reg Anesth Pain Med* **25**(2), 113–116.
14. Hayashi N, Weinstein JN, Meller ST *et al.* (1998). The effect of epidural injection of betamethasone or bupivacaine in a rat model of lumbar radiculopathy. *Spine (Phila Pa 1976)* **23**(8), 877–85.
15. Lee HM, Weinstein JN, Meller ST *et al.* (1998). The role of steroids and their effects on phospholipase A2. An animal model of radiculopathy. *Spine (Phila Pa 1976)* **23**(11), 1191–96.
16. Khanapure SP, Garvey DS, Janero DR *et al.* (2007). Eicosanoids in inflammation: biosynthesis, pharmacology, and therapeutic frontiers. *Curr Top Med Chem* **7**(3), 311–40.
17. Spicarova D, Palecek J (2008). The role of spinal cord vanilloid (TRPV1) receptors in pain modulation. *Physiol Res 57 Suppl* **3**, S69–77.

18. Abdi S, Datta S, Trescot AM *et al.* (2007). Epidural steroids in the management of chronic spinal pain: a systematic review. *Pain Physician* **10**(1), 185–212.

19. George R, Jeba J, Ramkumar G *et al.* (2008). Interventions for the treatment of metastatic extradural spinal cord compression in adults. *Cochrane Database Syst Rev* Issue 4, CD006716.

20. Behar M, Magora F, Olshwang D *et al.* (1979). Epidural morphine in treatment of pain. *Lancet* **1**(8115), 527–29.

21. Yaksh TL, Rudy TA (1976). Analgesia mediated by a direct spinal action of narcotics. *Science* **192**(4246), 1357–58.

22. Yaksh TL (1981). Spinal opiate analgesia: characteristics and principles of action. *Pain* **11**(3), 293–346.

23. Kedlaya D, Reynolds L, Waldman S (2002). Epidural and intrathecal analgesia for cancer pain. *Best Pract Res Clin Anaesthesiol* **16**(4), 651–65.

24. Dickenson AH (1991). Mechanisms of the analgesic actions of opiates and opioids. *Br Med Bull* **47**(3), 690–702.

25. Onofrio BM, Yaksh TL (1990). Long-term pain relief produced by intrathecal morphine infusion in 53 patients. *J Neurosurg* **72**(2), 200–9.

26. Vella-Brincat J, Macleod AD (2007). Adverse effects of opioids on the central nervous systems of palliative care patients. *J Pain Palliat Care Pharmacother* **21**(1), 15–25.

27. Markham A, Faulds D (1996). Ropivacaine. A review of its pharmacology and therapeutic use in regional anaesthesia. *Drugs* **52**(3), 429–49.

28. Grant GJ, Barenholz Y, Bolotin EM *et al.* (2004). A novel liposomal bupivacaine formulation to produce ultralong-acting analgesia. *Anesthesiology* **101**(1), 133–37.

29. Kalso E, Heiskanen T, Rantio M *et al.* (1996). Epidural and subcutaneous morphine in the management of cancer pain: a double-blind cross-over study. *Pain* **67**(2–3), 443–49.

30. Vainio A, Tigerstedt I (1988). Opioid treatment for radiating cancer pain: oral administration vs. epidural techniques. *Acta Anaesthesiol Scand* **32**(3), 179–85.

31. Waterman NG, Hughes S, Foster WS (1991). Control of cancer pain by epidural infusion of morphine. *Surgery* **110**(4), 612–4.

32. Hassenbusch SJ, Pillay PK, Magdinec M *et al.* (1990). Constant infusion of morphine for intractable cancer pain using an implanted pump. *J Neurosurg* **73**(3), 405–9.

33. Crawford ME, Andersen HB, Augustenborg G *et al.* (1983). Pain treatment on outpatient basis utilizing extradural opiates. A Danish multicentre study comprising 105 patients. *Pain* **16**(1), 41–7.

34. Driessen JJ, de Mulder PH, Claessen JJ *et al.* (1989). Epidural administration of morphine for control of cancer pain: long-term efficacy and complications. *Clin J Pain* **5**(3), 217–22.

35. Samuelsson H, Malmberg F, Eriksson M *et al.* (1995). Outcomes of epidural morphine treatment in cancer pain: nine years of clinical experience. *J Pain Symptom Manage* **10**(2), 105–12.

36. Ballantyne JC, Carwood CM (2005). Comparative efficacy of epidural, subarachnoid, and intracerebroventricular opioids in patients with pain due to cancer. *Cochrane Database Syst Rev* Issue 2, CD005178.

37. Shir Y, Shapira SS, Shenkman Z *et al.* (1991). Continuous epidural methadone treatment for cancer pain. *Clin J Pain* **7**(4), 339–41.

38. Christo PJ, Mazloomdoost D (2008). Interventional pain treatments for cancer pain. *Ann NY Acad Sci* **1138**, 299–328.

39. Smith HS, Deer TR, Staats PS *et al.* (2008). Intrathecal drug delivery. *Pain Physician* **11**(2 Suppl), S89–S104.

40. Hassenbusch SJ, Portenoy RK, Cousins M *et al.* (2004). Polyanalgesic Consensus Conference 2003: an update on the management of pain by intraspinal drug delivery—report of an expert panel. *J Pain Symptom Manage* **27**(6), 540–63.

41. Rauck RL, Cherry D, Boyer MF *et al.* (2003). Long-term intrathecal opioid therapy with a patient-activated, implanted delivery system for the treatment of refractory cancer pain. *J Pain* **4**(8), 441–7.

42. Gestin Y, Vainio A, Pegurier AM (1997). Long-term intrathecal infusion of morphine in the home care of patients with advanced cancer. *Acta Anaesthesiol Scand* **41**(1 Pt 1), 12–7.

43. Sallerin-Caute B, Lazorthes Y, Deguine O *et al.* (1998). Does intrathecal morphine in the treatment of cancer pain induce the development of tolerance? *Neurosurgery* **42**(1), 44–9.

44. Penn RD, Paice JA (1987). Chronic intrathecal morphine for intractable pain. *J Neurosurg* **67**(2), 182–86.

45. Paice JA, Penn RD, Shott S (1996). Intraspinal morphine for chronic pain: a retrospective, multicenter study. *J Pain Symptom Manage* **11**(2), 71–80.

46. Devulder J, Ghys L, Dhondt W *et al.* (1994). Spinal analgesia in terminal care: risk versus benefit. *J Pain Symptom Manage* **9**(2), 75–81.

47. Schultheiss R, Schramm J, Neidhardt J (1992). Dose changes in long- and medium-term intrathecal morphine therapy of cancer pain. *Neurosurgery* **31**(4), 664–69.

48. Follett KA, Hitchon PW, Piper J *et al.* (1992). Response of intractable pain to continuous intrathecal morphine: a retrospective study. *Pain* **49**(1), 21–5.

49. Madrid JL, Fatela LV, Lobato RD *et al.* (1987). Intrathecal therapy: rationale, technique, clinical results. *Acta Anaesthesiol Scand Suppl* **85**, 60–67.

50. Brazenor GA (1987). Long term intrathecal administration of morphine: a comparison of bolus injection via reservoir with continuous infusion by implanted pump. *Neurosurgery* **21**(4), 484–91.

51. Nitescu P, Sjöberg M, Appelgren L *et al.* (1995). Complications of intrathecal opioids and bupivacaine in the treatment of 'refractory' cancer pain. *Clin J Pain* **11**(1), 45–62.

52. Bennett G, Serafini M, Burchiel K *et al.* (2000). Evidence-based review of the literature on intrathecal delivery of pain medication. *J Pain Symptom Manage* **20**(2), S12–36.

53. Smith TJ, Coyne PJ, Staats PS *et al.* (2005). An implantable drug delivery system (IDDS) for refractory cancer pain provides sustained pain control, less drug-related toxicity, and possibly better survival compared with comprehensive medical management (CMM). *Ann Oncol* **16**(5), 825–33.

54. Du PS, Du PA, Hillyer J (2006). Intrathecal hydromorphone for intractable nonmalignant pain: a retrospective study. *Pain Med* **7**(1), 10–5.

55. Anderson VC, Cooke B, Burchiel KJ (2001). Intrathecal hydromorphone for chronic nonmalignant pain: a retrospective study. *Pain Med* **2**(4), 287–97.

56. Johansen MJ, Satterfield WC, Baze WB *et al.* (2004). Continuous intrathecal infusion of hydromorphone: safety in the sheep model and clinical implications. *Pain Med* **5**(1), 14–25.

57. Ramsey CN, Owen RD, Witt WO *et al.* (2008). Intrathecal granuloma in a patient receiving high dose hydromorphone. *Pain Physician* **11**(3), 369–73.

58. Jacobson L, Chabal C, Brody MC *et al.* (1990). Intrathecal methadone: a dose-response study and comparison with intrathecal morphine 0.5 mg. *Pain* **43**(2), 141–8.

59. Hogan Q, Haddox JD, Abram S *et al.* (1991). Epidural opiates and local anesthetics for the management of cancer pain. *Pain* **46**(3), 271–9.

60. Smitt PS, Tsafka A, Teng-van de ZF *et al.* (1-11-1998). Outcome and complications of epidural analgesia in patients with chronic cancer pain. *Cancer* **83**(9), 2015–22.

61. Saito Y, Kaneko M, Kirihara Y *et al.* (1998). Interaction of intrathecally infused morphine and lidocaine in rats (part I): synergistic antinociceptive effects. *Anesthesiology* **89**(6), 1455–63.

62. Kopacz DJ, Sharrock NE, Allen HW (1999). A comparison of levobupivacaine 0.125%, fentanyl 4 microg/mL, or their combination for patient-controlled epidural analgesia after major orthopedic surgery. *Anesth Analg* **89**(6), 1497–503.

63. Walker SM, Goudas LC, Cousins MJ *et al.* (2002). Combination spinal analgesic chemotherapy: a systematic review. *Anesth Analg* **95**(3), 674–715.

64. Sjoberg M, Nitescu P, Appelgren L *et al.* (1994). Long-term intrathecal morphine and bupivacaine in patients with refractory cancer pain. Results from a morphine: bupivacaine dose regimen of 0.5:4.75 mg/ml. *Anesthesiology* **80**(2), 284–97.

65. Sjoberg M, Appelgren L, Einarsson S *et al.* (1991). Long-term intrathecal morphine and bupivacaine in 'refractory' cancer pain. I. Results from the first series of 52 patients. *Acta Anaesthesiol Scand* **35**(1), 30–43.

66. van Dongen RT, Crul BJ, van EJ (1999). Intrathecal coadministration of bupivacaine diminishes morphine dose progression during long-term intrathecal infusion in cancer patients. *Clin J Pain* **15**(3), 166–72.

67. Baker L, Lee M, Regnard C *et al.* (2004). Evolving spinal analgesia practice in palliative care. *Palliat Med* **18**(6), 507–15.

68. Dahm P, Nitescu P, Appelgren L *et al.* (1998). Efficacy and technical complications of long-term continuous intraspinal infusions of opioid and/or bupivacaine in refractory nonmalignant pain: a comparison between the epidural and the intrathecal approach with externalized or implanted catheters and infusion pumps. *Clin J Pain* **14**(1), 4–16.

69. Nitescu P, Appelgren L, Linder LE *et al.* (1990). Epidural versus intrathecal morphine-bupivacaine: assessment of consecutive treatments in advanced cancer pain. *J Pain Symptom Manage* **5**(1), 18–26.

70. Bannister K, Bee LA, Dickenson AH (2009). Preclinical and early clinical investigations related to monoaminergic pain modulation. *Neurotherapeutics* **6**(4), 703–12.

71. Eisenach JC, DuPen S, Dubois M *et al.* (1995). Epidural clonidine analgesia for intractable cancer pain. The Epidural Clonidine Study Group. *Pain* **61**(3), 391–9.

72. Niemi G, Breivik H (2002). Epinephrine markedly improves thoracic epidural analgesia produced by a small-dose infusion of ropivacaine, fentanyl, and epinephrine after major thoracic or abdominal surgery: a randomized, double-blinded crossover study with and without epinephrine. *Anesth Analg* **94**(6), 1598–605, table.

73. Coombs DW, Saunders RL, Fratkin JD *et al.* (1986). Continuous intrathecal hydromorphone and clonidine for intractable cancer pain. *J Neurosurg* **64**(6), 890–4.

74. Tumber PS, Fitzgibbon DR (1998). The control of severe cancer pain by continuous intrathecal infusion and patient controlled intrathecal analgesia with morphine, bupivacaine and clonidine. *Pain* **78**(3), 217–20.

75. Gu X, Zhang J, Ma Z *et al.* (2010). The role of N-methyl-D-aspartate receptor subunit NR2B in spinal cord in cancer pain. *Eur J Pain* **14**(5), 496–502.

76. Wong CS, Liaw WJ, Tung CS *et al.* (1996). Ketamine potentiates analgesic effect of morphine in postoperative epidural pain control. *Reg Anesth* **21**(6), 534–41.

77. Lauretti GR, Gomes JM, Reis MP *et al.* (1999). Low doses of epidural ketamine or neostigmine, but not midazolam, improve morphine analgesia in epidural terminal cancer pain therapy. *J Clin Anesth* **11**(8), 663–8.

78. Vranken JH, Troost D, Wegener JT *et al.* (2005). Neuropathological findings after continuous intrathecal administration of S(+)-ketamine for the management of neuropathic cancer pain. *Pain* **117**(1–2), 231–5.

79. Benrath J, Scharbert G, Gustorff B *et al.* (2005). Long-term intrathecal S(+)-ketamine in a patient with cancer-related neuropathic pain. *Br J Anaesth* **95**(2), 247–9.

80. Wermeling DP (2005). Ziconotide, an intrathecally administered N-type calcium channel antagonist for the treatment of chronic pain. *Pharmacotherapy* **25**(8), 1084–94.

81. Staats PS, Yearwood T, Charapata SG *et al.* (2004). Intrathecal ziconotide in the treatment of refractory pain in patients with cancer or AIDS: a randomized controlled trial. *JAMA* **291**(1), 63–70.

82. Wallace MS, Kosek PS, Staats P *et al.* (2008). Phase II, open-label, multicenter study of combined intrathecal morphine and ziconotide: addition of ziconotide in patients receiving intrathecal morphine for severe chronic pain. *Pain Med* **9**(3), 271–81.

Chapter 6

Neuraxial (epidural and intrathecal) infusions II: Patient selection, epidural versus intrathecal, equipment, description of the technique, complications, national use

Joan Hester

The anatomy of the epidural and intrathecal routes, and the pharmacokinetics of the drugs that may be used, have been described in Chapter 5. This chapter covers:

- patient selection
- comparison of epidural and intrathecal routes
- a description of the two techniques
- equipment
- choice of mode of delivery
- preparation of the patient
- risks and side effects
- management of complications
- outline of the national use of this technique
- future developments

Patient selection

There are no hard and fast rules for selecting patients for neuraxial infusions, but it is generally accepted that they should be considered when:

- pain is unrelieved by oral and systemic opioids with adjuvants (1, 2)
- there are unacceptable side effects from oral and systemic analgesics, especially drowsiness
- there is a large, permanent increase in dosage of oral and systemic opioids (3)
- there are concerns about dependency and addiction (2)

There are situations where difficult pain can be predicted and where a neuraxial infusion might be beneficial. These are:

- pathological fracture awaiting fixation or radiotherapy
- spinal tumours causing radicular pain

- brachial and lumbar plexopathy
- advanced intra-abdominal cancer, especially pancreatic cancer, carcinoma of the cervix, uterus and bladder
- visceral tumours causing autonomic dysfunction, gut motility disorders, pseudo obstruction or bowel obstruction
- intraspinal slowly growing tumours such as cordoma
- mesothelioma
- carcinoma of the lung invading the chest wall
- widespread painful bony metastases
- possibly head and neck cancer (see Chapter 2)
- where aggressive chemotherapy may be considered as the patient's performance status will be preserved for a longer period of time
- in cancer survivors who develop complex regional pain syndrome secondary to cancer treatment (implanted system)

Case study

A better than more oxycodone

A lady of 72 years had advanced cancer of the pancreas. The tumour enclosed the coeliac plexus and was invading retroperitoneal tissue anterior to the L1 and L2 vertebral bodies. She was bed-bound, drowsy and incoherent on large doses of oral Oxycontin and Oxynorm. A tunnelled epidural catheter was inserted at T10 with an infusion of 2 ml/h bupivacaine 0.25% with diamorphine 25 mg in 250 ml bupivacaine. Oral opioids were halved. The next day she became alert and mobile, getting out of bed to pass urine and to walk short distances with her husband. The epidural continued until she died, giving excellent pain relief from both her visceral and somatic pain. She required escalating doses of both epidural and systemic opioids in the last week of life, but for approximately three months she was pain free and could talk freely with her husband and family.

Learning point

Pancreatic cancer can cause severe visceral and somatic pain, both of which will often respond to a low thoracic epidural.

Burton *et al.* 2004 (1) have developed a decision-making algorithm for treating refractory cancer pain (Fig. 6.1).

Epidural or intrathecal?

The epidural space is easily accessed via the back in the lumbar and thoracic region, but flow of drugs within the space varies with anatomy, presence of epidural adhesions and the level at which the catheter is inserted, as explained in Chapter 5. It may also be accessed via the caudal route, although this carries a greater risk of infection, and the cervical route is technically more challenging as the epidural space is narrow.

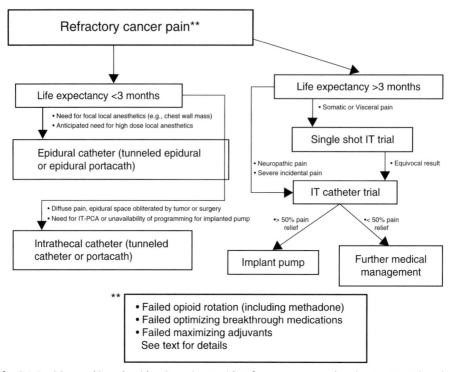

Fig. 6.1 Decision-making algorithm in patients with refractory cancer-related pain. Reproduced from (1) with permission. IT-PCA, intrathecal patient-controlled analgesia.

A particular advantage of the epidural route is that it is highly effective where the pain is localised, such for managing pain arising from a chest wall tumour, since the catheter tip can be sited in the epidural space at the level of the lesion, for example at T10–12 for pain in the flank and lower abdomen, or T6–8 for pain in the chest wall radiating to the upper abdomen. The combination of local anaesthetic with opioid delivered at the appropriate level will block the relevant nerves and provide more effective pain relief than opioid alone. This is even more important in opioid non-responsive pain, particularly neuropathic pain, where the analgesic effect of the local anaesthetic is of great importance.

There is evidence that epidural fibrosis may develop after long-term catheter placement (4). Pain on injection is a common side effect of intermittent bolus injection of opioid (5), which sometimes responds to prior application of a local anaesthetic, to a very slow injection or to injection of steroid. Continuous infusions are more commonly used in cancer pain management and this side effect is rarely seen.

Obstruction or displacement of the catheter from the epidural space is common, and the catheter has to be replaced. Very rarely the catheter might migrate from the epidural space into the intrathecal space, where the effect of the infused drugs is more pronounced. Increasing weakness and sensory loss should alert carers to this possibility; the pump should be stopped and urgent specialist review requested. Catheters can also migrate out of the neural foraminae, causing unilateral block or loss of effect, or into a vein, where the local anaesthetic bupivacaine can cause signs of toxicity. Convulsions or cardiac arrest are known extreme side effects of high dose intervascular injection although this is very unlikely from a low-rate infusion; we have never seen this complication.

The intrathecal route may offer advantages, especially for long-term use or for home care as the infusion rate is lower (0.5–4 ml/h) and pump reservoirs are refilled less frequently.

An intrathecal catheter is more likely to stay patent, it is less commonly displaced, the dose of drugs administered is less and their effect more predictable over time. Intrathecal infusions are favoured over epidurals where the pain is diffuse and poorly localized, although the catheter tip is still approximated to the level of the lesion(s). Burton advocates the intrathecal route in cases where there is pathology, such as tumour, in the epidural space or where the epidural space has been surgically obliterated (1).

Disadvantages of the intrathecal route include spinal headache after insertion, although specially designed catheters may help to overcome this problem (see section on equipment). It is often assumed that there is more potential for serious complications such as respiratory depression and meningitis, but comparative studies have shown that, in long-term use, intrathecal morphine administration may give better pain relief, with lower doses of morphine and fewer side effects, than epidural administration (6, 7). Dahm also reported better pain relief, fewer treatment failures and fewer system-related complications with the intrathecal approach in a cohort of non-cancer pain patients with both externalized and implanted systems (7).

Long-term hormonal effects have been demonstrated in the management of chronic non-cancer pain with intrathecal opioids. These include depression of the hypothalamic–pituitary axis, reduced libido and sexual function, hypogonadism, lowered testosterone blood levels in men and lowered oestradiol levels, oligomenorrhoea and amenorrhoea in women. Abs et al. demonstrated hypogonadotrophic hypogonadism in the majority of men and all women receiving intrathecal opioids for an average of 26 months (±16 months), with about 15% developing hypocorticism and 15% growth hormone deficiency (8). The significance of these findings in the cancer population has not been assessed.

Rarely, development of an intraspinal granuloma has been reported after intrathecal morphine. This can lead to neurological deficit and requires surgical removal. It appears to be associated with infusion of high concentrations of morphine, and is unlikely to occur in a cancer patient with a limited life prognosis (see below).

Ballantyne and Carwood, in a Cochrane review, compared the efficacy of epidural, intrathecal and intracerebroventricular opioids in patients with pain due to cancer, and found that all routes provided effective pain relief (9). There was more sedation and respiratory depression in the intracerebroventricular route.

Nitescu compared epidural versus intrathecal morphine–bupivacaine in advanced cancer pain, and found the intrathecal route gave more satisfactory pain relief with lower daily doses (10).

Burton et al. found no difference in pain scores or reduction of opioid-related side effects in a group of 87 cancer patients, 61 of whom received intrathecal and 26 epidural analgesia (1).

Baker, Lee and Regnard reviewed 100 neuraxial infusions performed in St Oswald's Hospice, Newcastle upon Tyne over a 15-year period (11). During this time there was a major shift in practice from epidural to intrathecal lines, arising 'from a better understanding of the safety and efficacy of intrathecal analgesia'. They cite evidence that intrathecal lines are safer than epidurals if an infusion needs to be *in situ* for longer than three weeks. In their series, 67% patients had a clinical improvement in pain, and adverse effects were reported as low when compared to other series.

Crul *et al.* reported a 5% complication rate with intrathecal catheters compared with a 55% rate with epidural catheters, mostly related to obstruction and dislocation of the catheter (4).

More recent reviews tend to favour the intrathecal route, with a trend to the use of more implanted drug delivery systems (2). The infection rate is much lower in totally implanted systems (2, 8).

The choice of route ultimately depends on more practical issues such as the availability of equipment, the skills of the practitioner, the anatomy of the individual patient and the familiarity of the staff looking after the patient after the block. It is much better to do a familiar technique well than an unfamiliar one badly. If a needle, intended to be placed epidurally, in fact penetrates the dura and cerebrospinal fluid appears—a so-called 'spinal tap'—the block should be converted into an intrathecal without hesitation.

It also has to be accepted that the first attempt may not be the definitive procedure: a second or third procedure may sometimes be necessary. This should not be regarded as a 'failure'. The high level of skill required should not be underestimated. Even an experienced anaesthetist, familiar with epidurals for obstetrics, surgery and chronic pain may find a cancer patient challenging. Patients are very ill, turning on the side is difficult, tissues can be oedematous and anatomy distorted, and there may be unknown tumour deposits in the epidural space. Unfamiliar surroundings and lack of skilled assistance also add to the stress of the situation. Two anaesthetists are often required in a hospice setting, one to sedate and look after the patient while the other performs the block. Monitoring and resuscitation equipment and drugs should be available, as described in Chapter 7.

There is no substantial difference in the overall complication rates for the 2 techniques. The advantages and disadvantages of the epidural versus the intrathecal routes are summarised in table 6.1.

Thoracic and cervical epidurals and intrathecals

The anatomy of these approaches is described in Chapter 5.

Epidurals can be performed under X-ray guidance in the thoracic spine to provide relief of chest-wall pain. A catheter can be threaded cephalad from T1-3 into the cervical spinal canal for the relief of shoulder and arm pain. It is tunnelled over the shoulder to the anterior chest wall and connected to an external pump, as described below. Caution is required in patients with compromised respiratory function, but good pain relief can be obtained with careful management.

Baker describes six cases of an 18-g intrathecal catheter inserted at T3/4 or T4/5 and threaded cephalad, with good pain relief and no meningitis (12). There was one instance of respiratory depression in this small series, one of arm weakness and one of leg weakness. All patients were in the terminal phase of their illness.

Table 6.1 Comparison of the epidural and intrathecal routes

	Epidural route	Intrathecal route
Advantages	May give better pain relief for localized pain in a specific neuronal distribution, especially when local anaesthesia is used	Greater potency of drugs allowing lower infusion rates
	More familiar	Less likely to become blocked or displaced
		More predictable over time
		Low infection rates in totally implanted systems
Disadvantages	Catheters more prone to blocking and displacement	Spinal headache, leak of CSF, hygroma
	Less predictable over time	Long-term endocrine effects
	Unilateral block	
	Pain on injection	Rarely, intraspinal granuloma
	Epidural fibrosis	

The authors' recommendation would be to use the epidural route for managing pain in the thoracic and cervical regions.

Methods of delivery of neuraxial drugs

There are three methods for delivery of neuraxial drugs:

1 Percutaneous epidural or intrathecal catheter, with or without subcutaneous tunnelling. This may be injected intermittently (bolus injection) or connected to an infusion pump (see Figs 6.22, 7.1, and 7.2, Plates 29 and 30).

2 Totally implanted catheter with a subcutaneous injection port (access port) (see Fig. 6.4). This may be injected intermittently or connected to an infusion pump (see Figs 6.4 and 6.5).

3 Totally implanted catheter and pump. The pump is either manually activated, or gas driven at constant flow, or is a battery driven, constant flow or programmable infusion pump. Fig. 6.2 shows a Medtronic Synchromed II fully programmable pump *in situ*.

Advantages and disadvantages of the methods of drug delivery

The percutaneous catheter is quick, cheap and easy to insert. The catheter is attached to an antibacterial filter, but the risk of local infection is greater than with a totally implanted system. Tunnelling the catheter away from the back, usually to the upper abdomen or chest wall, reduces the risk of infection spreading to the meninges. Handling of the connecting tubing and multiple injections increase the risk of contamination. Catheters are easily dislodged and may kink or leak at the connection site. The procedure can be performed in the patient's bed in the hospice, home or palliative care unit at minimal cost, and takes 20–30 minutes.

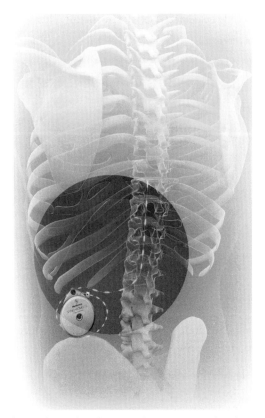

Fig. 6.2 Medtronis Synchromed Intrathecal Drug Delivery Pump and catheter in situ. Also appears in colour in the colour plate section, Plate 9.

The subcutaneous injection port reduces the likelihood of displacement of the catheter or of the patient inadvertently pulling it out. If an intermittent bolus injection technique is used, the drugs have to be drawn up and delivered by a carer or the patient, if at home. The port membrane must be able to withstand a thousand or more injections without disintegrating. Some ports become too easily disconnected from the catheter or may leak. The patient has an external device to carry around if a continuous infusion is used.

Gourlay *et al.* compared intermittent bolus with continuous infusion of morphine via epidural catheters for the relief of cancer pain (13). The mean duration of treatment was about 150 days in both groups. There was no significant difference in pain relief; both methods provided satisfactory pain control. No comment was made on the infection rate in the two groups.

Totally implanted pumps should be considered if life expectancy is longer than three months. These pumps have a much lower infection potential. Programmable pumps are more expensive but are much more versatile and responsive to fluctuating pain levels. Modern pumps can be provided with a patient- or carer-operated device giving as-required boluses for breakthrough pain. Constant-flow pumps, which are gas driven, are less versatile in responding rapidly to changes in analgesic requirement. There is a minimal risk of pump failure or overdose. Technology is improving all the time to minimize these risks.

Equipment

Skin cleaning

For skin decontamination prior to spinal procedures, 0.5% chlorhexidine in 70% alcohol or 10% povidone–iodine is recommended (14); if local surgical skin preparation guidelines exist, these should be followed. Chlorhexidine skin preparation should be coloured to ensure it cannot be confused with other medicines. At the current time there is insufficient evidence to support the efficacy or safety of Chloraprep (2% chlorhexidine in 70% alcohol) for this purpose. The solution must dry before any needles are inserted. The solution should be carefully checked for date of expiry and should not be more than six months old.

Catheters

There are several catheters manufactured for epidural and intrathecal use. The commercially available devices for epidural and intrathecal access include ports and three categories of catheter:

- short-term catheters made from polyamide, polyurethane and nylon, with friction adaptors attached to their distal end (Portex, Braun)
- non-kinking, wire-supported epidural catheters, with friction adapters that, under ideal clinical conditions, may be used for prolonged epidural access (Agilecath, Codman)
- long-term silicone rubber catheters with fixed integrated Luer-Lock adapters (DuPen, CR Bard)
- implantable epidural and intrathecal ports (CR Bard, Portacath)

Stiffness may play a role in catheter migration from epidural to intrathecal spaces or in the reverse direction; stiffness may also result in pressure and nerve root paraesthesiae. Device selection is an individual choice. The practitioner should select the apparatus with which he or she is most adept and comfortable; this usually results in the most predictable outcomes.

Short-term catheters

Percutaneous epidurals are usually performed using catheters designed for temporary use (Portex). These are manufactured from a clear blend of polyether block amide and are blunt-tipped with three holes in the side wall of the catheter tip. Manufacturing technology developed in the 1970s allowed the drilling of small holes in the catheter, and more recent technology has allowed them to become closer together (1-mm separation) and much closer to the tip. In the USA, Portex nylon, teflon and wire-reinforced catheters are available, but not in the UK. Portex catheters are made in 16-G and 18-G diameter, are 915 mm long and are marked at 1-cm intervals to facilitate accurate catheter positioning. A 19G × 650 mm version is made for paediatric use.

Catheters may be supplied separately or in a kit that includes a Tuohy needle, loss-of-resistance syringe and filter.

Medium-term use

Both Arrow International Inc. and Codman (Johnson and Johnson) produce a polymer catheter reinforced with a spiral-wound stainless steel metal wire down its length. This prevents kinking. It has the advantage of ease of insertion and infrequent paraesthesiae and bleeding from epidural veins (15). It has a single open-end hole and SnapLock adapter, and is supplied with a wire introducer.

Examples of epidural catheters

Arrow: FlexTip Plus epidural catheter 19g
Codman: Agilecath epidural catheter
Codman: Surestream Intraspinal catheter 19g (Fig. 6.3)

Long-term use

The DuPen epidural catheter was designed by Stuart L. DuPen from Seattle, when he recognized the limitations of using a temporary catheter for long-term use, these limitations include a high incidence of infection, kinking and dislocation (16). He adapted technology from vascular access catheters, such as the Hickman line, which are designed to reduce infection risk even after multiple punctures. His catheter consists of an epidural segment, placed percutaneously into the epidural space, an exteriorized line equipped with an external Luer connector and subcutaneous Dacron cuff, which can be anchored and serves as a barrier to bacteria. There is a small splice to join the two catheter segments, which is inserted through a small incision in the back. This is now made of radio-opaque silicone and includes a 0.22 μm filter, pre-attached injection cap, a yellow band for colour coding and a SureCuff tissue ingrowth cuff to provide catheter fixation.

DuPen's original series of 58 catheter insertions showed no infections in 3891 catheter-days of use. Williams 1990 reported a series of 400 catheter insertions with a 5% infection rate requiring removal of the system (17). There was no meningitis in her series. Dislodgement was rare and the patients could be nursed at home.

The DuPen catheter has now been discontinued by Bard Access systems.

Intrathecal catheters

Portex epidural catheters, which are made of polyamide nylon, may be used for short-term intrathecal use, but are relatively stiff, although they have been shown to cause fewer nerve root/spinal cord injuries than soft silicon catheters inserted with a guide wire (7). The same review article found a rate of postdural puncture headache of 22% with externalized nylon intrathecal catheters with an outer diameter of 1.2 mm inserted through a 17g Tuohy needle. This was comparable to the 20% and 31% reported in two studies using silicone catheters with an outer diameter of 1.2 mm inserted through a 16g Tuohy needle (6, 18).

The Surestream by Codman is made for intrathecal use (Fig. 6.3). This is a 19 g polyurethane catheter with titanium coil, with length 105 cm and internal diameter of 0.5 mm.

Important Features-Surestream

• **With inner titanium coil to prevent kinking, tearing & bunching**

    – Catheter can be tied in knots and drug will still flow

    – Stainless steel guide wire and inner titanium coil allow for easy guide wire
      removal (metal on metal)

    – Less prone to bunching during guide wire removal due to more rigid material

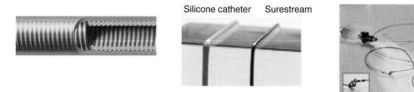

Silicone catheter   Surestream

• One hole, located at catheter tip (open tip)

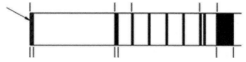

Fig. 6.3 Codman Surestream Intraspinal catheter 19g. Also appears in colour in the colour plate section, Plate 10.

It is inserted through a 17 g Tuohy needle and is designed for externalized systems. It has an anchor, which can be sewn to the spinal ligaments to prevent dislodgement, and a SnapLock Flushing adaptor. Nitescu *et al.* suggested that suturing the catheter hub to the skin and leaving less than 0.5 cm exposed after tunnelling would reduce the likelihood of displacement (18).

Catheters for implanted systems

These catheters are made by Medtronic and Codman to fit their implantable pumps. They are made of silicone with a guidewire, which is supplied with appropriate connectors, Tuohy needle and anchors. The specifications for two Medtronic catheters are shown in Table 6.2.

    The intrathecal catheter creates a pathway for medication flowing from the pump to the drug delivery site. Medtronic intrathecal catheters come in one- and two-piece models. The silicone, radiopaque catheter body is elastic, flexible and trimmable.

Filters

Cousins reviewed the effectiveness and frequency of changing antibacterial filters on intrathecal catheters (20). Most UK anaesthetists use the Portex epidural flat filter, which is a 0.2-μm mesh (micropore) filter that the manufacturers recommend is changed every 96 h. However, De Cicco *et al.* tested the Portex filter over a 60-day period, with intermittent flushing of a *Streptococcus milleri* suspension after 7, 14, 28 and 60 days (21). They concluded that the filter maintained antimicrobial function for 60 days. This was supported by Nitescu *et al.*, who also discussed the efficiency of two filters, changing the distal filter

Table 6.2 Comparison of intrathecal catheter models 8709SC and 8731SC (Medtronic Ltd)

	Model 8709SC	Model 8731SC
Total length	89 cm	104.1 cm
Spinal segment	81.4 cm	38.1 cm
Pump segment or SC interface	7.6 cm	66 cm
Connector pin	Yes	Yes
Pin type	Sutureless	Suture grooves
Introducer needle	15-gauge Tuohy	15-gauge Tuohy
Needle length	9.3 cm	11.4 cm/9.3 cm
Numeric markings	Yes	Yes
Trimmable segments	Spinal	Spinal/pump end

every day and the proximal filter once per week and found this offered no advantage (19, 22). A positive trend between the number of filter changes and the incidence of hub contamination has been found (20).

Bupivacaine has a antibacterial effect against commonly encountered skin organisms, which increases with concentration and the addition of diamorphine (23). Racemic bupivacaine has a more potent antibacterial effect than levobupivacaine (24). It therefore seems reasonable to recommend monthly filter changes on externalized catheter systems where bupivacaine 0.25% is being used, to minimize the risk of contamination via handling of the hub.

Subcutaneous ports

A subcutaneous injection port can be used with an epidural or intrathecal catheter (as shown in Fig. 6.4), which is tunnelled to the anterior chest wall. This is demonstrated in Fig. 6.5. A non-coring gripper needle is inserted into the port and this can then be attached to the infusion pump. A subcutaneous port is shown in Fig 6.4. Positioning of the port is shown in Fig 6.5.

De Jong *et al.* (25) retrospectively analysed the technical complications of epidural catheters with or without subcutaneous injection ports, used for the treatment of cancer pain during a 3.5-year period. There were no dislodgements in the injection port group and no early infections within the first 70 days of treatment.

Holmfred *et al.* 2006 (26) reported an incidence of infection of 2% using intrathecal catheters with subcutaneous ports, inserted under strict aseptic conditions but without antibiotic prophylaxis. The infections appeared more than 2 weeks after insertion of the catheters, and the median treatment time was 71.5 days (range 4–150 days).

It seems that subcutaneous port systems confer the advantage of fewer catheter dislodgements and a lower infection rate than simple tunnelled catheters, but require suitable expertise to insert them and thorough aseptic conditions. Care needs to be taken in managing the injection port. Reinsertion of the non-coring needle that punctures the port membrane must also be performed with careful aseptic technique.

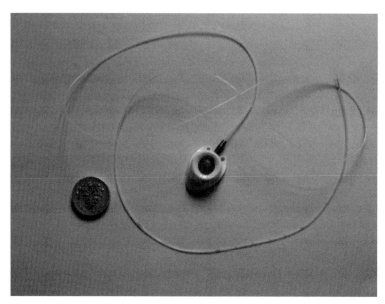

Fig. 6.4 Subcutaneous port attached to catheter. Also appears in colour in the colour plate section, Plate 11.

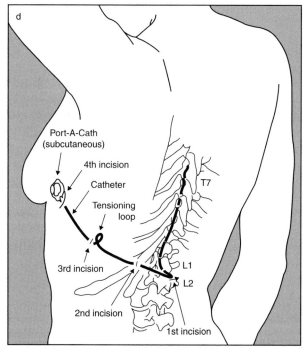

Fig. 6.5 Positioning of subcutaneous port.

Implanted pump and catheter systems

The intrathecal route is used for fully implanted systems, since the infused volume required using this route is low enough to prevent the need for very frequent refills. Two types of pump are available, a constant-flow pump driven by compressed gas, which expands at a constant rate (Archimedes, Codman; see Figs 6.6 and 6.7) or a battery-powered fully programmable pump (Synchromed, Medtronic; see Figs 6.2 and 6.8 and Codman, not illustrated).

They are used for both cancer and non-cancer pain. In fact there is more experience worldwide with their use in non-cancer pain, as short life prognosis, late referral to a specialist for assessment, lack of awareness of the possible benefits, ongoing chemotherapy and radiotherapy, and patient preference often preclude the timely use of this option in cancer pain. However, several sources (see below) have stated that the technique is underused as an option for severe cancer pain when other options have been tried and have not had the desired effect.

Constant flow drug delivery system: compressed gas

This type of pump has no battery and does not need to be replaced as does a battery-powered pump. The Codman Archimedes Pump (Figs 6.6 and 6.7) is divided into inner and outer chambers by accordion-like bellows. The inner chamber contains the drug that is to be infused. The outer chamber contains the propellant, permanently sealed inside. When implanted, the patient's body temperature warms the propellant, causing it to expand. This exerts a constant pressure on the bellows and allows the drug to flow out of the inner chamber through a filter and flow restrictor down the catheter into the cerebrospinal fluid.

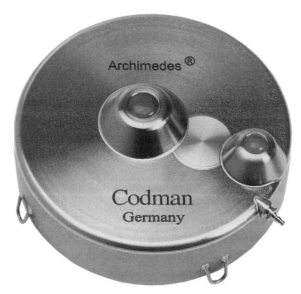

Fig. 6.6 Codman Archimedes Pump. Also appears in colour in the colour plate section, Plate 12.

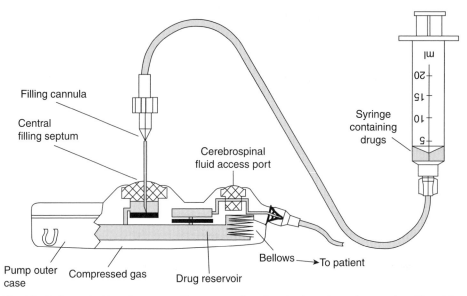

Filling cannula

Central
filling septum

Cerebrospinal
fluid access port

Syringe
containing
drugs

ml

20

15

10

5

Pump outer
case

Compressed gas

Drug reservoir

Bellows

To patient

Fig. 6.7 Codman Archimedes Pump. Also appears in colour in the colour plate section, Plate 13.

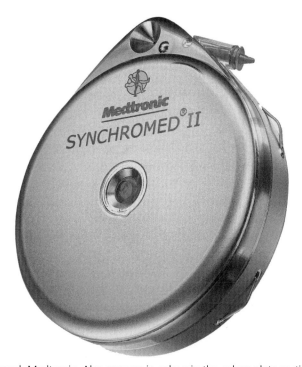

Fig. 6.8 Synchromed, Medtronic. Also appears in colour in the colour plate section, Plate 14.

Codman pumps are manufactured in three reservoir sizes: 16, 30 and 50 ml. The flow rate is pre-set as high, medium, low and ultra-low, but in order to change the daily dose delivered to the patient, the pump has to be refilled with a new concentration of drug(s). With the fluctuating analgesic requirements of a patient with cancer pain, this may not provide sufficient flexibility to adequately control pain and the patient may need frequent pump refills. Patient-delivered doses are not possible with this system. The refill process itself is not easy as the drugs have to be injected into the drug reservoir under pressure. However, the reservoir size can be larger and, if the pain level is constant, there can be a longer time interval between top-ups. This type of pump is considerably cheaper than a programmable pump.

Programmable pump: battery powered

Battery-powered programmable pumps (e.g. those made by Medtronic Ltd; see Fig. 6.8) contain a drug reservoir of 20 or 40 ml, which is accessed via a filling port, felt just under the skin. The pump is positioned subcutaneously, in a surgically created pocket in a convenient place, usually on the abdominal wall. The pump also contains a battery, pumping mechanism and a side port that allows direct aspiration of, or injection into, the CSF. This can be useful if catheter migration is suspected when dye can be injected down the catheter under X-ray screening to see the position of the catheter tip and distribution pattern of the injectate. The battery life of the system varies between 5 and 8 years.

The pump is programmed via a handheld computer and a telemetric head, which is held over the pump to interrogate, programme or re-programme it. The pump can be programmed to deliver a continuous infusion, intermittent boluses, background infusion with boluses at intervals or variable doses at specified times of the day or night.

There is also an option of a patient-delivered bolus for breakthrough pain in cancer patients, called My Personal Therapy Manager (PTM; Fig. 6.9). The PTM is a handheld device about the size of a cell phone. Patients use the PTM by pressing a button, which triggers the delivery of medication after the device software verifies that the 'lockout interval', the length of time during which the patient no longer receives additional doses of medication. A 'lockout interval' can be programmed into the pump which prevents the delivery of excessive amounts of medication or the delivery of a requested bolus too rapidly after the previous one. The physician can set a safe maximum of doses per 24 h. Rauck and Cherry, in an open-label study of 119 patients implanted with a patient-activated device, reported overall success in over 83% over a four-month period (27).

Programmable systems allow versatility in dosing, but the patient is dependent on a specialist physician for the dose to be changed. However, the drug reservoir does not need to be emptied and refilled for the dose to be changed, and the programmer clearly states when the top-up date is due. An alarm sounds when the reservoir reaches a preset limit, typically 2 ml, and issues a more urgent repeat alarm at shorter time intervals when the reservoir has only 0.5 ml remaining. The programmer is handheld and can be used in a hospice or home setting. Pump refills can only be performed by a specially trained healthcare professional, with full aseptic precautions in a clinical area.

Drugs licensed for use in Medtronic programmable pumps include: preservative-free morphine sulphate, hydromorphone, baclofen, clonidine, bupivacaine, ropivacaine

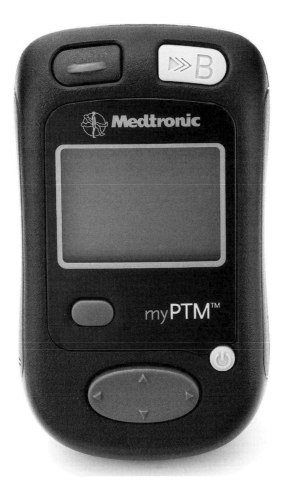

Fig. 6.9 A patient-delivered bolus, My Personal Therapy Manager. Also appears in colour in the colour plate section, Plate 15.

and ziconotide. Diamorphine is not recommended for use in the Synchromed pump as there have been two case reports of precipitation of diamorphine when used in high concentrations, leading to malfunction and stopping of the pump. Diamorphine can be used in constant-low-flow pumps where its high solubility is valuable. The pharmacockinetics and use of these drugs has been explained in Chapter 5.

Wal is pictured in his garden with his PTM remote control in Fig. 6.10. See Case study p 98.

Evidence for effectiveness of implanted intrathecal drug-delivery systems

The British Pain Society comments in its guidance on intrathecal drug delivery (ITDD) that it 'currently appears to be particularly underused in cancer pain in the UK' (28). This comment is a consensus opinion of the authors, based on several case series, one comparator study, a systematic review and, in particular, on the findings of Smith *et al.*, a multicentre, international, randomized controlled trial that showed improved quality of

Case study

Living a little longer

Wal is 64. He has a pleomorphic leiomyosarcoma anterior to the right side of the sacrum, where it is wrapped around the 5th lumbar and 1st sacral nerve roots, giving him intense burning pain in the right leg, with numbness over the dorsum of the foot and a partial foot drop. He is very sensitive to oral opioids, which make him drowsy, confused and nauseated, and can tolerate a maximum of oxycodone 80 mg bd and gabapentin 2,700 mg daily, but without relief of his symptoms. Increasing his oxycodone leads to unacceptable drowsiness. He was referred to King's for consideration of an intrathecal pump, and a PTM has been inserted by the neurosurgeons, with a background infusion of 4 mg morphine/day intrathecally, and optional boluses of 0.5 mg up to four times per day. He is glad to be back at home with his wife and family and to have the freedom that the pump gives him to move around and get on with his life, despite his serious illness. As his wife said, 'we thought we were at the end of the road and there was no hope; this has given us fresh hope that we can live a little longer and be still able to do things together'.

Learning point

Some patients really can not tolerate the side effects of opioids, even if they are very carefully titrated and used in combination with other types of analgesics. Intrathecal delivery of low doses of opioids can be life transforming.

life, sustained pain control and significantly less drug-related toxicity with intrathecal drug delivery compared to comprehensive medical management (29). Survival in the ITTD arm at 6 months was 53% compared with 32% of the conventional medical management group, results that were obtained using an intention-to-treat analysis technique. The British Pain Society comments that there may be several reasons for this increase in longevity, including improved mobility and alertness, and the dose-related effect of morphine in causing inhibition of the immune system. These effects have not been fully quantified in humans.

A review by Stearns *et al.* also concludes that ITDD offers an effective pain-control approach for the small number of patients whose pain is not otherwise controlled or who develop analgesic-related toxicities (2). They found that reductions of up to 200% in the amount of parenteral and oral medication is achieved, and improved pain relief results in fewer hospital admissions for pain control.

The evidence for the effectiveness of the different drugs used in both externalized and internalized systems is explained in Chapter 5.

Cost effectiveness

Cost-effectiveness studies have not been performed in cancer patients. Externalized systems are relatively cheap and the cost of the equipment will be offset quickly by the

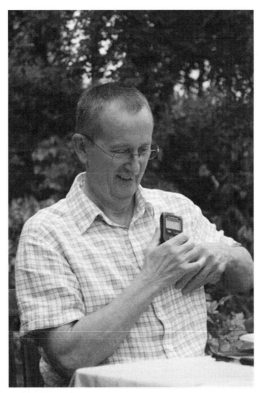

Fig. 6.10 Wal is pictured in his garden with his PTM remote control. Also appears in colour in the colour plate section, Plate 16.

savings achieved in reducing doses of oral and systemic opioids and adjunct agents. 'Normal' practice is to immediately halve oral and/or systemic opioids once a neuraxial system is established.

A further reduction may be achieved as the dose of neuraxial opioid is increased. There is the cost of the time of trained personnel to perform the procedure and to look after the patient more intensively afterwards. Pump-bag refills are often not available commercially and have to be made up as a special order (see Chapter 7). Training costs also have to be factored into the equation, and there is also the cost of possible readmission to a specialist unit for catheter replacement or management of complications.

Implanted pumps are costly (between £2500 and £7500, depending on the type used) and there is a cost associated with the surgical procedure and hospital stay. Cost-effectiveness analyses have been performed that show that, beyond three to six months, ITDD systems are more cost-effective than systemic medication for cancer pain (30, 31). More recent data are not available. Burton advises that implanted pump systems should be reserved for patients with a life expectancy of more than six months, who have refractory pain not adequately controlled by other forms of analgesia (1).

Maintenance of implanted systems is not labour intensive, depending on the refill interval, and the volume and daily dose of drugs used is comparatively extremely low.

The cost of the refill kit and time of the healthcare professional performing the refill should be taken into consideration, but this is offset by frequent patient visits for titration of oral and systemic medication, and the cost of the drugs needed to control side effects.

Some opioid preparations, especially oral oxycodone, transdermal and oral transmucosal fentanyl, and injected diamorphine and alfentanil, are also very expensive when monthly dose costs are calculated. Towards the end of life, drug doses tend to escalate by whatever route they are given, and a combination of intrathecal, oral and systemic drugs may be needed.

Insertion and maintenance of implanted pumps requires a high level of expertise, available from fully trained pain medicine physicians and their teams, working in close liaison with neurosurgeons, oncologists and/or palliative medicine teams.

Choice of method of delivery

The choice between an external catheter, subcutaneous port and fully implanted system depends largely on prognosis and where the patient is likely to spend his/her last weeks or months of life. If the prognosis is very short (days to weeks) an external catheter can be inserted quickly and cheaply in the patient's bed in hospice or hospital and, provided trained nursing care is available, can be managed successfully and effectively. Patients can return home provided adequate nursing, pharmacy and medical support are available (see Chapter 7).

If the prognosis is of medium length (a few weeks to six months) a subcutaneous port can be considered to prevent dislodgement and to reduce infection risk, while allowing the patient to return home, provided adequate nursing, pharmacy and medical support are available (see Chapter 7).

If the prognosis is longer than six months, a fully implanted system should be considered as this will not restrict any activity, will give greater freedom to the patient and regular nursing care is not needed.

The procedure

The procedure for inserting an externalized catheter is shown in Figs 6.11–6.22 (Plates 17–28).

Preparation of the patient

The pain specialist, in collaboration with the referring doctor(s)—usually an oncologist, primary care physician or palliative care consultant—will make a thorough assessment of the patient, as described in Chapter 3, and will consider the pros and cons of the routes of delivery before making the decision to perform an epidural or intrathecal.

Consent

The procedure will be discussed with the patient and his/her relatives in a way they can understand, including the expected benefits, risks and possible complications. Their own preferences and decisions must be respected. As an externalized line will require an

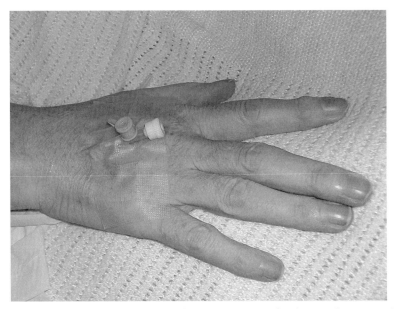

Fig. 6.11 An intravenous cannula is inserted for administration of sedation. Also appears in colour in the colour plate section, Plate 17.

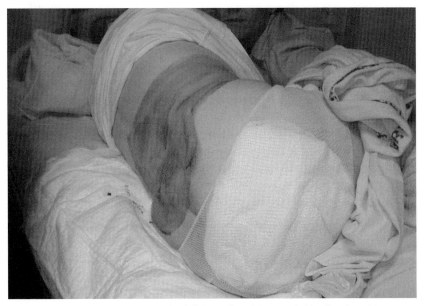

Fig. 6.12 Positioning of the patient in the left lateral position, and skin cleaning. Also appears in colour in the colour plate section, Plate 18.

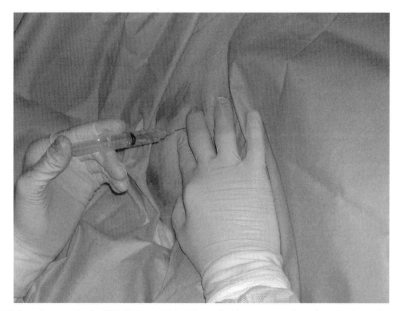

Fig. 6.13 Local anaesthetic (1% Lidocaine) is injected. Also appears in colour in the colour plate section, Plate 19.

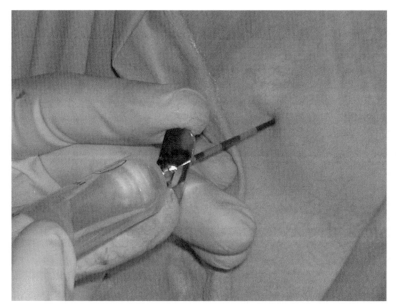

Fig. 6.14 Insertion of a 16g Tuohy needle. Also appears in colour in the colour plate section, Plate 20.

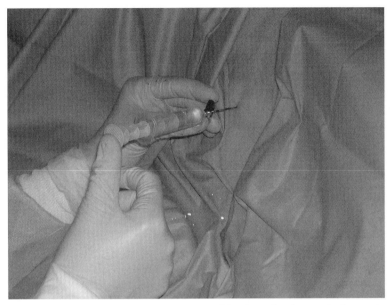

Fig. 6.15 Testing for loss of resistance to saline. A sudden loss of resistance indicates that the epidural space has been entered. Also appears in colour in the colour plate section, Plate 21.

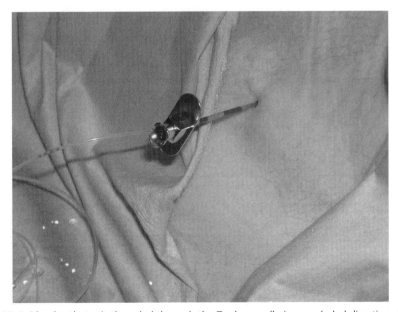

Fig. 6.16 Epidural catheter is threaded through the Tuohy needle in a cephalad direction. Also appears in colour in the colour plate section, Plate 22.

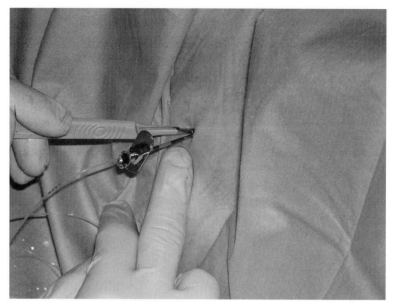

Fig. 6.17 A small incision is made in the back adjacent to the Tuohy needle for tunnelling. Also appears in colour in the colour plate section, Plate 23.

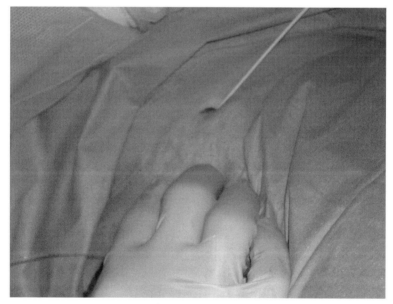

Fig. 6.18 The tunneller (16g long Abbocath®-T , Hospira) is inserted subcutaneously from front to back. Also appears in colour in the colour plate section, Plate 24.

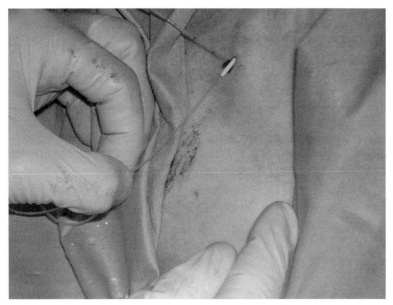

Fig. 6.19 The epidural catheter is threaded through the tunneller from back to front. Also appears in colour in the colour plate section, Plate 25.

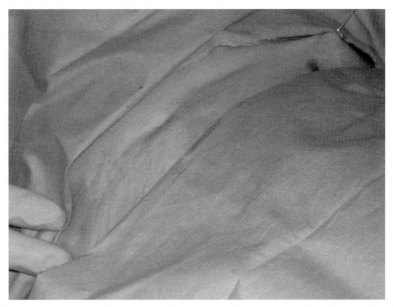

Fig. 6.20 Two or three tunnellings are performed until the catheter reaches the anterior chest or abdominal wall. Also appears in colour in the colour plate section, Plate 26.

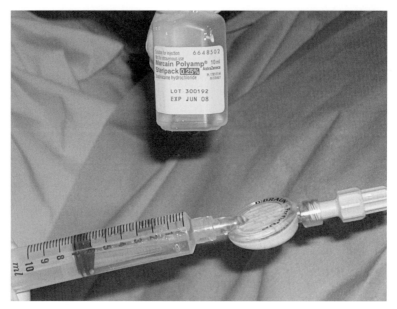

Fig. 6.21 A filter is placed on the end of the epidural catheter and a test dose of 2 ml 0.25% bupivacaine is given. Also appears in colour in the colour plate section, Plate 27.

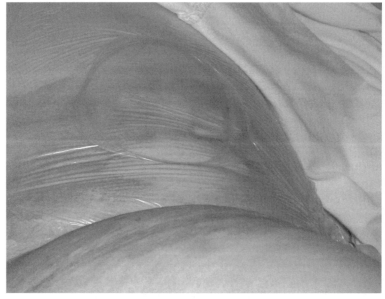

Fig. 6.22 The epidural catheter is looped around and secured with Tegaderm transparent dressings. Also appears in colour in the colour plate section, Plate 28.

enhanced level of care after the procedure, how this is going to be delivered is an important part of the discussion and will involve carers as well as the patient. An implanted system will require a stay in hospital while it is inserted, and the patient will be dependent on the pain physician and his/her team for top-ups, which may entail long journeys by car or other transport.

Consent is an important part of discussion and decision making. Guidance is available from the General Medical Council (32). Having made the decision to proceed, informed consent must be obtained in writing. Benefits and risks are explained and documented, and the form is signed and dated both by the patient and the doctor who is going to perform the procedure, or delegated to a suitably trained and qualified person. The consent process will include the sedation (if any) that will be used. Most patients with advanced cancer will require sedation in order to lie in the required position, usually the lateral position, without discomfort.

A patient with advanced cancer might be too physically weak to sign the consent form but still have the capacity to consent. A relative may sign the form as a witness to appropriate explanation having been given in these circumstances. If the patient lacks capacity to consent, GMC guidance should be followed.

Environment and facilities

Ideally, all epidural and intrathecal procedures would be performed in a theatre type of environment, where monitoring equipment, imaging, resuscitation and post-procedure care facilities are available. The level of asepsis available should be equal to that needed for open surgery, and trained assistance must also be available.

However, it is recognized that many patients with advanced cancer will be cared for in hospices, and the risk of transferring the patient to a hospital might outweigh the potential benefits of the procedure. In these circumstances a tunnelled and externalized catheter may be inserted in a patient's bed, provided that intravenous access, oxygen, monitoring, necessary equipment to perform aseptic technique, resuscitation equipment, post-procedure care and trained assistance are available.

Subcutaneous ports and implanted pumps require a theatre environment for insertion.

Fluoroscopy

Cervical, high thoracic and caudal epidurals should be performed under fluoroscopic guidance. There is risk of perforating the dura and damaging the spinal cord in the cervical and high thoracic region, and the procedure requires a high level of expertise. Studies indicate that a significant number of caudal epidurals (30%) may not be in the right place if done blindly, and El-Khoury *et al.* make a case for fluoroscopic control (33).

Fluoroscopic guidance would be preferred for epidurals in the low thoracic and lumbar regions, but if the patient is very ill and frail the risk of transferring to a hospital setting with X-ray facilities might outweigh the potential benefit of the procedure.

Intrathecals can be performed without fluoroscopy, as the catheter will be inserted below the level of the spinal cord and the flow of CSF indicates that the catheter has successfully entered the theca. In patients with difficult anatomy, fluoroscopy in the anterior–posterior and lateral planes is used to guide entry into the theca. For implanted pumps, fluoroscopy is used to accurately position the tip of the catheter.

Contraindications

Absolute contraindications

The following are contraindications to both epidural and intrathecal catheter insertion:

- the presence of an infected lesion on the back at the site of needle entry
- irreversible severe clotting abnormality

Low platelet count (<50,000)—a platelet transfusion may be given after consulting a haematologist, if the procedure is necessary

Anticoagulants

Clopidogrel, which irreversibly inhibits platelet aggregation and binding between platelets and fibrinogen, should be stopped for seven days before a neuraxial injection. Low molecular weight heparin (LMWH) in prophylactic dose should not be given for 10–12 h before the procedure, and, if the patient is receiving a treatment dose, for 24 h before the procedure. Warfarin should be stopped for four to five days before a planned procedure and INR checked immediately beforehand. INR should be 1.3 or less. LMWH can be given in prophylactic dose to cover this period, if necessary. A haematologist may be consulted for advice if necessary. It is safe to continue oral low-dose aspirin.

Relative contraindications

Infected lesions close to the needle entry or exit site, for example a sacral pressure sore, may be a contraindication and will require an assessment of benefit versus risk of infection. If MRSA is present advice should be sought from a microbiologist. Colonization of the skin will be present if a colostomy or fistula is present, and this will require greater care, but is not a total contraindication.

Previous back surgery and/or radiotherapy are relative contraindications, as these may distort the anatomy at the site of needle insertion. Severe scoliosis or other spinal deformity may also make the procedure very difficult. Fluoroscopy can be helpful in these circumstances.

An imminent course of chemotherapy or radiotherapy need not be a contraindication, although there will be an increased infection risk and, in the case of chemotherapy, bone marrow depression and potential risk of bleeding. This risk can be monitored and appropriate action taken if necessary. The effect of radiation or of planned radiation on the skin should be considered and the catheter should be tunnelled away from the affected skin. Neuraxial infusions can offer worthwhile pain relief on a temporary basis while awaiting the beneficial effect of prophylactic chemotherapy and radiotherapy. Liaison with the oncologist is advised.

Test dose

A bolus injection or temporary infusion of intrathecal drugs is recommended before consideration of an implanted pump.

Antibiotic prophylaxis

There is no published guidance to enable an informed choice. It is suggested that local surgical practice guidelines for antibiotic prophylaxis should be followed.

Risks and complications

The risks and complications applicable to both epidural and intrathecal injections/infusions are as follows:

- ◆ failure
  - not possible to enter epidural or intrathecal spaces
  - administered drugs fail to relieve the pain
- ◆ bleeding
  - increased pain, bruising, back pain
  - bleeding from epidural vessels
  - epidural haematoma
- ◆ infection
  - superficial
    - o at exit site of catheter
    - o subcutaneous port infection
    - o tracking along tunnelling track
    - o pump-pocket infections
  - deep
    - o epidural abscess
    - o meningitis
- ◆ neurological damage
  - damage to spinal cord or nerve roots
  - intrathecal granuloma
- ◆ technical complications
  - catheter
    - o dislodgement
    - o kinking/obstruction
    - o disconnection
    - o fracture
  - pump
    - o failure
    - o programme error
    - o overfill
    - o incorrect refill

- pump pocket
  - pump movement
  - erosion of skin over the pump
  - discomfort
- related to intrathecal
  - postdural puncture headache
  - cerebrospinal fluid leaks
  - hygroma
- related to the infused drugs (see Chapter 5).

Failure

Spinal epidural metastases may be present, although often not diagnosed (34), and the failure rate may be as high as 30% (35). The anatomy of the epidural space may be distorted or bleeding may occur, resulting in failure to place the catheter in the intended position.

Bleeding

Bruising of the ligaments and/or lumbar muscles can occur during traumatic needle insertion, especially if there are repeated attempts to enter the right space. This depends on the skill and experience of the operator. A 'bloody tap' occurs commonly during epidural catheter insertion because of the presence of epidural blood vessels, which are traumatized by the needle and/or catheter. In cancer patients this proportion may be higher because of the presence of epidural metastases. The catheter is withdrawn and re-inserted at a different level.

Epidural haematoma

Bleeding from epidural vessels can lead to epidural haematoma formation; this can also occur following trauma or spontaneously. Aprili, writing in a review article, quotes the risk of haematoma in cancer pain patients as 0.9% based on a single case with bleeding in the post-operative period (36). An extensive post-operative epidural audit conducted by the Royal College of Anaesthetists in 2008 showed an incidence of epidural haematoma of approximately 1 in 60,000, mostly during thoracic epidural insertion in older patients with coagulation derangement (37). Delays in diagnosis led to irreversible harm in most of the cases.

Unexplained and advancing leg weakness was the most common presenting symptom; early MRI is needed to confirm the diagnosis, followed by prompt surgical removal of the clot. MRI of an epidural haematoma is shown in Figure 6.23.

The true incidence of epidural haematoma in a cancer pain population is unknown.

Bleeding in the tunnelling track and pump pocket usually settles with a pressure dressing. Occasionally surgical removal of the clot may be required. No case of intrathecal bleeding leading to harm is reported in the literature.

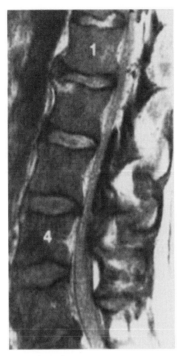

Fig. 6.23 Epidural haematoma extending from L2 to L4.

Infection

In a recent review article by Aprili *et al.* the incidence of superficial infection associated with external intrathecal catheters for cancer pain was 2.3% (95% CI 0.8–6.1) and deep infection was 1.4% (95% CI 0.5–3.8) (36). The authors calculated that every 71st patient had a deep infection after an average catheter duration of 54 days. These risks seem to be quite low and comparable to reported infection rates for chronic indwelling epidural catheters, 4.6% for superficial and 1.2% for deep infection (38).

Holmfred reported superficial infection rates of 6% (CI 0–12.6) and deep infection rates of 2% (CI 0–5.8) in intrathecal catheters attached to subcutaneous ports in patients with severe cancer-related pain (26). De Jong *et al.* studied the complication rate in 250 epidural catheters for the treatment of cancer pain (25). In 52 patients a subcutaneous port was used and in 198 the catheter was inserted percutaneously and fixed with adhesive dressing. Forty-one of the percutaneous catheters were tunnelled a short distance from the midline. The overall incidence of infections was the same in both groups (13.6%) but no injection port became infected in the first 70 days of treatment, and when infection was linked to catheter days there were half as many infections in the injection port group. In the percutaneous group the complication rate was equally high in the tunnelled and non-tunnelled catheter groups.

The subcutaneous port does offer an advantage in terms of lowered infection rate. A review of infections in fully implanted drug-delivery systems was conducted by Follett *et al.* who found one deep infection every 7620 device months in a largely non-cancer pain population (39). Most (60–80%) infections in these patients related to the pump-pocket site, occurring in up to 5% of cases. Preparation of the patient by washing with an antiseptic agent the night before surgery, not removing hair unless absolutely necessary and meticulous surgical technique, are important in preventing infection.

Staphylococcus aureus is the most common organism to infect ITDD systems; the next most common is *Pseudomonas*, but it only affects 3% of cases. *Staphylococcus epidermidis* infections can occur as a result of refills or can occur in the pump pocket. It remains unclear if the use of prophylactic antibiotics influences the rate of infection. When there are signs of infection, antibiotics should be started at the first possible opportunity and removal of the pump and/or catheter may be necessary. Treatment of established infection is almost always successful.

Epidural abscess and meningitis

Aprili's meta-analysis of both cancer and non-cancer pain patients calculated the risk for deep infection with externalized catheters to be 1.4% (36); in these studies the deep infection appears to be meningitis rather than epidural abscess. Burton *et al.* report two cases of epidural abscess and one case of bacterial meningitis in their series of 84 patients with refractory cancer pain (1). The abscess patients both had non-healing wounds from recent surgery close to the exit site of the tunnelled epidural catheter and were subjected to frequent wound debridements. The meningitis patient had an externalized intrathecal catheter, and it was postulated that the infection might have been introduced at the time of a bag change.

Epidural abscess can occur spontaneously, and it is also reported following epidural insertion in the perioperative period, where the incidence is 1 in 47,000 (37). Risk factors may be diabetes and immunological compromise. Unexplained back pain, fever, raised inflammatory markers and increasing neurological deficit should raise the possibility of epidural abscess. It is unlikely to occur without superficial signs of infection. Suspicion should prompt transfer of the patient to a neurological centre for MRI scanning, withdrawal of the catheter and surgical drainage. However, it has to be remembered that there may be other causes of sepsis in the cancer patient, as illustrated in the case study 'Sepsis may not be the fault of the epidural . . .' at the end of this chapter.

The rate of deep infection in a fully implanted system is much less than that of an externalized pump system. Follett quotes one infection in every 7620 device months in a non-cancer population (39). With the short life prognosis of the cancer patient this risk must be very small.

Neurological damage

Damage to the spinal cord and nerve roots

It is possible for both nerve roots and the spinal cord to be damaged by traumatic insertion of a needle and/or catheter. The risk is greater in the cervical and thoracic regions, where the epidural space is narrower and the spinal cord lies within the dura. For this reason imaging is advised for these approaches (see below), which should be performed only by (or under supervision by) an experienced operator.

Undiagnosed tumour may be present in advanced cancer within the spinal column, epidural space or dura, and this can make procedures difficult, and can lead to increased risk of bleeding and failure. Baker reports two spinal cord compressions in her series of 76 intrathecal catheter patients, but it is not known if these were related to the disease or to the therapeutic procedure (11). Sjöberg's post-mortem study (see below) would indicate that tumour infiltration is common (40). His series showed microscopic neuropathological changes in the nerve roots in 9 out of 15 patients and spinal cord lesions in 5 out of 15, including a spinal artery thrombus caused by tumour infiltration of the vertebral bodies. In most cases the aetiology of these changes was unclear, the changes could have been caused by tumour, radiotherapy or chemotherapy, but in two to three cases the insertion technique could not be excluded as a cause.

It is clear that damage to nerve roots and the spinal cord can indeed occur, especially as we do not know exactly what lies beneath the needle. The art is in understanding when the benefits are likely to outweigh the risks.

Intrathecal granuloma

This rare complication of the infusion of drugs via an intrathecal catheter has been reported in non-cancer pain.

An intrathecal granuloma is an inflammatory mass that forms at the tip of an intrathecal catheter in response to the administration of medications, and was first reported in 1991 by North (41). The risk may increase with implantation time and higher concentrations of opioids. It has been reported after both morphine and hydromorphone administration, and, more recently, after baclofen. Clonidine may have a protective effect as seen in animal studies. Granulomas are unrelated to infection and are sterile masses; many theories have been postulated to explain their origin, perhaps the most plausible being that a mitogen-activated protein kinase cascade that increases lymphocytic activity is the underlying aetiology (42).

No cases of intrathecal granuloma have been reported during intrathecal drug therapy for cancer pain. Sjoberg, in a fascinating and meticulous study, reported post-mortem findings on 15 cancer patients who had received intrathecal morphine (with preservative) and bupivacaine for up to 274 days through a tunnelled nylon epidural catheter (40). It appeared that a fibrous reaction around the catheter occurred in the epidural space in 12 of the 15 cases, and in 2 cases there was subdural fibrosis and granulation tissue where the catheter entered the dura, but otherwise the nylon catheters showed complete biological inertness in the subarachnoid space. There was no apparent neurotoxicity from morphine with preservative. There were changes associated with the paraneoplastic process, in the vertebrae, epidural space and dura, which were often much more extensive than had been anticipated.

The Medicines and Healthcare Products Regulatory Agency (MHRA) issued a medical device/equipment alert in June 2008 (43), after a study by Deer quoted the incidence of intrathecal granuloma to be 3%, higher than previously cited, and occurring after baclofen as well as morphine (44).

The symptoms and signs of possible inflammatory mass formation are:

◆ decreased therapeutic response
◆ pain (either new onset or loss of analgesic effect)
◆ neurological deficit/dysfunction.

Inflammatory mass formation may result in permanent neurological impairment. The measures advised by MHRA to manage this complication include:

◆ decreasing or discontinuing drug infusion into the intrathecal space in order to reduce the size of the mass
◆ withdrawal or repositioning of the catheter
◆ surgical intervention to remove the mass.

MRI scanning is essential if this complication is a possibility, as is referral to a neuro-surgical unit.

Technical complications

Catheter complications

Both epidural and intrathecal catheters may obstruct, leak, dislodge, migrate or acciden-tally fall out. Dahm reviewed 21 studies on the use of epidural and intrathecal catheters for the administration of opioids and/or local anaesthetics in refractory non-cancer pain (7). There were differences between epidural and intrathecal catheters, as has already been described. In fully implanted systems with internalized catheters there were no acci-dental withdrawals of the catheter. Catheter complication rates as assessed by Dahm are shown in Table 6.3.

Nitescu looked at 200 adults with refractory cancer pain treated for 1–575 days (45). Seventy-nine of these patients were treated at home with intrathecal nylon catheters and reported perfect function in 93%. The complication rates in this series are shown in Table 6.3.

There have been case reports of epidural catheters knotting or looping around a nerve root, migrating into the subdural space or subarachnoid space, or into an epidural vein, and McIntyre recommends the use of epidural contrast studies and local anaesthetic test dosing to reduce the risk (46). It is possible for an intrathecal catheter to migrate out of the intrathecal space into the subdural space or into the dural sleeve of a nerve root. However, these are very rare events.

Table 6.3 Catheter complication rates

Catheter complication rates	Epidural	Intrathecal
Dislodgement	13/126 (10%)	6/150 (4%)
Leakage	5/51 (10%)	1/116 (<1%)
Obstruction	21/75 (28%)	1/101 (<1%)

After Dahm 1998 (7).

Table 6.4 Technical complications rates of intrathecal catheters

	Complication rate (%)	
	Nitescu: series of IT catheters, 200 patients	Range reported in literature
Epidural haematoma (from injury to unknown epidural tumour)	0.5	0–6
Skin breakdown at insertion site	2	2–50
Spinal headache	15.5	10
External leakage of CSF	3.5	4–27
CSF hygroma	1.5	4–6.25
Pain on injection:	0	3–36
Continuous infusion Intermittent injections	4.5	
Catheter tip dislodgement	1.5	6–33
Occlusion	1	3–12
Accidental catheter withdrawal	4	3–22
Leakage	1.5	2.1–26.6
All mechanical complications	8.5	10–44

After Nitescu 1995 (46).

MRI scanning and injection of contrast through the side port of an implanted pump may be required in order to establish the exact position of the catheter tip and the direction of flow of the injection.

Overall, for long-term use in cancer pain, the intrathecal route appears to be associated with fewer catheter complications.

Pump complications

Technical problems with external pumps are addressed in the manufacturers' manuals and should be obvious. If a patient is sent home with a pump, training the patient and carer in troubleshooting the pump will be necessary, as explained in Chapter 7. Complications with implanted pumps are potentially serious. Some are drug related or caused by filling errors, such as using the wrong drug, using the wrong concentration or failing to correctly fill the reservoir itself. A pump refill has been described where the practitioner failed to inject the refill dose through the port into the drug reservoir and, instead, injected 20 ml of concentrated morphine subcutaneously, with fatal consequences. It is imperative to follow the manufacturer's instructions carefully and only to allow trained personnel to perform refills. The correct equipment must be used.

Programming errors can also occur. It is important to work with a trained assistant who will check the programming recipe. 'Failsafe' questions have been built into the Medtronic programmer to assist this process.

Pump failure has also been reported. In a systematic review, Williams quotes a high incidence of mechanical failure—up to 20%—and in one case malfunction of an infusion device resulted in the spontaneous discharge of the reservoir's contents (morphine) into the patient (48). Many of these problems with pumps have now been overcome with newer models, and there are no recent reports in the quoted case series of pump failures, but pump malfunction remains a risk.

Complications related to pump pockets

Implanted pumps have to be carefully positioned in a cancer patient so that the skin can heal over the pump. In a cachexic patient the skin might break down over the pump. Implantation may not be acceptable to a very thin or small patient, because the pump would be protuberant, and is better not attempted.

Seroma is not of any consequence unless it becomes infected. The size of the seroma is related to the size of the pocket fashioned, the elasticity of adjacent tissue and surgical wound healing. It usually resolves within one to two weeks.

Pump-pocket infection is in direct contact via the catheter track to the CSF and should be treated vigorously with antibiotics. If it does not resolve, the pump has to be removed.

If not fixed to the fascia the pump can move sideways, making it more difficult to refill. It will occasionally turn face down, requiring surgical revision.

Pain in the pump pocket may be a sign of infection or may occur spontaneously.

CSF leak and hygroma

CSF leaks through the hole made by insertion of the needle (usually a Tuohy needle) through the dura because the pressure within the CSF is higher than that in the epidural space. The amount of leakage depends on several factors. The first factor is the size of the needle—the larger the diameter of the needle the greater the potential leak. This is why spinal anaesthetics are delivered through a fine needle of 25–27gauge. Secondly, there is the question of whether the dura is perforated more than once, and whether it is a 'clean' perforation. A dural tear is more likely to produce a headache that is more severe and lasts a long time. In spinal anaesthesia a 'pencil point' needle is used to reduce the risk of dural tear and to enable the dural fibres to close after the needle is withdrawn. The last factor is the CSF pressure, which could be affected by the presence of tumour within the spinal canal. The pressure is higher in the lumbar region than the thoracic and cervical region and is, to some extent, posture dependent.

As the intrathecal catheter is threaded through a needle that is a wider diameter than the catheter, it is inevitable that some CSF loss will occur after the needle is withdrawn. This is often observed, and can cause a palpable collection of fluid under the skin in the back where the needle was inserted, known as a CSF hygroma, or pseudomeningocoele. Alternatively, it can track along the catheter track to the exit point of the catheter or accumulate in the pump pocket. The leak usually stops within a few days, but it can be persistent. Williams quotes the incidence as 10% (47). Hygromas are usually small, self-limiting and of no clinical importance, but if they became large the infused analgesics may be redistributed and this will reduce pain relief. A skin fistula is a possibility, with potential infection risk. Under these circumstances the catheter has to be withdrawn. Very rarely surgical repair may be necessary.

Post-dural puncture headache

This is a 'low pressure' headache, caused by CSF leak and lowering of intracranial pressure, especially when in an upright position, and is eased by lying down. A pounding headache can be accompanied by diplopia (from sixth cranial nerve irritation), tinnitus, dizziness, photophobia, nausea and vomiting. This can be very unpleasant and last for several days until the leak heals. It is well described after diagnostic lumbar puncture, myelography, therapeutic intrathecal injections, accidental dural tap during epidural insertion (c. 2%) and spinal anaesthesia.

The incidence of headache after accidental dural puncture with a Tuohy needle during epidural anaesthesia is estimated to be 50% (48). The fine pencil point needles used for spinal anaesthesia make very small holes in the dural and the incidence of headache following their use is about 0.5%.

In cancer patients this complication seems to be rarely reported; Baker reported no spinal headache in her series of 100 patients, and postulated this was due to the opioids they were already taking, but perhaps it is more related to low CSF pressure and recumbent position (11). The paramedian approach to the dura and use of the Arrow FlexiTip catheter and needle are reputed to lower the risk of postdural puncture headache.

Prevention and management of headache

The patient should be warned of this possibility. Performing the procedure in the lateral position is helpful; the patient is kept lying down for several hours post-procedure and is kept well hydrated. A gradual return to sitting, and then standing, ensuring that there is no headache before going to the next stage, is advised. If headache occurs the patient should lie down again immediately.

Various manoeuvres have been used to try and stop the leak when symptoms become persistent and troublesome: an epidural blood patch, fibrin glue and even surgical repair of a dural tear. To apply an epidural blood patch, an epidural needle is inserted into the epidural space at the level of the leak and 20 ml of the patient's own blood is taken from a vein, aseptically, and injected down the epidural needle, where it forms a clot to seal the hole. This cannot be performed in the presence of a catheter, but could be used after an intrathecal catheter has been removed. It is remarkably effective; instant relief of headache is often reported.

Overall risk of complications

It is hard to quantify the overall risk of complications of neuraxial infusions for cancer pain. The literature reports a variety of catheter and pump techniques and there are no comparative studies apart from Smith et al., who compared ITDD through an implanted pump with comprehensive medical management (29). Of the 100 patients who were implanted with a pump, 15 had technical problems with the catheter, pump pocket, seroma, etc., and a further 12 with minor infections, lumbar site and wound healing. However, the drug-related toxicities decreased by 50% and quality of life also improved. The benefits and risks have to be carefully weighed up and discussed with the patient and his/her family and friends.

Outline of the national use of neuraxial infusions for cancer pain in UK

Petrovic and Hester surveyed palliative care units in the UK in 2006 (pers. commun.). While 96% had access to specialist pain services, only 14% had regular input, and between one and ten invasive procedures were performed each year, equating to a total of 1000 procedures in the whole of the UK. A working group from the British Pain Society (BPS) conducted an audit into current practice in the use of intrathecal drug therapy for the management of pain and spasticity in adults alongside the production of BPS guidelines. These were published in December 2008 (49). A total of 37 hospitals in UK perform ITTD procedures, and only 13 of these centres for cancer pain. One hundred and fifty-one procedures were performed for cancer pain, of which 132 were externalized catheters and only approximately 20 were implanted pumps. Indications for ITTD were described as failure of conventional therapy and/or unacceptable side effects from current therapy. A wide variety of intrathecal drugs and dosages and antibiotic prophylaxis regimes are used. The audit did indicate that the pumps themselves were reliable, and most complications were related to the catheter systems.

Many centres had local guidelines. The BPS has provided national guidelines, which will be revised at regular intervals. There appears to be a large gap between the number of patients whose quality of life could be improved by the use of neuraxial infusions and the number that are currently inserted in UK.

The future

Stearns *et al.*, in their 2005 review of intrathecal drug delivery for the management of cancer pain, a multidisciplinary consensus of best clinical practices, conclude that 'increased understanding of the options available for truly effective pain management in the oncology and palliative care arena and the benefits of multidisciplinary cooperation will translate into genuine improvements in patient quality of life and a measurable decrease in the number of patients who suffer needlessly in their final days' (2).

This should apply to any specialist intervention in cancer pain management. We have a better idea now of what works and what doesn't, we have the expertise, but too little of it. Cancer pain is immensely complex and it is only by lifelong learning that we can begin to understand what to do, put into place the means to do it and teach others to do the same.

Case study

Sepsis may not be the fault of the epidural . . .

Mary was a plucky lady in her late 50s. She had advanced pelvic cancer from an anorectal tumour that had been treated with surgery and chemotherapy. She had a colostomy, and bilateral ureteric stents inserted for ureteric obstruction from the recurrent tumour. She was said to have a 'fistula', but she had only scanty vaginal mucous discharge and was passing urine successfully through the urethra.

She hated the smell of her colostomy and the thought of any further surgery filled her with dread. She had had unsuccessful back surgery in the past and her daughter suffered a cauda equina syndrome, which had only partially been relieved by surgery. This weighed heavily on her mind. Her husband was often away from home and coped with the situation by cracking inappropriate jokes. Despite all this Mary maintained appearances and liked to dress well and put on make-up. She was finding it very difficult to walk though: she had severe pain in the buttock and left leg, with episodic fever and weakness. She also found it painful to sit upright as her perineum was very sore. She became very drowsy on her opioids and the pain team was asked if we could offer an alternative form of pain relief.

Mary had several types of pain: neuropathic pain from tumour invading the lumbar plexus at L3 and L4 on the left side, visceral pain from pelvic tumour and somatic pain from infiltration of the perineum. I offered her a lumbar epidural infusion, which she accepted and she became very comfortable after it was established. A constant infusion of bupivacaine 0.25% 4 ml/diamorphine 0.4 mg/h gave excellent pain relief. However, two days after the epidural was established Mary became drowsy and showed signs of sepsis. She was transferred to King's as a 'suspected epidural infection' although she had no back pain and the epidural site was clean. Antibiotics helped and the epidural was left *in situ*.

Subsequent CT scan of her pelvis showed a large necrotic mass and abscess, hydronephrosis, liver metastases and very large (asymptomatic) bilateral pulmonary emboli. An immediate desire on the part of the FY2 doctor to give her large doses of anticoagulants was discouraged and we decided the priority was to drain the pelvic collection under CT, which helped her to feel much better, and her fever subsided. The epidural was then removed and her leg pain did not come back for a few weeks.

Mary's perineal pain was helped considerably by an intrathecal injection of phenol in glycerol, 1 ml, given at L5/S1 with her in the sitting position. She returned to the hospice. Anticoagulants were tried but produced brisk haematuria, so they could not be used. Mary then developed with hypercalcaemia and her left leg became oedematous. When the leg pain returned she did not want another epidural as she associated this with being unwell and in hospital and she did not want to go back there. Her pain was managed with transdermal fentanyl topped up with an alfentanil spray.

Learning point

In the absence of back pain and localised signs of infection pyrexia is unlikely to indicate a catheter related infection in patients with indwelling neuraxial infusions. Appropriate non invasive investigation of patients with a pyrexia and pain may demonstrate a lesion which can be drained in order to relieve symptoms.

References

1. Burton A, Rajagopal A, Shah HN *et al.* (2004). Epidural and intrathecal analgesia is effective in treating refractory cancer pain. *Pain Med* **5**(3), 238–46.

2. Stearns L, Boortz-Marx R, Du Pen S *et al.* (2005). Intrathecal drug delivery for the management of cancer pain: a multidisciplinary consensus of best clinical practices. *J Support Oncol* **3**(6), 399–408.

3. Naumann C, Erdine S, Koulousakis A *et al.* (1999). Drug adverse events and complications of intrathecal opioid delivery for pain: origins, detection, manifestations, and management. *Neuromodulation* **2**(2), 92–107.

4. Crul BJP, Delhaas EM (1991). Technical complications during long-term subarachnoid or epidural administration of morphine in terminally ill cancer patients: a review of 140 cases. *Regional Anesthesia* **16**(4), 209–213.

5. Talu GK, Erdine S (2001). Epidural neuroplasty against fibrous mass formation during long-term use of epidural route: case report. *Agri* **13**(1), 21–24.

6. Krames ES, Lanning RM (1993). Intrathecal infusional analgesia for non-malignant pain: analgesic efficacy of intrathecal opioid with or without bupivacaine. *J pain Symptom Manage* **8**(8), 539–548.

7. Dahm P, Nitescu P, Appelgren L, Curelaru I (1998). Efficacy and technical complications of long-term continuous intraspinal infusions of opioid and/or bupivacaine in refractory non malignant pain: a comparison between the epidural and intrathecal approach with externalised or implanted catheters and infusion pumps. *Clin J Pain* **14**(1), 4–16.

8. Abs R, Verhelst J, Maeyaert J *et al.* (2000). Endocrine consequences of long-term intrathecal administration of opioids. *J Clin Endocrinol Metab* **85**(6), 2215–22.

9. Ballantyne JC, Carwood CM (2005). Comparative efficacy of epidural, subarachnoid, and intracerebroventricular opioids in patients with pain due to cancer. *Cochrane Database of Systematic Reviews* **1**(2), CD005178.

10. Nitescu P, Appelgren L, Linder L-E *et al.* (1990). Epidural versus intrathecal morphine-bupivacaine: assessment of consecutive treatments in advanced cancer pain. *J Pain Symptom Manage* **5**(1), 18–26.

11. Baker L, Lee M, Regnard C (2004). Evolving spinal analgesia practice in palliative care. *Pall Med* **18**(6), 507–515.

12. Baker L, Balls J, Regnard C (2007). Cervical intrathecal analgesia for head and neck/upper limb cancer pain: 6 case reports. *Pall Med* **21**(6), 543–45.

13. Gourlay G, Plummer J, Cherry D *et al.* (1991). Comparison of intermittent bolus with continuous infusion of epidural morphine in the treatment of severe cancer pain. *Pain* **47**(2), 135–40.

14. Faculty of Pain Medicine of the Royal College of Anaesthetists (2011). *Recommendations for good practice in the use of epidural injection in the management of pain of spinal origin in adults.* www.rcoa.ac.uk/docs/epiduralinjections.pdf.

15. Banwell BR, Morley-Foster P, Krasue R (1998). Decrease incidence of complications in parturients with the Arrow (FlexTip Plus) epidural catheter. *Can J Anaesth* **45**(4), 370–2.

16. Du Pen S, Peterson D, Bogosian A *et al.* (1987). A new permanent exteriorised epidural catheter for narcotic self-administration to control cancer pain. *Cancer* **59**(5), 986–93.

17. Williams A, Beaulaurier K, Seal D (1990). Chronic cancer pain management with the Du pen epidural catheter. *Cancer Nursing* **13**(3), 176–82.

18. Chambers FA, MacSullivan R (1994). Intrathecal morphine in the treatment of chronic intractable pain. *Irish J Med Sci* **163**(7), 318–21.

19. Nitescu P. Appelgren L, Hultman E *et al.* (1991). Long term open catheterisation of the spinal subarachnoid space for continuous infusion of narcotic and bupivacaine in patients with refractory cancer pain. A technique for catheterisation and its problems and complications. *Clin J Pain* **7**, 143–61.

20. Cousins K, Duggan G, Panizza N *et al.* (2003). Intrathecal catheters: developing consistency in filter use and dressings in Perth, Australia. *Int J Palliat Nursing* **9**(7), 308–314.

21. De Cicco M, Matovic M, Castellani G *et al.* (1995). Time-dependent efficacy of bacterial filters and infection risk in long-term epidural catheterization. *Anesthesiology* **82**(3), 765–70.

22. Nitescu P, Hultman E, Appelgren L, Linder L, Curelaru I (1992). Bacteriology, drug stability and exchange of percutaneous delivery systems and antibacterial filters in long-term intrathecal infusions of opioid drugs and bupivacaine in 'refractory' cancer pain. *Clin J Pain* **8**(4), 324–36.

23. Cook TM, James PA, Stannard CF (1998). Diamorphine and bupivacaine mixtures: an in vitro study of microbiological safety. *Pain* **76**(1–2), 259–63.

24. Hodson M, Gajraj R, Scott NB (1999). A comparison of the antibacterial activity of levobupivacaine vs. bupivacaine: an in vitro study with bacteria implicated in epidural infection. *Anaesthesia* **54**(7), 699–702.

25. De Jong P, Kansen P (1994). A comparison of epidural ports with or without subcutaneous injection ports for treatment of cancer pain. *Anesth Analg* **78**(1), 94–100.

26. Holmfred A, Vikerfors T, Berggren L, Gupta A (2006). Intrathecal catheters with subcutaneous port systems in patients with severe cancer-related pain managed out of hospital: the risk of infection. *J Pain Symptom Manage* **31**(6), 568.

27. Rauck RL, Cherry D, Boyer M *et al.* (2003). Long-term intrathecal opioid therapy with a patient-activated, implanted delivery system for the treatment of refractory cancer pain. *J Pain* **4**(8), 441–47.

28. The British Pain Society (2008). *Intrathecal drug delivery for the management of pain and spasticity in adults: recommendations for best clinical practice.* http://www.britishpainsociety.org/pub_professional.htm#itdd.

29. Smith TJ, Staats P, Deer T *et al.* (2002). Randomised clinical trial of an implantable drug delivery system compared with comprehensive medical management for refractory cancer pain: impact on pain, drug-related toxicity and survival. *J Clin Oncol* **20**(19), 4040–49.

30. Kumar K, Hunter G, Demeria DD (2002). Treatment of chronic pain by using intrathecal drug therapy compared with conventional therapies: a cost effectiveness analysis. *J Neurosurg* **97**, 803–810.

31. Mueller-Schwefe G, Hassenbusch SJ, Reig E (1999). Cost effectiveness of intrathecal therapy for pain. *Neuromodulation* **2**(2), 77–87.

32. General Medical Council (2008). *Consent: patients and doctors making decisions together.* National Library of Guidelines, UK. GMC/CMDT/0408. ISBN:978-0-901458-31-5.

33. El-Khoury GY, Ehara S, Weinstein JN *et al.* (1988). Epidural steroid injection: a procedure ideally performed with fluroscopic control. *Radiology* **168**(2), 554–57.

34. Appelgren L, Nordborg C, Sjöberg M, Karlsson P-A, Nitescu P, Curelaru I (1997). Spinal epidural metastasis: implications for spinal analgesia to treat 'refractory' cancer pain. *J Pain Symptom Manage* **13**(1), 25–42.

35. Chubrasik J, Chubrasik S, Friedrich G, Martin E (1992). Long-term treatment of pain by spinal opiates: an update. *Pain Clinic* **5**(3), 147–56.

36. Aprili D, Bandschapp O, Rochlitz C, Urwyler A, Ruppen W (2009). Serious complications associated with external intrathecal catheters used in cancer pain patients: a systematic review and meta-analysis. *Anesthesiology* **111**(6), 1346–55.

37. NAP (2009) 3: Report and findings of the 3rd National Audit Project of the Royal College of Anaesthetists. http://www.rcoa.ac.uk/docs/NAP3_web-large.pdf.

38. Ruppen W, Derry S, McQuay H, Moore A (2007). Infection rates associated with epidural indwelling catheters for seven days or longer: systematic review and meta-analysis. *BMC Palliat Care* **6**, 3.

39. Follett K, Boortz-Marx R, Drake J *et al.* (2004). Prevention and management of intrathecal drug delivery and spinal cord stimulation system infections. *Anesthesiology* **100**(6), 1582–94.

40. Sjöberg M, Karisson P-A, Nordborg C *et al.* (1992). Neuropathologic findings after long-term intrathecal infusion of morphine and bupivacaine for pain treatment in cancer patients. *Anesthesiology* **76**(2), 173–86.

41. North RB, Cutchis PN, Epstein JA *et al.* (1991). Spinal cord compression complicating subarachnoid infusion of morphine: case report and laboratory experience. *Neurosurgery* **29**(5), 778–84.

42. Hassenbusch S, Burchiel, K, Coffey RJ *et al.* (2002). Management of intrathecal catheter-tip masses: a consensus statement. *Pain Med* **3**(4), 313–23.

43. Medicines and Healthcare Products Regulatory Agency (2008). *Warning issued to all manufacturers re implantable drug pumps for intrathecal therapy.* MDA/2008/038. www.mhra.gov.uk/publications/safetywarnings/medical.

44. Deer TR (2004). A prospective analysis of intrathecal granuloma in chronic pain patients: a review of the literature and report of a surveillance study. *Pain Physician* **7**(2), 225–28.

45. Nitescu P, Sjöberg M, Appelgren l, Curelaru I (1995). Complications of intrathecal opioids and bupivacaine in treatment of 'refractory' cancer pain. *Clin J Pain* **11**(1), 45–62.

46. McIntyre P, Deer T, Hayek S (2007). Complications of spinal infusion therapies .Techniques in regional anesthesia and pain management. *Anesthesia Pain Manage* **11**(3), 183–92.

47. Williams JE, Louw G, Towlerton G (2004). Intrathecal pumps for giving opioids in chronic pain: a systematic review. *Health Technol Assess* **4**, No 32.

48. Gaiser R (2006). Postdural puncture headache. *Curr Opin Anaesthesiol* **19**(3), 249–53.

49. Williams JE, Grady K (2008). *Intrathecal drug delivery for the management of pain and spasticity in adults: a national audit. Pain News The British Pain Society Winter* 2008. www.britishpainsociety.org/patient_pain_news.htm.

Chapter 7

Practical nursing management of epidural and intrathecal infusions

Julie O'Neill

Introduction

Aim of chapter

This chapter will discuss the practical management of continuous epidural and intrathecal infusions, predominantly in a palliative care inpatient unit (IPU) setting. The role of the nurse and involvement and role of other healthcare professionals in the management of patients with these infusions will be discussed. The aim is to provide guidance in maintaining a safe, viable service to patients, with particular consideration of the nursing issues involved. Patients and those close to them, particularly the ones who are also informal carers, are an integral part of the team (1). There will be discussion of how to meet their needs as part of the wider challenges of achieving the discharge of a patient with a neuraxial (epidural or intrathecal) infusion to their home, and the successful maintenance of the infusion in the home setting.

Setting

The author draws on her experience of working in a palliative care IPU of a hospice where there is a weekly service provided by pain specialists from a local NHS trust hospital. Key to the success of this service is collaboration between the interventional pain specialists from the hospital and the palliative care medical and nursing team at the hospice. Referral of IPU patients to the service arises from discussion at the multidisciplinary (MD) ward round or initial assessment on admission. Some patients are seen on an outpatient basis following assessment at home by a hospice clinical nurse specialist (CNS) or palliative physician. The procedure may take place in the hospice ward or under radiographic screening at the hospital, depending on its level of technical difficulty.

Frequency of use of epidural and intrathecal infusions in palliative care

How often patients have epidural or intrathecal infusions within this setting and the implications and consequences of this are important to consider. Even in a large specialist palliative IPU, any given registered nurse (RN) is only occasionally likely to care for one of these patients. This is in contrast to RNs working, for example, on a surgical unit where they may care for several patients with these infusions on a daily basis. Achieving a maximum level of competency, knowledge and skills for the RNs, who may have limited practical experience can cause a number of dilemmas (2, 3). This is due to the unpredictable nature of the frequency at which RNs will encounter these infusions. The challenge is nonetheless to ensure that a safe and competent service is provided for patients with epidural and intrathecal infusions (4).

Competencies

RNs working within the IPU come from a variety of nursing backgrounds and have differing levels of knowledge and skills. Some will have had experience with epidural and intrathecal infusions and others little or none. It is important to recognize this when planning any education programme, in order to ensure that specific levels of competency and skills are achieved (5–7). An organizational policy and guidance that is regularly updated, for example every three years (with recognition that changes may need to be made within this time), is essential. Although RNs will be the primary members of the MD team involved in the practical management of these infusions, the policy and guidance must be compiled by various professions within the team. This ensures that all aspects of managing the service are taken into consideration and also reflects the principles of MD working. In particular it is valuable to have input from a pharmacist when compiling the policy and guidance.

In order for the policy and guidance to be effective they need to be promoted so that the staff they are intended to inform and guide are aware of and comply with them (4, 5). In the author's organization, all senior staff nurses are required to become competent in the care and management of epidural and intrathecal infusions. Translating policy and guidance into meaningful, safe, competent practice can be challenging but is nonetheless achievable. A key way of doing this is to hold workshops and regular updates for RNs who are competent or working towards competency (5–7). In the author's setting, RNs attend an epidural workshop regardless of their previous experience and competence. The content of these workshops includes familiarizing RNs with the organizational policy, a revision of the anatomy and physiology of the spine and spinal nerves, as well as the rationale for use of this intervention with the specific patient group. The workshops include a practical element so that the RNs have dedicated time to learn about the functions and management of the infusion pumps that are used (8). In this part of the workshop time is also spent on troubleshooting and advice in regard to the care and management of the skin, infusion line, filter and pumps (5, 9–11).

It is important to make sure that the information presented in these workshops is particularly relevant to palliative care patients as, although the procedures and management should be more or less the same as within an acute setting, the circumstances are different. These circumstances include the fact that the intention is to maintain the epidural or intrathecal infusion for as long as possible in order to relieve the patients' pain. This could mean anything from a day to weeks or months depending on the efficacy of the intervention as well as the patients' choice and, of course, their prognosis. As the duration of the infusion is expected to be longer than the usual 24–48 h following surgery, patients who have epidural or intrathecal infusions inserted in the palliative setting have their catheters tunnelled subcutaneously (12). This is done to help secure the catheter in place for a longer period of time and to reduce the incidence of infection. There is also the advantage that if infection does occur, it is detectable at the subcutaneous exit site first. In addition, it is more convenient for patients to have their catheter tunnelled, as dressing and washing are easier and they do not have to change their position when the nurse is checking the exit site.

In addition to the workshops, practical updates are a useful means of establishing and maintaining confidence, skills and knowledge. These can also provide an opportunity to encourage RNs who have been assessed as epidural and intrathecal competent to mentor RNs who are working towards competency, or who may have been assessed as competent but need to build up their experience or confidence (4, 6, 13). The workshops and practical updates are also an ideal setting for RNs to voice any concerns they may have in caring for patients with these infusions. It is important for the nursing staff co-ordinating these services to recognize the problems, real and perceived, that RNs can face and then to acknowledge and address them. Themes identified in discussions during these workshops and updates include concern about competence in managing the infusion pumps, worry about caring for the infusion itself, recognition of signs of infection, and troubleshooting problems. Part of being competent in neuraxial management is the ability to assess patients who are not known to the nurse, e.g. on other wards. This ability, along with the themes described, is built into the competencies that the nurses need to achieve in order to become fully competent in managing these infusions.

Preparing the patient: assessment of the physical, psychological and emotional state of the patient and family

Palliative care patients who require referral for interventional pain review have usually undergone a variety of treatments for both their cancer and their pain. They can often be exhausted and despondent as a result of their disease progression and the difficulties encountered in the symptom control of the pain that they are experiencing (14–17). Their family and friends will also have been affected by this and may influence the patient's decision on whether or not to consent to have the procedure. Careful explanation of the procedure, including the risks involved and the rationale for choosing this particular option, is needed. The patients family members and friends should be involved to the extent that the patient wishes them to be (18). It is often necessary to repeat this information subsequently as many patients are in so much distress beforehand that they do not assimilate all the information presented to them. They may be unhappy about having an infusion pump attached via an epidural or intrathecal line that they will need to carry with them, so it is important for nurses to be aware of this and any other practical as well as emotional issues that can affect the patient. Some patients may already have a urinary catheter and/or a colostomy or ileostomy bag, and the thought of having yet another attachment that they have to carry around and live with can be too much to tolerate. Other patients feel that it is an external reminder of what is happening inside their bodies as a result of their disease progression. In addition to RNs being aware of the physical and practical implications for patients an awareness of the emotional and psychosocial effects is also necessary (19). Patient information leaflets are extremely useful and can provide essential information for patients and their families but should not replace the role of the nurse and doctor in providing ongoing individual support and information (20, 21). If the patient and family's preferred place of care is at home the ideal is for this to be considered and discussed initially by the MP team prior to referral for pain specialist review, in order to assess the practical challenges involved in the individual case. In some cases it may not be possible or appropriate to have a MD discussion.

An example from clinical practice to illustrate this point is a patient who was in excruciating pain when seen on admission by a consultant at the hospice. This patient was admitted from the author's organization's own specialist community team and so the inpatient team clinicians already had detailed information on the nature of his pain, possible causes and the impact of all of the interventions thus far. His son had been carrying him from bed to chair at home because of the pain caused by attempts to walk. The patient and his close family were distraught as a result of the physical pain the patient was experiencing. The pain specialist was in the process of assessing referred patients in the hospice at the time, and the patient agreed to be assessed. He consented to have a continuous epidural infusion that afternoon (i.e. the day of his admission to the hospice) and within 24 h of insertion of the epidural catheter his pain control had improved so much that it was possible for him to move himself from bed to chair comfortably with the assistance of two nurses. As time went on his pain control was complex and needed continuous monitoring and titration. What is crucial in this man's case is the difference the intervention made to him and his family so soon after his admission following a difficult time trying to manage his pain at home (22, 23). It was fortunate that the pain specialist was available at the right moment, but the case is also a reminder of the importance of being able to make a prompt assessment as to whether or not interventional analgesic techniques are appropriate.

Preparing the equipment
Setting and sterility
The majority of interventional pain procedures are carried out in the IPU of the hospice, and this means that most patients and their families do not have the added burden of having to transfer to a hospital setting for the procedure. It also means that RNs and other health-care professionals have experience of caring for patients before, during and immediately following their procedures. This in turn adds to the necessity of ensuring that the policy and guidance are clear, informative and accessible to staff and that all staff adhere to this guidance (24). An adequate supply of the relevant equipment needs to be maintained along with the drugs required to perform the procedure. Support from a pharmacist is invaluable and should include information on where to access infusion bags containing specific drugs required by the specialist pain consultants for this particular group of patients.

Ideally the patient should be in a single room, but in practice the procedure is often carried out within a shared four-bedded area. Regardless of the environment, strict aseptic techniques should be used before and during the procedure (including use of sterile gowns and drapes) with thorough skin preparation (25–29). A sterile dressing trolley should be

Table 7.1 Equipment required for insertion of epidural/intrathecal catheter and infusion

Chlorhexidine in 70% alcohol
Local anaesthetic
Selection of needles and syringes
Sterile dressing pack(s)
Sterile surgical gloves
Sterile drape/s and gown/s
Tuohy needle and assorted gauge spinal needles
'Loss of resistance' syringe
Epidural/intrathecal catheters
Bacterial filter
Transparent dressing (waterproof, adhesive and breathable)

prepared prior to the procedure. A separate epidural/intrathecal equipment trolley is useful so that all necessary equipment and drugs are stored in this and made readily available at the patient's bedside during the procedure.

The procedure

The nurse's role and levels of competency and responsibility

There are several levels of responsibility that need to be identified when considering the nurse's role, and it is useful to have these clearly defined, in particular when considering policy and guidance (4). In order to demonstrate the varied responsibilities of RNs that encapsulate their role, there follows a brief description of each area of competence and responsibility.

All registered nurses

Any RN on the ward team may be responsible for the care of a patient with an epidural/intrathecal infusion and will therefore need to be aware of the frequency with which they need to monitor patients' observations and any signs and symptoms of complications following the procedure (23). They will also be responsible for observing the skin around the epidural/intrathecal site and checking that the dressing remains intact. As with all other patients in their care they will assess and manage their pain and symptom issues, and should be aware of the signs of any complications following these interventions (8, 30, 31). It is not necessary for RNs to have attended any workshops or other updates in order to carry out these responsibilities as it is part of their code of professional practice (4). It is, as stated before, very important to ensure they subsequently attend the relevant sessions.

Registered nurses who have been assessed as 'epidural and intrathecal competent'

As well as the above responsibilities, these RNs will deal with infusion bag and rate changes (as per policy) and any troubleshooting in regard to the infusion pumps, lines

Table 7.2 Drugs that should be available when epidural/intrathecal interventions are undertaken

Item	Use
Adrenaline injection 1mg in 10 ml	For treatment of anaphylaxis, hypotension or cardiac arrest
Bupivacaine injection 0.25%	Long-acting local anaesthetic
Bupivacaine injection 0.5%	Long-acting local anaesthetic
Chlorhexidine 2% spray	Skin preparation
Ephedrine injection 30 mg	For treatment of hypotension
Flumazenil injection 500 µg	To reverse benzodiazepine (midazolam) sedation
Lignocaine injection 1%	Local anaesthetic (for the skin)
Lignocaine injection 2%	Local anaesthetic (for the skin)
Methylprednisolone (Depo-medrone injection 40 mg in 1 ml)	Steroid
Midazolam injection 10 mg in 2 ml	Benzodiazepine sedation, has an amnesic effect however prolongs recovery and can increase the risk of respiratory depression
Naloxone 400 µg	To reverse opioid induced respiratory depression
Propofol injection 10 mg in 1 ml (20 ml amps)	Very short-acting (general) anaesthetic, used due to fast recovery time after administration, but can cause cardiovascular instability
Povidone iodine solution 10%	Skin preparation
Povidone iodine spray 10%	Skin preparation

The stock list of drugs has been agreed with the pain specialists at the acute hospital trust who review patients during their weekly visits. The stock is checked and topped up each week by pharmacy staff. A supply of 250-ml bags of bupivacaine 0.125% and bupivacaine 0.25% are kept as stock in addition to the above items.

and other equipment. They will assess if the dressings covering the entry and exit site need to be renewed. On evening and night shifts in particular they are expected to assess patients with epidural or intrathecal infusions on other wards depending on the competence levels and experience of the staff on those wards. They are encouraged to share their knowledge with the RNs who are not yet experienced in the care of these infusions so that information is cascaded on a practical level as well as in the more formal educational settings (6, 13). If any nurse has any concerns in regard to the patient or the condition and care of the skin at the entry and exit sites or the infusion pumps they need to report these as soon as possible to a senior nurse and/or the doctor as appropriate (11, 26, 32).

Epidural management team

As well as the responsibilities of all RNs and all upper band 5 epidural-competent nurses, the IPU also has a third group of more senior nurses called the epidural management team. One nurse from this team attends the weekly interventional pain consultant's round during discussions with patients, their families and medical staff. They ensure that the RN responsible for caring for each patient is involved in any discussions and procedures. Involvement of the RN at this point provides an opportunity for them to ask questions, understand more about the complexities of pain assessment and management, and also to contribute to the discussions, particularly if they have been caring for the patient for some time.

Healthcare assistants

Within the palliative care setting of this hospice IPU, healthcare assistants (HCAs) are an integral part of the nursing team and must therefore be aware of the needs of patients with epidural/intrathecal infusions, even if they will not be responsible for these patients' care and management. They will be involved in the patients' daily nursing care and should not be excluded from the sharing of relevant information and advice. If a patient is immobile and requires full assistance with their wash, the RN caring for this patient should carry out their hygiene needs with the HCA so that they can observe the infusion site. The HCAs need to be aware of when they should inform an RN of any problems or concerns with regards to the patient and these infusions.

Care before, during and immediately following the procedure

Patients are usually allowed clear fluids only from about 3 h prior to the scheduled time of the procedure. Oral medications are taken as prescribed so that symptom control is not compromised. The RN caring for them needs to ensure that the patient, their family members and other nurses involved are aware of this restriction and that they understand the rationale, namely that the patient will possibly have sedation prior to and during the procedure. Baseline observations need to be taken prior to the procedure, including a record of bladder and bowel function and control, so that a comparison can be made when carrying out post-insertion observations and assessments (23).

Owing to the use of sedation, the patient will receive oxygen therapy throughout the procedure. A pulse oximeter is used to monitor the oxygen saturation, and blood pressure is checked regularly. Following the procedure, temperature, pulse, blood pressure and respirations are recorded regularly, with the frequency of observations reducing over the next few hours. The patient's bladder function is also kept under review (some patients will already have urinary catheters *in situ*, unrelated to this procedure). The frequency and duration of these observations will be dependent on the policy and guidelines, the condition of the patient following the procedure and the specific recommendations of the pain specialist following the procedure. Following insertion into the epidural or intrathecal space and subcutaneous tunnelling of the catheter, several transparent dressings are applied to the skin for protection, and also as a means to prevent the catheter from falling out (12, 25).

Care of the skin and sites

Transparent dressings are used so that the area of skin around the sites can be monitored for signs of infection or inflammation and the position of the catheter as it comes out at the subcutaneous exit site can be seen clearly. Dressings also need to be waterproof, adhesive and breathable, so that they allow good oxygen and moisture exchange while protecting the skin from outside contamination (26). Protection from contamination is only assured if the dressing is intact and this should be checked regularly. Nurses in the IPU are advised to check the dressing at least once per shift so that if the edges of the dressing start to become detached an extra dressing can be overlaid to secure it. This avoids unnecessary changes of dressings, therefore reducing the risk of contamination of the skin. The clear dressing covering the entry site (i.e. where the catheter has been inserted via the skin into the epidural/intrathecal space) remains in place until it is obvious that the area around the puncture site has healed. This needs to be checked at least twice per day until healed to ensure the dressing is intact.

In this particular palliative care unit, the policy does not state a specific time limit on how often the dressings around the subcutaneous exit site should remain in place in between dressing changes. What it does recommend is careful observation and monitoring so that RNs are making decisions on clinical assessment rather than a fixed time frame (4, 33). As long as the integrity of the clear dressing is intact, it is better that an RN applies an extra dressing to secure it in place and then ask for assistance or advice from a nurse with more experience. When a dressing does need to be changed it should be carried out by two RNs, one of whom should either be assessed as 'epidural and intrathecal competent' or have changed a dressing before with supervision (3). Aseptic technique is used (25), and as one nurse carefully removes the dressings, the other nurse secures the catheter to the skin using her hands while wearing sterile gloves. If the catheter has started to mark the skin it is advisable to alter its position on the skin, taking care not to pull on it as there is a risk that the catheter could be accidently displaced during this process. It is usually better to do this whilst the patient is lying on their side, with another nurse helping them to get into position comfortably.

The considerable amount of time that may be required to remove and renew the dressings can be tiring for the patient, so the change needs to be planned for a time when it is convenient for both patient and nurses. When these infusions are successful it makes a real difference to the pain management and quality of life of the patient and those close to them. The approach to management of dressings that has been described here is intended to ensure that the infusion line stays in place for as long as possible (30, 33).

It is useful to take a photograph (see Figs 7.1 and 7.2) of the exit site, as it will not always be the same nurse or doctor assessing the site and a picture allows comparison. The rationale for taking photographs should be explained to patient and family and written consent obtained before proceeding. The photographs should be kept with the patient's documents. This is extremely useful when a patient is being discharged home so that health professionals in the community have a point of reference when observing the skin and site. It is advisable to take a new photograph one or two days prior to discharge if a considerable amount of time has passed since the first one was taken, especially as the position of the catheter on the skin may have been slightly altered and the dressing will probably have been renewed.

If there is a small amount of leakage of fluid from the entry or exit site for a few days following insertion, it can cause the transparent dressing to lift off. As long as the leakage is judged not to be due to infection it is better to leave the transparent dressing intact and apply several folded gauze squares over it at the site of the leakage to maintain sufficient pressure to stop the dressing from coming away. The leakage will usually stop after a few

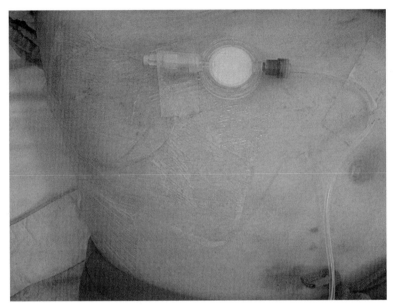

Fig. 7.1 The tunnelled epidural catheter as it comes out at the skin (exit site) showing attached filter and transparent dressing. Patient at St Christopher's Hospice, by permission. Also appears in colour in the colour plate section, Plate 29.

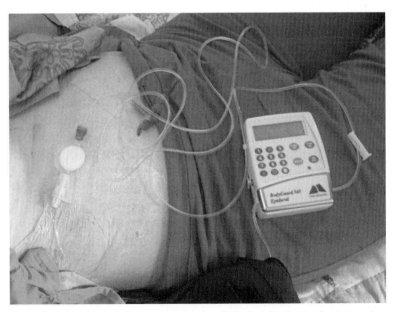

Fig. 7.2 Illustration showing infusion pump and site. Patient at St Christopher's Hospice, by permission. Also appears in colour in the colour plate section, Plate 30.

days but this must be observed each shift and the gauze renewed. If necessary, the transparent dressing should be replaced as described above (12, 25).

Patients are advised to only have showers or very shallow baths, taking care with the transparent dressings. The area needs to be patted dry carefully and checked for any lifting of the edges of the dressings as this would be the opportune time to fix extra dressings to keep them in place.

Any concerns about signs of infection should be reported to a senior nurse and a doctor as soon as possible and the RN should check the patient's temperature and other observations. Once the site has been re-checked by the senior nurse and/or the doctor a swab is taken from the site (following the same method described previously in regard to careful renewal of the dressings). If the infection is present only at the subcutaneous exit site the infusion can usually be continued whilst the patient has oral or intravenous antibiotics (27). This decision will depend on the individual circumstances of the patient affected and there is often a discussion between the palliative physician and the interventional pain specialist in order to decide the best course of management (10). If, for example, it is believed that the patient's prognosis is a matter of days and their pain control has been substantially relieved by having this catheter *in situ* it would be appropriate to keep the infusion running (31). This would be done with the agreement of the patient concerned or, if they were unable to give consent, on the basis of a best interests judgement in consultation with their healthcare proxy, family or significant other (34).

Case study

Managing an epidural infection

A patient who had distressing symptoms of pain that had since been relieved by the insertion of an epidural catheter developed an infection around his subcutaneous exit site. He did not want to have the catheter removed and the opinion of the medical and nursing team caring for him was that if this were done his pain management would become difficult. He was aware that he was at the end of his life and that his pain had been complex and difficult to manage. It was decided to continue the epidural infusion as before. In addition to this the RNs changed his transparent dressing daily, cleaning with chlorhexidine solution and applying an antimicrobial cream to the subcutaneous exit site. There was no evidence that the infection had spread further than the exit site and this man died several days later without an exacerbation of his pain. The epidural catheter tip was sent to microbiology following removal and no organisms were detected. This is an example of how one occurrence of infection was managed within the palliative care IPU, but each case should be considered individually, preferably with the involvement of the patient.

Learning point

Infection does not always require the removal of an epidural catheter.

Managing complications

During the procedure there are potential risks of respiratory depression caused by the administration of intravenous sedation and, as mentioned, oxygen therapy is given and appropriate antagonist drugs are available. Airways and an Ambubag are stored in the equipment trolley that is taken to the patient's bedside during these procedures. Patients referred for these procedures within this palliative care setting are not opioid naïve and have often been taking adjuvant medications that can include sedatives. As a result they may require a substantial amount of medication to achieve the desired level of sedation. Following initial assessment by the pain specialist, either in the clinic or in the palliative care IPU, the procedure may be carried out within the acute NHS trust hospital if radiological guidance is considered necessary (10, 33).

After insertion, catheter migration and infection are the key complications of these procedures. If the infusion ceases to relieve the pain, the nurse should check the exit site of the tunnelled catheter. The appearance of any blue markings (at 10, 15 and 20 cm from the tip) indicates that migration has occurred and effectively the catheter has come out. If the catheter is not tunnelled and comes straight out of the back, the 15- and 20-cm markings will normally be visible and, following the insertion, the pain specialist should have recorded in the notes the length of catheter left in the epidural space and the distance between the skin and catheter tip within the epidural space. If there is any uncertainty as to whether the catheter has moved out of the epidural space a doctor can give a bolus dose of bupivacaine, which, if effective, shows that no significant migration has occurred. If the bolus is ineffective it is likely that the catheter is no longer in the epidural space and re-siting will be necessary (10).

Sometimes the pain blockade is effective on one side but not the other, a situation that might be helped by turning the patient onto the side that is inadequately relieved. Should this manoeuvre not work on its own a bolus can be given, but if there is still no result the catheter may well need to be re-sited. Migration of an epidural catheter through the dura into the cerebrospinal fluid (CSF) effectively converts the procedure into an intrathecal. Because the medication doses in the infusion will be higher than those needed for an intrathecal, having been intended to be used epidurally, the result is increasing numbness and weakness of the legs occurring over 30–60 min, giving rise to a sensory level that extends progressively up the body. If the nurse suspects that this is happening, the infusion should be stopped and the doctor or pain specialist alerted immediately. On the other hand intrathecal catheters can only come out of the CSF, in which case the infusion simply stops working (10, 23, 33).

The presence of redness or pus around the exit site of the catheter may indicate local infection, but on its own does not imply any central spread of infection. A central infection is potentially much more hazardous, giving the possibility of an epidural abscess or, in the case of an intrathecal infusion, meningitis. A risk of central infection would be suggested by tracking of redness from the exit site back along the path of the catheter, or a complaint of back pain, especially if either of these is accompanied by the onset of pyrexia. If any sign of infection is present the doctor should be informed. In the case of a local infection it is usually appropriate to give an oral antibiotic and observe the site. However, if there is evidence of central spread of infection, an epidural catheter should be removed and consideration given to intravenous antibiotics (11, 32). In consultation with the palliative medicine consultant and the pain specialist an intrathecal catheter may be left in place, as it allows samples of CSF to be obtained for microbiology. It can also be used for spinal administration of antibiotics. This is, however, rarely necessary.

Training: developing and maintaining competency

The challenges that exist in developing nurses' competencies have already been discussed earlier in this chapter. The varying degrees of responsibility that the RNs in this setting undertake have also been described. Palliative care nurses are used to dealing with many challenging and complex issues in regard to the patients in their care and the family and friends who are affected by the patient's illness and prognosis. Learning to develop skills and knowledge that some nurses perceive to be more akin to acute nursing can have as much to do with attitude and beliefs as ability, competence and confidence (5, 7).

RNs who have had the opportunity to witness the significant difference that an epidural or intrathecal infusion can make to the comfort of some of the patients are excellent advocates for encouraging their colleagues to be competent in managing epidurals. As well as the workshops and the practical updates described earlier in the chapter, all RNs within the IPU attend a one hour session in regard to managing epidurals and intrathecals as part of their mandatory annual update days. This 'refresher' is a crucial message to staff on the importance of palliative care specialists being competent to manage this sort of intervention for pain (4). The session on the annual update day is also the opportunity for case studies to be presented. The knowledge that this intervention can make a significant improvement in the patient's quality of life is very encouraging for nursing staff who are struggling with the technical knowledge required to become competent.

Discharge planning

When planning a patient's discharge it is necessary to consider what support there will be at home, at both professional and personal levels (35–37). It is not always possible to predict how a patient and their informal carers will cope with and manage the continuous infusion. It is essential to establish the supply route for the drugs that will be needed in the community (Box 7.1). It is vital to explore these issues prior to discharge with the patient and their family, as they are a crucial part of the caring team (38, 39). Exploring their concerns and fears can help to form a more individualized plan that can be incorporated into the information provided in the standard guidance for the professionals and informal carers in the community (21, 40).

Healthcare professionals in the community do not get regular experience in caring for patients with an epidural/intrathecal infusion (even less often than RNs working in the IPU). As a result it is difficult to develop and maintain their competence, and hence many professionals in the community feel inadequately informed or prepared to manage these infusions (2, 10). The challenge is ensuring that these professionals and the patients and their families and carers are sufficiently prepared so that they have confidence that they will be able to manage. In order to make this possible, there needs to be a system in place within the IPU to provide this information and support on a continuing basis. This in itself adds to the responsibilities and resources that are necessary within an IPU to ensure the practical management of epidural and intrathecal infusions.

There needs to be a system that can support the community professionals, out of hours as well as at other times. Any written information provided for the patient, family and community professionals that is sent home with the patient should be duplicated and kept where it will be accessible for nursing staff on the IPU, if they are the first point of contact for community professionals. An agreed plan of action (after discussion with relevant members of the medical and nursing team) should also be included with this information (41, 42). The following case study shows an example of how discharging a patient home can be achieved in a situation where the patient's wife was very clear that she wanted to be able to manage the infusion when her husband returned home. This case study also demonstrates the importance of planning, communicating with colleagues and sharing information with all relevant parties.

Case study

Going home with an epidural

Mr A was a 61-year-old man with prostate cancer and metastases in his right femur who was admitted to a ward in the IPU for pain specialist review. Five days after admission he consented to an insertion of an epidural catheter and a continuous infusion was commenced. Approximately two weeks later Mr A's pain was well controlled and he wanted to go home. Following discussion with him (43), his wife and the ward manager it was agreed that the ward manager would teach Mrs A how to manage and care for the infusion and the skin around the exit site of the epidural. A spare infusion pump with basic written instructions was given to Mrs A to read through.

The following day the ward manager continued with more structured teaching and gave further information about managing and troubleshooting the pump. The ward manager and other RNs who were epidural competent continued to build on the information and teaching on a daily basis over the next ten days. This included Mrs A changing the infusion bags with supervision and also question and answer sessions with the ward manager. Mrs A changed the infusion bag on the day of discharge and the plan was for the ward manager to meet the district nurse and community palliative care clinical nurse specialist at Mr and Mrs A's home two days later so that they could observe the next time the infusion bag was due to be changed. The infusion line and filter were also due to be changed and the clear dressing over the epidural exit site needed to be renewed on the same day. Mrs A wanted to do this herself with supervision, if needed, from the ward manager and she was happy for the district nurse and clinical nurse specialist to observe.

This was an opportunity for the community staff to see the skin around the exit site, the type of dressing used and the infusion pump, and to recognize that Mr and Mrs A felt secure and that she could care for the infusion. It also was a good time to stress that the community team were there to continue to support them with any other problems they might encounter in regard to Mr A's symptoms and disease progression. There was some concern initially from the community professionals over whether Mrs A was able to manage the infusion and the fact that they were unable to do so (mainly due to lack of resources rather than a lack of ability) (44). It became clear that it was extremely important for the couple that Mrs A managed the epidural but that she had support from the clinical nurse specialist and the district nurses and, when needed, the key nursing staff on the hospice IPU.

The ward manager was required to go out to see Mr A twice during the several weeks that he was able to spend at home. This was necessary because the rate of infusion needed to be changed following review by the community palliative medicine consultant. On each occasion the ward manager was met at Mr A's home by either the clinical nurse specialist or the palliative medicine consultant to discuss the plans and then alter the rate of infusion. Each time this happened the information was updated in the plan that was kept in the senior nurse bleep folder (as first point of contact for community staff), and the medical team in the hospice were kept updated in case there were any calls out of hours (41).

During his time at home, Mr A and his family were able to spend significant birthdays and anniversaries together (45). This probably would not have been possible without having the epidural in place and planning and maintaining the safe management of the infusion at home (46, 47). Although this was challenging for Mr A, and in particular for Mrs A, they both felt that the positive aspects outweighed the potential negative challenges they faced.

Learning point

In reality it is not always possible to ensure long-term discharge for patients with these infusions, and quite often hospice readmission is needed for reassessment of pain and other symptoms. Sometimes patients go home to die and it is even more important that a system is put in place to enable them to spend their last few days at home. When this has happened it has entailed careful planning of who will go out with the clinical nurse specialist and meet with the district nurses at the patient's home to renew infusion bags or change rates. This can tax staff resources and time management for both IPU and community nursing teams, but if it is possible to work out a practical way of achieving this for a patient the rewards to all involved are considerable.

The decision to teach an informal carer (that is a patient's spouse, partner or other family member or friend) is not taken lightly. The nurse initiating the training needs to be sure that the informal carer is able to take on this responsibility, whether it involves just agreeing to be at home with the patient with no supervision between visits from professionals, or involvement such as happened with Mr and Mrs A.

Before commencing training it is agreed between the nurse, the patient and their informal carer what can be managed. Once the training sessions, some examples of which were given in the case study, have been carried out there needs to be signed consent from the patient, their informal carer and the RN who has initiated the training. It is advisable also to have a second RN to witness this (41). At present, the Epidural Management Nursing Team initiate this training, with contributions from other RNs. The rationale for this is that the same information and process are carefully applied in each case.

Suggested models for practice: what are the options?

When planning or maintaining an interventional pain service that relies on collaborative working between MD team members, several components need to be considered. In the author's unit the service has been established for over 30 years, with the pain specialists attending on a weekly basis to assess or review patients. In the past, a specialist registrar from the IPU would accompany the pain specialist on the round as it was recognized as a learning opportunity and often part of their learning objectives (i.e. knowledge of interventional pain management techniques). It was noted that over a period of time the nurses' involvement was becoming less obvious and that many RNs did not feel they had a role despite the fact that they were the professionals who would be directly involved in caring for these patients over a 24-h period. They would be more likely to be the first to encounter problems with pain control and troubleshooting and there was a need for them to be able to assess the situation prior to informing senior nurses and/or medical staff (2, 3).

It was then agreed that a nurse from a core group of nurses who were 'epidural and intrathecal competent' would accompany the pain specialists each week and their role and responsibilities were identified as described earlier in this chapter. A specialist registrar would take part in the review of patients if they had specific learning objectives in regard to interventional pain methods. This now ensures that the relevant MD team members' learning needs and professional development are catered for and also improves ongoing care of the patients undergoing these procedures. A senior nurse who is epidural and intrathecal competent co-ordinates the overall training and development of staff, and ensures that there is a designated epidural co-ordinator nurse on the interventional pain assessment round each week.

It is important that medical staff new to the unit have input from a lead nurse on the practical management of these infusions. It is helpful to have a joint session from a lead nurse and one of the palliative medicine consultants so that there is a greater potential to address any questions. Medical staff need to know how to manage titration of medication and rates of the infusions in order to optimize pain control for any patient who has one. The pain specialists will have discussed and documented a plan for each patient immediately following insertion of the epidural/intrathecal catheter. Nurses should continue to monitor and assess the patient's pain and alert the doctor as soon as they have any concerns so that any plans in regard to titration can be initiated rapidly and their effectiveness assessed and noted (10).

The pain specialists have overall responsibility for the management of these infusions and are available for consultation by telephone in between the weekly visits. It is good practice to have a plan in place so that if there are any particular concerns about a patient's pain management the pain specialist is contacted within 'normal hours'. This is so that a clear plan of action for that patient can be agreed and documented and then, if there are further difficulties out of hours, the MD team are all aware of what can be done to address them.

In order for collaborative team work such as this to be effective, it is helpful and necessary for the key members to meet as regularly as is practical for all concerned. This does not need be a fixed arrangement in regard to frequency; rather it should be as flexible as possible whilst still ensuring that all relevant healthcare professionals attend and that it identifies subjects pertinent to the professionals, the patients and the service that is being provided. There needs to be open communication between all the key members of this MD team in order to guarantee the best possible service for the patients involved. It is worthwhile investing time in developing a good working relationship so ideas can be shared between these key members of the team.

Earlier in this chapter, considerations in regard to managing infusions for patients who wish to be cared for at home were highlighted. In the author's place of work patients have been successfully cared for at home over several days or weeks. The input provided in particular by the lead nurse and other members of the epidural management team of nurses has been intensive and time-consuming and absolutely necessary to ensure these individual successes (48, 49). It is, however, recognized that there is a need for ongoing education, support and provision of information for the patients, their families and community professionals (50). More patients could be discharged home if this is their preferred place of care and their informal carer (i.e. spouse, daughter, son, etc.) feels able to cope if supported by healthcare professionals (51–54). These infusions are an added responsibility for the carers, who will have varying information and support needs. A supportive pharmacist is a vital part of the team, especially in the procurement, storage and delivery of drugs for neuraxial (epidural/intrathecal) infusions in the home setting.

It is necessary to audit the service that has been provided so far for patients that have been discharged home, and also to develop the written information that is provided and offer workshops for the community professionals. Other options in the future could include a system where each community team has a link nurse identifiable to the IPU epidural management team that can be contacted at the initial stages of discharge planning. There is also great potential to train and develop upper band 5 RNs who can be included in the team of epidural management nurses to go out to patients' homes to provide teaching and support. These prospective ideas fall under the umbrella of an outline for an epidural outreach service that could be developed over time.

A lead nurse would need to orchestrate the various concepts and functions of this service, ensuring the development of other nurses in contact with the patients on the IPU and in the community. In addition, members of the MD team involved with the patient will be vital in ensuring the key function of this service in supporting patients, families and healthcare professionals. The aim would be to disseminate information and skills to enable the continuing care of these patients in their homes over periods that may range from days to weeks to several months.

Box 7.1 Drugs for neuraxial infusions

Margaret Gibbs, specialist senior pharmacist, St Christopher's Hospice, London

Obtaining a reliable supply of the drugs required for continuous infusion presents practical difficulties to nursing and pharmacy staff. The specific combination and concentration of local anaesthetic and opioids used in palliative care patients is not routinely used in other therapeutic areas, so although infusions are available commercially, they are mainly intended for obstetrics and surgery and are of lower concentrations. To make matters worse, there are limitations on the range of infusion products that can be made up in most hospital pharmacy manufacturing units for individual patients, and also issues with supplying to patients who are not resident in the hospital wards.

Regional, licensed pharmacy manufacturing units (listed in the back of the BNF) and 'specials' manufacturers can supply some items to order, although there may be a time lag between ordering and supply, and shelf-life can be an issue, especially if the bag contains more than one ingredient. The infusion bags need to be compatible with the chosen pump and the nurse trainers who work for the pump manufacturers can be supportive in advising on this when setting up a new service or purchasing new pumps.

On an inpatient unit, one option is to purchase bags of local anaesthetic (e.g. bupivacaine) from a company or pharmacy unit and then add the prescribed opioid using the aseptic technique in the ward treatment room. Although this is not ideal, it may be the only practical option, especially if the dose is being titrated and may change. Once the patient's pain reaches a satisfactory level and a dose and rate have become established, infusion bags containing local anaesthetic plus opioid can be obtained from one of the commercial specials companies in the UK. Some of these are registered as pharmacies and can accept FP10 prescriptions.

If a patient wishes to go home with a neuraxial infusion in place, negotiation needs to take place, not just between the patient and carers, but also with homecare teams and primary care. GPs may feel unable to support a patient with such specialist needs, and it is likely that the specialist team would continue to take responsibility for the ordering and supply of the bags as well as the overall management of the patient. There are two commercial pharmacy companies (ITPharma (www.ithpharma.com) and Hospira (www.hospira.co.uk)) who can supply and deliver infusion bags by courier to patients' homes and this has been crucial to the success of the discharges (55).

Conclusion

In summary, offering epidural and intrathecal intervention is an important part of delivering a high-quality specialist palliative care service. Preparation of the patient and family is key. For a patient where discharge is a possibility, the ongoing management needs to be thought through from the outset.

Case study

A coeliac plexus failure

Paul had been living with the diagnosis of primary hepatoma for years. He had just moved, and was in the process of setting up a family home for his wife, two children and kitten, in the full knowledge he had a very limited life expectancy. Treatment options had come to an end, and his disease was clearly rapidly advancing. Approximately six months before we saw him, he had had a very successful coeliac plexus block, which had given him good control of his upper abdominal pain. Pain had returned and was now over a much more extensive area.

Detailed assessment confirmed that in fact the nature of his pain had changed—he had significant lower thoracic back pain radiating to his upper abdomen, combined with a generalized 'heavy dull ache' which he found difficult to localize. There was slight, but consistent, alteration of sensation bilaterally at L1. We reviewed his imaging and it was clear that he now had spread of disease into the posterior abdominal wall, and considered that this was probably responsible for the somatic component to his pain.

He wanted to avoid analgesics at all costs, having previously suffered very nasty hallucinations and sedation, and was requesting another coeliac plexus block, since that had worked so well previously. We carefully discussed the possibilities with him, explaining that in all probability a further coeliac plexus block would be technically difficult to undertake due to anatomical difficulties and that his principal pain (back ache) was probably now arising from invasion of different nerves. He was happy to undergo insertion of a low thoracic epidural, which gave him good pain control and minimal motor block. He learned to manage the infusion himself very quickly, returning home pain free and taking no oral analgesics.

Learning point

If the patient is keen, willing and able consider the possibility of teaching them to manage their own infusions.

For nursing staff with adequate training and encouragement it is possible to make and maintain the competency of managing epidural and intrathecal infusions for all Senior Staff nurses.

References

1. Smith P (2001). Who is a carer? Experiences of family caregivers in palliative care. In: Payne S, Ellis-Hill, C (eds). *Chronic and Terminal Illness: New Perspectives on Caring and Carers.* Oxford University Press, Oxford.
2. Mackin tyre P, Ready L (2001). Epidural and intrathecal analgesia. In: Macintyre P. Ready, L (eds). *Acute Pain Management. A Practical Guide* 2nd edn. W.B. Saunders, London.
3. Hall J (2000). Epidural analgesia management. *Nursing Times* **96**(28), 38–9(40).
4. NMC (2008). The Code: Standards of Conduct, Performance and Ethics for Nurses and Midwives. *Nursing and Medical Council,* London.

5. Redfern S, Norman L, Calman L *et al.* (2002). Assessing competence to practise in nursing: a review of the literature. *Res Papers Educ* **17**(1), 51–77.

6. Neary M (2000). *Teaching, Assessing and Evaluation for Clinical Competence: a Practical Guide for Practitioners and Teachers.* Stanley Thornes, Cheltenham.

7. Bradshaw A (2000). Competence and british nursing: a view from history. *J Clin Nursing* **9**(3), 321–9.

8. Dougherty L, Lister S (eds) (2008). *The Royal Marsden Hospital Manual of Clinical Nursing Procedures* **7th edn.** Wiley-Blackwell, Oxford.

9. Day R (2001). The use of epidural and intrathecal analgesia in palliative care. *Int J Palliat Nursing* **7**(8), 369–74.

10. Royal College of Anaesthetists (2004). *Good Practice of Continuous Epidural Analgesia in the Hospital Setting.* Royal College of Anaesthetists, London.

11. Murdoch J (2005). Ensuring prompt diagnosis and treatment of epidural abscess. *Nursing Times* **101**(20), 36–8.

12. Baker L, Lee M, Regnard C *et al.* (2004). Evolving spinal analgesia in practice in palliative care. *Palliat Med* **18**(6), 507–15.

13. Alsop, A (2000). *Continuing Professional Development: A Guide for Therapists.* Blackwell Science, Oxford.

14. Ballantyne JC, Carwood CM (2005). Comparative efficacy of epidural, subarachnoid and intracerebroventricular opioids in patients with pain due to cancer. *Cochrane Database of Systemic Reviews* Issue 2, **(1): CD005178.**

15. Burton AW, Rajagopal A, Shah HN *et al.* (2004). Epidural and intrathecal analgesia is effective in treating refractory cancer pain. *Pain Medicine* **5**(3), 239–47.

16. Chapman S, Day R (2001). Spinal anatomy and the use of epidurals. *Professional Nurse* **16**(6), 1174–7.

17. Stevens RA, Ghazi SM (2000). Routes of opioid analgesic therapy in the management of cancer pain. *Cancer Control* **7**(2), 132–41.

18. Thoms GM, McHugh GA, Lack, JA (2002). What information do anaesthetists provide for patients? *Brit J Anaesth* **89**(6), 917–9.

19. Morgan A (2001). Protective coping: a grounded theory of educative interactions in palliative care nursing. *Int J Pall Nursing* **7**(2), 91–9.

20. Nicklin J (2002). Improving the quality of written information for patients. *Nursing Standard* **16**(49), 39–44.

21. Sanford RC (2000). Caring through relation and dialogue: A nursing perspective for patient education. *Adv Nurs Sci* **22**(3), 1–15.

22. Wallace MS (2002). Treatment options for refractory pain: the role of intrathecal therapy. *Neurology* **59**(5Suppl 2), S18–S24.

23. Wheatley R, Schug S, Watson D (2001). Safety and efficacy of postoperative epidural analgesia. *Brit J Anaesth* **87**(1), 47–61.

24. Bibby P (2001). Introducing ward-based epidural pain relief. *Professional Nurse* **16**(6), 1178–81.

25. Preston RM (2005). Aseptic technique: evidence-based approach to patient safety. *Brit J Nursing* **14**(10), 540–5.

26. Robinson SJ (2005). A systematic review of effectiveness of skin preparation and dressings in patients receiving epidural analgesia. *Acute Pain* **7**(4), 177–83.

27. Dawson S (2001). Epidural catheter infection. *J Hosp Infect* **47**(1), 3–8.

28. Rothwell M, Pearson D, Wright K, Barlow, D (2009). Bacterial contamination of PCA and epidural infusion devices. *Anaesthesia* **64**(7), 751–3.

29. Parker LJ (2004). Decontamination of medical devices: legislation and compliance to practice. *Brit J Nursing* **13**(17), 1028–32.

30. Du Pen A (2005). Care and management of intrathecal and epidural catheters. *J Infus Nursing* **28**(6), 377–81.

31. Muir MR, Sullivan FL, Dear G, Ginsberg B (1997). Monitoring practices following epidural analgesics for pain management, a follow-up survey. *J Pain Symptom Manage* **14**(1), 36–44.

32. Follett KA (2003). Intrathecal analgesia and catheter-tip inflammatory masses. *Anesthesiology* **99**(1), 5–6.

33. Dickson D (2004). Risks and benefits of long-term intrathecal analgesia. *Anaesthesia* **59**(7), 633–5.

34. Morris SM, Thomas C (2002). The need to know: informal carers and information. *Eur J Cancer Care* **11**(3), 183–7.

35. Department of Health (2006). *Our Health, Our Care, Our Say: a New Direction for Community Services*. DH, London.

36. Department of Health (2008). *End of Life Care Strategy: Promoting High Quality Care for All Adults at the End of Life*. DH, London.

37. Higginson I (2003). *Priorities and preferences for end of life care in England, Wales and Scotland*. The National Council for Palliative Care, London.

38. National Institute for Health and Clinical Excellence (NICE). (2004). *Improving Supportive and Palliative Care for Adults with Cancer*. National Institute for Health and Clinical Excellence, London.

39. Hirst M, Arksey H (2000). Informal carers count. *Nursing Standard* **14**(42), 33–4.

40. Harding R, Higginson I (2003). What is the best way to help caregivers in cancer and palliative care? A systematic literature review of interventions and their effectiveness. *Pall Medicine* **17**(1), 63–74.

41. NMC (2005). *Guidelines for records and record keeping*. Nursing and Medical Council, London.

42. Tarling M, Jauffur H (2006). Improving team meeting to support discharge planning. *Nursing Times* **102**(26), 32–5.

43. Erickson E, Lauri S (2000). Informational and emotional support for cancer patients' relatives. *Eur J Cancer Care* **9**(8), 8–15.

44. Sheldon F, Turner P, Wee B (2001). The contribution of carers to professional education. In Payne S, Ellis-Hill C (eds). *Chronic and Terminal Illness: new Perspectives on Caring and Carers* 83–98, Oxford University Press, Oxford.

45. Hudson P (2004). Positive aspects and challenges associated with caring for a dying relative at home. *Int J Pall Nursing* **10**(2), 58–64.

46. Mercadante S, Arcuri E, Ferrera P *et al.* (2005). Alternative treatments of breakthrough pain in patients receiving spinal analgesics for cancer pain. *J Pain Symptom Manage* **30**(5), 485–91.

47. Exner HJ, Peters J, Eikermann, M (2003). Epidural analgesia at end of life: facing empirical contraindications. *Anesth Analg* **97**(6), 1740–2.

48. Adam J (2000). Discharge planning of terminally ill patients home from an acute hospital. *Int J Pall Nursing* **6**(7), 338–46.

49. Murray AM, Miller T, Fiset V *et al.* (2004). Decision support: helping patients and families to find a balance at the end of life. *Int J Pall Nursing* **10** (6), 270–7.

50. O'Neill J (2008). Preparing carers to look after palliative care patients at home. *End Life Care J* **2**(3), 14–24.

51. Ingleton C, Payne S, Nolan M, Carey, I (2003). Respite in palliative care: a review and discussion of the literature. *Palliat Med* **17**, 567–75.

52. Broback G, Bertero C (2003). How next of kin experience palliative care of relatives at home. *Eur J Cancer Care* **12**, 339–46.

53. Osse BH.P, Vernoojj-Dassen MJFJ, Schade E, Grol RPTM (2006). Problems experienced by the informal carers of cancer patients and their needs for support. *Cancer Nursing* **29**(5), 378–88.

54. Morris SM, Thomas C (2001). The carer's place in the cancer situation: where does the carer stand in the medical setting?. *Eur J Cancer Nursing* **10**, 87–95.

55. ITPharma tel : 020 8838 8260 http://www.ithpharma.com/Hospira tel: 0207 365 9096 www.hospira.co.uk/english/custommanufacturingservices.aspx.

Chapter 8

Peripheral blocks, plexus blocks, and intrathecal neurolysis

Sue Peat, Kevin Fai, and Joan Hester

Introduction

In this chapter we will consider blockade of the somatic nerves at points after they have left the spinal canal, and the use of neurolytic block of somatic nerves. It has been estimated that up to 8–10% of palliative care patients may benefit from peripheral nerve blocks (1). It is clear that these techniques have a significant place in the management of cancer patients, particularly in a terminal care setting, although many patients with advanced disease experience pain at multiple sites, which does limit the usefulness of individual peripheral nerve blocks (2, 3). Their usual place is as part of a multimodal analgesic regime, i.e. as a technique for managing one component of the patient's pain, particularly in situations were pain is localized and severe. They can be very helpful when pain affects, or prevents delivery of, specific nursing care or localized treatments such as physiotherapy.

The types of blocks used range from simple application of local anaesthetic onto or into the skin over the site of the pain (e.g. lidocaine plasters) to the perineural infusion of local anaesthetics via catheters inserted into defined anatomical spaces around nerves (e.g. continuous plexus blocks). Peripheral perineural infusions have three principal advantages over epidural or intrathecal infusions:

- they specifically target small localised areas of severe pain
- the degree of neurological deficit caused is limited
- they do not cause autonomic side effects

The infusion rates required are often low, and simple elastomeric pumps, some of which have variable infusion rates and a patient control facility, are idea for use in these situations. The pumps are convenient, light and non-electronic.

The successful use of peripheral techniques demands accurate patient assessment, a detailed knowledge of the relevant regional anatomy, and application of the agents used onto all of the nerves involved. They are particularly useful for the management of unilateral pain. In theory it should be possible to provide good analgesia for any well-localized somatic pain, providing the area does not have a complex nerve supply.

Most of the commonly described techniques are regularly used in an acute post-operative setting, to provide short-term post-operative pain control. They will be familiar to many anaesthetists, particularly for peri-operative management in orthopaedic surgery. In these situations, only short-term anaesthesia/analgesia of a specific and well-defined site is required. However, the use of peripheral nerve blocks for alleviating cancer pain is technically more difficult than their use in patients requiring short-term post-operative pain relief. The presence of oedema can make palpation of pulses and bony prominences (used to assist needle location) difficult or impossible, and the neuro-anatomy can be distorted by contractions, tumour or scarring in or near the nerves to be blocked. Hence the 'landmarks' traditionally used for needle and catheter placement during these procedures are often lost or unreliable. For example, it may not be possible to palpate the femoral artery whilst attempting a femoral nerve block.

General principles

Assessment

Pain assessment in cancer patients is often complicated by the coexistence of many types of pain in multiple sites (see Chapter 3). It should be remembered that presence of 'somatic' pain can indicate progressive disease at the affected site and/or at sites related to the nerves supplying it, particularly when it is progressively resistant to commonly used local treatments. An example is worsening chronic post-thoracotomy pain (4).

When considering the use of peripheral neural blockade in the management of cancer pain, it is important to recognize that the area in which the patient reports the pain may be distal to the site of the pathology causing it. The intervention has to be undertaken proximal to the site of pathology if it is to be completely effective. Inadequate assessment and the use of blocks that are too peripheral are likely to result in failure, and this needs to be carefully explained to the patient and his or her carers. A simple example is as follows: pressure on the ulnar nerve will cause a perception of pain in the little finger. Blockade of the digital nerves can be used to provide analgesia, and even highly effective surgical anaesthesia for the digit, but it will not relieve the perception of pain caused by ulnar nerve compression. Blockade of the appropriate part of the brachial plexus will be needed if this is to be achieved. Clinical examples of this principle include shoulder and hand pain secondary to an apical lung tumour.

In patients with chronic pain, particularly if it is longstanding, central mechanisms may well be the cause of pain perceived to be in the periphery, in which case peripheral nerve blocks will not usually be effective. An extreme example of this is thalamic pain, where typically the patient experiences pain in one side of the body due to a lesion in the thalamus. However, the complexity and plasticity of the human nervous system does offer the possibility that exceptions to the above principle will occur, and topical lidocaine has been successfully used in the treatment of what was thought to be central pain (5).

Careful consideration must be given to the expected duration of action of the drugs used, and the consequences of inducing motor block and systemic toxicity. 'Single-shot' injections of commercially available local anaesthetic agents are unlikely to give good analgesia for longer than 12 h, and will need to be repeated to maintain effect. However, they can be of vital assistance in situations where dense analgesia of short duration would be useful, e.g. for patient transport, to enable the patient to participate more fully in special events, positioning for radiotherapy, fracture management or whilst alternative strategies are being discussed.

There are few contraindications to the use of peripheral nerve blocks, but particular care should be taken to explain the risks and potential benefits to patients at risk of developing infection or haematoma at the injection sites, especially if the use of catheters is being considered.

Nerve localization

Traditionally, nerve localization has been achieved clinically, and was simply based on the use of anatomical 'landmarks' combined with the response to needle placement and injection. High-volume infusions or injections may compensate for inexact needle placement. The regular and increasing use of ultrasound and electrical stimulation to aid perineural needle and catheter placement has the potential to improve the efficacy of these techniques, leading to more reliable needle placement and a reduction in the amount of local anaesthetic agent needed to achieve analgesia, but this is by no means always so (6). It should be remembered that injections can be painful if adequate local anaesthesia is not used during needle placement, particularly when the area to be injected is already hypersensitive. Patients should be warned that parasthesia/muscle contraction induced by nerve stimulation can be painful.

The pharmacology of local anaesthetics

Local anaesthetics cause a reversible conduction block in the nerves with which they come into contact, via binding reversibly to sodium channels. They are divided into the amide type (lignocaine, bupivacaine, levobupivacaine, prilocaine and ropivacaine) and the ester type (benzocaine, cocaine and amethocaine). The amides are the most commonly used for peripheral neural blockade. Their action is terminated by uptake into the systemic circulation from the site of application. There is a considerable difference in the potency, duration of action and systemic toxicity of the local anaesthetics (7), so much so that combinations of different local anaesthetics have been used with the intention of providing safe analgesia with a rapid onset and prolonged action in the peri-operative setting (8).

The principal agents in current use are the long-acting amide-type local anaesthetics bupivacaine, levobupivacaine and ropivacaine. Of these, levobupivacaine and ropivacaine have less potential for inducing systemic toxicity, and ropivacaine induces less motor block than does bupivacaine in equipotent doses. In clinical practice the latter two agents may well offer little significant practical advantage over bupivacaine, provided that care is taken with the doses used and accidental intravascular injection is avoided (9).

In the future, the use of specialized formulations of local anaesthetics may well offer considerable advantages to patients with cancer pain. It has been demonstrated that prolongation of the action of local anaesthetics can be achieved following 'single-shot' administration of formulations using 'encapsulation' of local anaesthetics. This makes perineural injection of large doses safe, since rapid systemic uptake is prevented and the local anaesthetic is released from the site of injection continuously and slowly. This can provide effective analgesia for days after the injection, and these formulations may well replace the need for continuous infusions (10).

In the chronic and cancer pain setting the steroid preparation methylprednisolone (Depomedrone) is commonly combined with local anaesthetic. In addition to the expected local anti-inflammatory action, it is thought to obtund transmission via C fibres (11). An additional systemic analgesic effect may well occur.

Neurolytic agents (phenol and alcohol) are now rarely used on peripheral nerves due to the possibility of inducing intractable neuropathic pain and unwanted muscle weakness, but there is a definite but limited place for these agents in patients with a known short prognosis (12).

Side effects and toxicity

Motor block will occur if local anaesthetics are applied to motor nerves. This can be highly significant in patients who already have a motor weakness for other reasons, and will occur at doses much lower than would be expected in patients with previously good motor function. Although ropivacaine does offer a theoretical advantage in this regard, it may not be clinically significant unless very fine dose adjustment is undertaken (7). The possibility of unintentionally blocking motor nerves in the area of injection must be considered, particularly if this will induce clinically significant effects, e.g. phrenic nerve paresis is common following some types of brachial plexus block, and care needs to be taken in order to minimize this (13).

Systemic anaesthetic toxicity can result from intravascular injection or systemic absorption from the injection site. Symptoms include alteration in consciousness, sedation, circum-oral paraesthesia and muscle twitching. This may progress to convulsions and cardiovascular collapse, which will occur rapidly following direct accidental intravascular injection (e.g. during attempted brachial plexus or femoral nerve block) or less rapidly following systemic absorption from the injection site (e.g. from the pleural space following intercostal nerve blocks). Peak arterial plasma concentrations from systemic absorption usually occurs within 30 min of injection, and hence close post-procedure monitoring should be undertaken for at least this length of time. Systemic uptake will be increased if these agents are injected into inflamed or infected areas. Uptake can be limited by the addition of low concentrations of adrenalin to the solution used, but care must be taken to avoid intravascular injection of adrenaline-containing solutions and they should not be injected into areas where vasoconstriction would compromise tissue viability.

Treatment of local anaesthetic systemic toxicity

Acute toxicity can be treated by immediate administration of intravenous lipid emulsion (an intralipid bolus of up to 2 ml/kg, followed by an infusion of up to 0.5 ml/kg/min) (14). It is advisable to establish reliable intravenous access and to have lipid solution available for early use before undertaking blocks likely to result in systemic toxicity, particularly in a setting where resuscitation facilities are not available.

Intralipid provides a 'lipid sink', which extracts the local anaesthetic from the aqueous component of plasma, and is an effective treatment in life-threatening situations (cardiac arrhythmia and convulsions) providing it is administered rapidly (14). The cardiac toxicity of local anaesthetics is dependent on their lipophilicity, and hence lipid emulsion may be most effective in the management of bupivacaine toxicity (15).

Patients with a low fit threshold may theoretically be at higher risk of convulsions if exposed to local anaesthetics. The use of regional blockade in patients with a history of seizure disorder has been investigated in the post-operative setting, where the doses used are liable to be higher than required in palliative care patients. The calculated incidence of local-anaesthetic-induced seizures was between 0 and 120 per 10,000 cases, indicating that regional anaesthesia is not contraindicated in these patients (16).

Levobupivacaine and ropivacaine are left-isomers and have a lower potential for inducing cardiovascular and central nervous system toxicity than does bupivacaine. They are probably the agents of choice when this is a high possibility, but by no means guarantee safety, particularly when large doses are used in situations where high systemic uptake is likely (e.g. for brachial plexus and interpleural blocks). Clinically evident toxicity is not simply related to dose or plasma levels. In a series of 13 patients receiving 0.25% ropivacaine at 6–14 ml/h via perineural catheters for 6–27 days, serum levels were recorded within the toxic range in two patients who had received a 300 mg bolus of 0.5% ropivacaine within the previous 24 h, although this was not associated with symptoms (17). However, acute toxicity has been reported following interscalene block with ropivacaine where normal doses were used, and intravascular catheter placement was ruled out (18).

Specific blocks

Extensive descriptions of anatomy, technique and indications for a wide range of peripheral nerve blocks are available in standard text books. Many of these are potentially useful in the management of individual patients, and reference to standard texts will be useful in assessing their application to particular situations. Brachial plexus block is a very useful technique for managing pain in the upper limb, and has considerable advantages over cervical epidural block, which is associated with many unwanted effects and is difficult to carry out and manage in a hospice setting. Hence this procedure will be covered in some detail. Lumbar plexus block has fewer potential applications, particularly since lumbar epidural or spinal block is relatively reliable and easy to carry out.

We will consider the following specific blocks, and their use in cancer patients:

◆ scar injections
◆ 'trigger point' injections
◆ intercostal nerve blocks
◆ interpleural block
◆ suprascapular block
◆ transverse abdominal plane (TAP) block

◆ brachial plexus block

◆ lumbar plexus block

Scar injections

Scars can be associated with disabling pain for years after surgery and scar pain typically occurs following surgery affecting the intercostal nerves, e.g. thoracotomy and mastectomy (4, 19). This may be due to neuroma formation in the scar tissue. Often the affected area is locally hypersensitive or 'numb but painful', making wearing tight-fitting clothing impossible, in particular bras and belts. Application of local anaesthetic to the affected area, and/or a course of injections of methylprednisolone (Depomedrone) and bupivacaine directly into the scar may give good and long-lasting relief. Injection of alcohol has been used to good effect in the past (20).

Trigger-point injections

Myofascial pain syndromes are very common in the chronic pain setting, having a quoted incidence ranging from 30% to 85% in patients attending pain clinics (21). They present as areas of acute myofascial pain, with tender 'trigger points', commonly affecting the muscles of the back, neck and shoulders. Although the exact aetiology and best treatment options remain unknown, injection of methylprednisolone (Depomedrone) and local anaesthetic into the affected area may give good results. Available data indicate that the process of 'needleing' is at least as important as any pharmacological effect from the substance injected (22). The painful points can be simply located by palpation, and injection is safe providing the operator is familiar with the underlying anatomy and care is taken that needles are not sited near any vital structures. A prospective assessment of patients under going breast surgery indicates that myofascial pain occurs in over 40% of those undergoing surgery that includes axillary dissection (23). Cancer patients with pain leading to alteration of posture and muscle tension/function may well develop myofascial pain not directly caused by their primary disease. If recurrent injection gives only short-term results, pulsed radio frequency may be an appropriate treatment for intractable myofascial pain (24).

Intercostal nerve blocks

The intercostal nerves are situated in the neurovascular bundles sited immediately inferior to each rib. Typically they supply sensory fibres to one dermatone and a contribution to adjacent dermatones. An intercostal nerve can be blocked at any point in its course, and can usually be located easily by palpation of the relevant rib and by 'walking' a needle off its inferior surface. On correct needle placement parasthesia will often be felt radiating in the distribution of the nerve. Potential side effects include pneumothorax, accidental intravascular injection and toxicity from high systemic uptake of local anaesthetic. These blocks are particularly effective for the management of pain arising from pathology in the ribs or costo-chondral joints (e.g. pathological fractures). They will not be effective for sternal pain unless bilateral block is undertaken, which carries the risk of inducing bilateral pneumothoraces. Although intercostal muscle function may be affected at the level the blocks are undertaken, respiratory compromise is unlikely to be significant, even when multiple blocks are used. Often the ability to take a deep breath is improved once pain control has been achieved, making coughing and chest physiotherapy possible. The appropriate use of intercostal blocks in cancer patients has been demonstrated to be successful in 80% of patients in one small series, with a reduction in systemic analgesic requirements in over 50% (25).

Case study

A non-invasive alternative to intercostal nerve block

Mr Smith enjoyed his cigarettes, and despite warnings that his emphysema was becoming critical declined any attempt to give up. When his diagnosis of lung cancer was finally made he was already on home oxygen and high-dose steroids. He suffered from recurrent chest infections and this one was worse than usual. He was familiar with the experience of 'cracking' ribs, which he had done on more than one occasion during fits of violent coughing. Usually what happened is that he got acute one-sided upper 'back' pain that resolved after a few days.

This time was worse than usual. He had had significant localized pain at mid-thoracic level for a number of weeks, and during a bout of coughing had felt a sudden sharp pain at the same site that was now stopping him from breathing without extreme pain.

On examination he was clearly cyanosed, not able to talk in sentences, distressed and certainly not able to cough. Palpation of the ribs proximal to the pain clearly indicated a fracture, and in view of his history this was in all likelihood pathological.

We considered the options for pain control. Intercostal blocks would carry a small, but very significant, risk of inducing a pneumothorax, and he would probably need at least four injections, to block the nerves above and below the (probable) two rib factures. The duration of analgesia would be relatively short, but would probably enable him to have chest physiotherapy. An interpleural block would present similar risks, and we were concerned that even minor compromise of respiratory muscle function induced by a thoracic epidural would be detrimental. In view of the potential risks and difficulty in obtaining consent, and in view of his deteriorating clinical condition we decided to start by applying generous amounts of EMLA (eutectic mixture of lidocaine 2.5% and prilocaine 2.5%) cream to the affected sites and covering them with a large occlusive dressing whilst we all considered what to do next. Somewhat surprisingly, this gave excellent analgesia within about 1 h, enabling him to cough. His respiratory rate slowed, and the affected part of the chest wall was now moving reasonably on inspiration. In view of the pain control achieved we abandoned the idea of neural blockade, and continued with twice-daily application of EMLA. Perhaps his cachexia and the thinning of the skin secondary to long-term high-dose steroid use contributed to this somewhat unexpected effect, but whatever the reasons it was clearly the safest and most effective option for him.

Learning point

Topical local anaesthetic cream can sometimes give surprisingly good results in cancer patients.

Interpleural blocks

Insertion of a catheter between the visceral and parietal layers of the pleura is relatively easy in patients with normal anatomy at the site of insertion, and can be undertaken with a standard epidural kit. Ideally, careful assessment of the position of tumours affecting the chest wall is required, and the results may be unpredictable in patients with chest wall pathology or in those who have previously undergone pleurodesis. Pneumothorax is an obvious complication, and the systemic uptake of local anaesthetic from the pleura is relatively high. However, this technique can give very good results (26, 27). Simple injection of bupivacaine into the interpleural space (30 ml of 0.25% bupivicaine) every 6 h has been demonstrated to provide analgesia equivalent to that provided by an infusion running at 6 ml/h in post-operative patients (28). Continuous interpleural infusion of bupivacaine can be managed in a home setting, and appears very effective in selected patients with advanced malignancy and pain not well controlled with opioids (29).

Suprascapular nerve block

The suprascapular nerve supplies pain fibres to the shoulder, and is entirely sensory. It runs in a 'notch' in the superior border of the wing of the scapula. Suprascapular block can be highly effective in controlling shoulder pain, with no loss of motor function. Pneumothorax is a significant risk. Catheter insertion and continuous infusion have given effective control of pain from a tumour in the shoulder (30).

Transversus abdominis plane block

The transversus abdominis plane (TAP) block is undertaken by injecting local anaesthetic between the internal oblique and transversus abdominis layers of the abdominal wall. It is usually undertaken using ultrasound guidance and can be used to effectively anaesthetize the abdominal wall. Relatively high does of local anaesthetic may be needed, particularly if bilateral blocks are required. This block is being increasingly used in a surgical setting, where initial results are encouraging. It will only provide analgesia for abdominal pain arising from pathology in the abdominal wall (31).

Brachial plexus block

The brachial plexus and brachial plexopathy

The brachial plexus supplies sensory, motor and autonomic fibres to the upper limb, being formed from the anterior rami of C5–T1. There is a degree of anatomical variation,

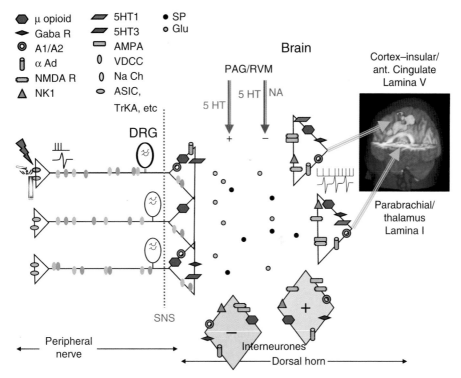

Plate 1 The diagram simplistically summarizes normal acute noxious input from the periphery, through the dorsal horn to the brain. From the left, noxious stimuli, such as heat, chemical or mechanical injury, are transduced via specific receptors, namely temperature coding receptors, acid sensing ion channels (ASIC), TrkA (inflammation) or pressure receptors. Transduction allows a flow of positive ions into the cell, which causes depolarization and action potentials. This is transmitted along the neurone via sodium (NaCh) and calcium (VDCC) channels to the dorsal root ganglion (DRG) and the dorsal horn. The sympathetic nervous system (SNS) lies close to the DRGs but is unaffected in acute noxious transmission. In the dorsal horn extensive modulation of the input can occur. Neurotransmitters such as substance P (SP) or glutamate (Glu) amongst others are released from the primary afferent and diffuse across the synapse. An array of receptors can be triggered, including N-methyl ᴅ-aspartate (NMDA), α-amino-3-hydroxy-5-methylisoxazole-4-propionic acid (AMPA), neurokinin 1 (NK1) and adenosine (A1/A2). Other inhibitory neurotransmitters are also released either locally, (such as enkephalins (μ opioid receptor) and gamma-aminobutyric acid (GABA)) or as a result of descending inhibition (noradrenalin (α Ad receptor) and serotonin). The overall modulated signal (either increased as shown or decreased) is transmitted to the brain via ascending pathways, predominately the spinothalamic from Lamina V, which terminates in the cortex, and the parabrachial from Lamina I, which terminates in the thalamic areas. Descending pathways arise from the brain and pass through the peri-aquaductal grey (PAG) and rostro-ventral medulla (RVM) areas before terminating in the dorsal horn. (See also Fig. 4.1).

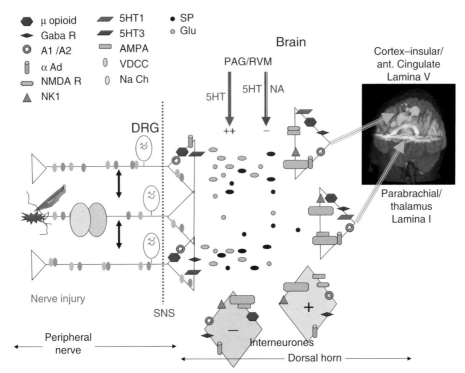

Plate 2 The same simplified diagram is used to summarize the changes that occur in the peripheral and central neuronal pathways following a peripheral nerve injury (nerve transection shown), resulting in chronic neuropathy. In the periphery, the nerve distal to the injury dies and regenerates in an abnormal manner. The sodium (NaCh) and calcium (VDCC) channels alter in expression (to be more responsive) and number (increase particularly around the area of damage). Aberrant transmission in the damaged nerve leads to spontaneous discharge and epiphatic cross-talk between damaged and undamaged neurones, and between DRG and SNS. This results in an increase in the receptive field size and spontaneous and lower threshold discharge of neurones, and can lead to the aberrant excitation of the sympathetic nervous system. Within the dorsal horn, glutamate (Glu) and substance P (SP) are released in increased and irregular amounts (not necessarily in response to a threshold stimuli), although there may be reduced or absent release in the damaged neurone termination. Increased excitatory amino acid release results in an overall excitation of the inter-neurones and increased transmission to the brain. This is further enhanced by the overall reduction in inhibition, by the loss of GABAergic neurones, the relative inactivation of μ opioid receptors and facilitation of descending serotonin–5HT3 excitation pathways. (See also Fig. 4.2).

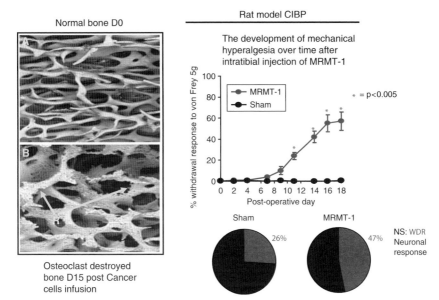

Normal bone D0

Rat model CIBP

The development of mechanical hyperalgesia over time after intratibial injection of MRMT-1

* = p<0.005

Osteoclast destroyed bone D15 post Cancer cells infusion

Sham   MRMT-1

26%   47%

NS: WDR Neuronal response

Plate 3 Results of intra-tibial injection of MRMT-1 breast cancer cells in rat model of CIBP. Left, two scanning electron microscope pictures of a normal rat tibia (top) and the pathological fracture (bottom) after d20. Note abnormal bone resorption (osteoclast action) and abnormal bone formation (osteoblast action). Right, the top panel demonstrates the withdrawal response to von Frey 5g filament over d0–d18 post MRMT1 injection (red) and sham injection (blue). Note the significant withdrawal from d11, indicating hyperalgesia in cancer model (CIBP). The bottom panel demonstrates the ratio of nociceptive specific (NS) to wide-dynamic range (WDR) in normal (or sham) and in CIBP (from d15 onwards). It can be seen that the percentage of WDR neurones increases from 25% to almost 50%. (See also Fig. 4.3).

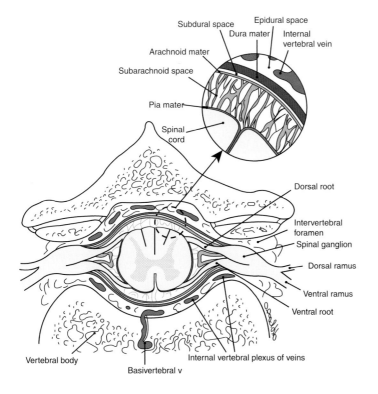

Plate 4 Cross section of a spinal cord. (See also Fig. 5.1).

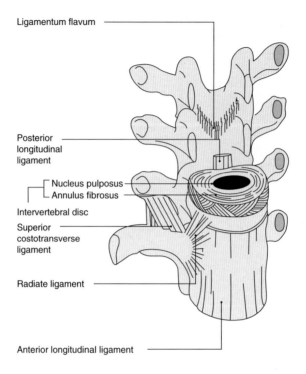

Plate 5 Anterior view of thoracic vertebrae. Bodies have been removed from upper two. (See also Fig. 5.3).

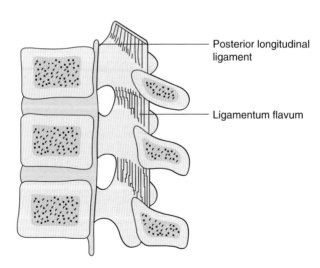

Plate 6 Lateral view of lumbar vertebrae excluding interspinous and supraspinous ligaments. (See also Fig. 5.4).

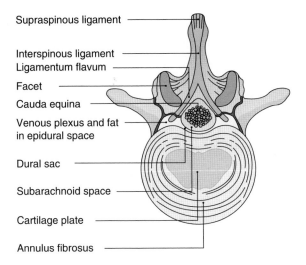

Supraspinous ligament

Interspinous ligament
Ligamentum flavum

Facet

Cauda equina

Venous plexus and fat
in epidural space

Dural sac

Subarachnoid space

Cartilage plate

Annulus fibrosus

Plate 7 Transverse section of an intervertebral disc, showing the subarachnoid space. (See also Fig. 5.5).

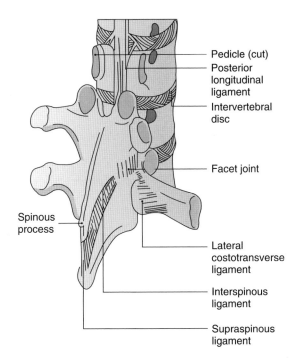

Pedicle (cut)

Posterior
longitudinal
ligament

Intervertebral
disc

Facet joint

Spinous
process

Lateral
costotransverse
ligament

Interspinous
ligament

Supraspinous
ligament

Plate 8 Dorsolateral view of the thoracic vertebrae and ligaments. The vertebral arch of the upper vertebra has been removed. (See also Fig. 5.6).

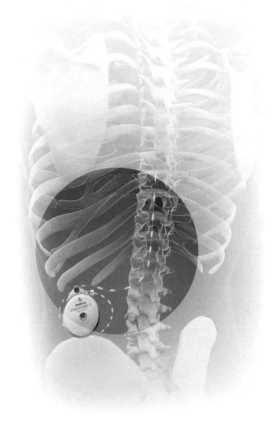

Plate 9 Medtronis
Synchromed Intrathecal Drug
Delivery Pump and catheter
in situ. (See also Fig. 6.2).

Important Features -Surestream

Codman
johnson-johnson

• **With inner titanium coil to prevent kinking, tearing & bunching**

  – Catheter can be tied in knots and drug will still flow

  – Stainless steel guide wire and inner titanium coil allow for easy guide wire removal (metal on metal)

  – Less prone to bunching during guide wire removal due to more rigid material

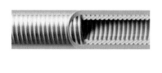

Silicone catheter   Surestream

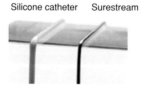

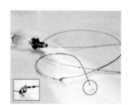

• One hole, located at catheter tip (open tip)

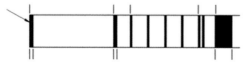

Plate 10 Codman Surestream Intraspinal catheter 19g. (See also Fig. 6.3).

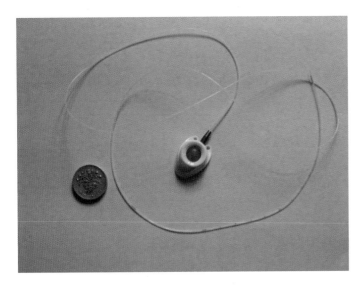

Plate 11 Subcutaneous port attached to catheter. (See also Fig. 6.4).

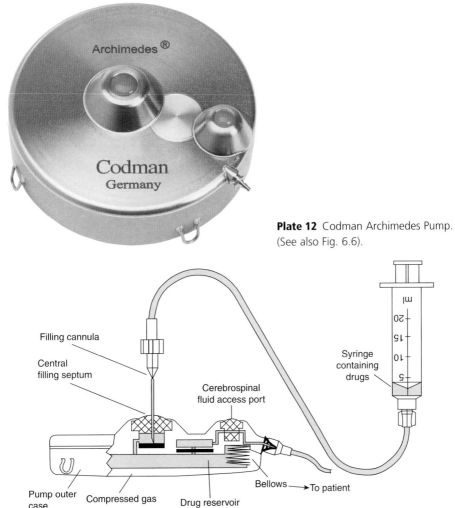

Archimedes ®

Codman
Germany

Plate 12 Codman Archimedes Pump. (See also Fig. 6.6).

Filling cannula

Central filling septum

Cerebrospinal fluid access port

Syringe containing drugs

ml
20
15
10
5

Pump outer case

Compressed gas

Drug reservoir

Bellows → To patient

Plate 13 Codman Archimedes pump. (See also Fig. 6.7).

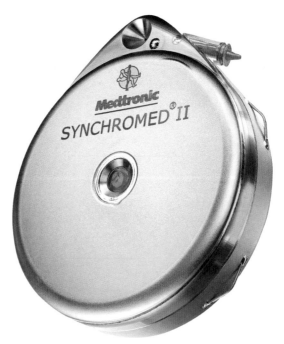

Plate 14 Synchromed, Medtronic Ltd. (See also Fig. 6.8).

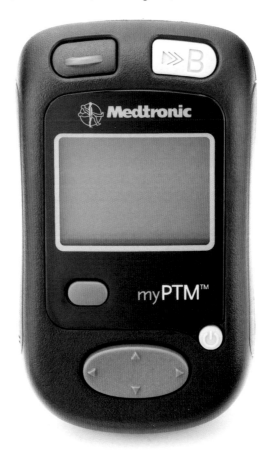

Plate 15 A patient-delivered bolus device, My Personal Therapy Manager, Medtronic Ltd. (See also Fig. 6.9).

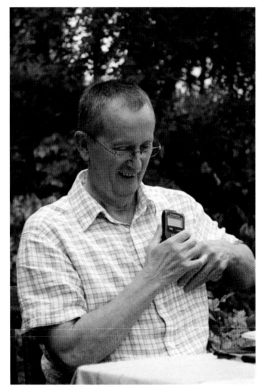

Plate 16 By permission Wal is pictured in his garden with his PTM remote control. (See also Fig. 6.10).

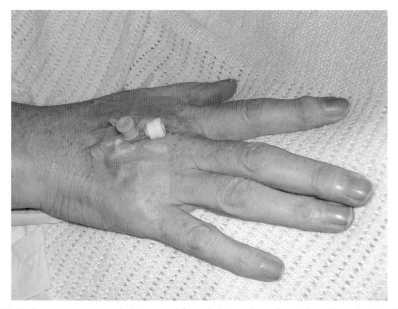

Plate 17 An intravenous cannula is inserted for administration of sedation. (See also Fig. 6.11).

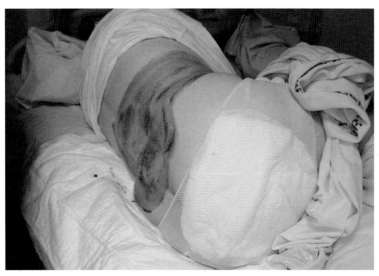

Plate 18 Positioning of the patient in the left lateral position, and skin cleaning. (See also Fig. 6.12).

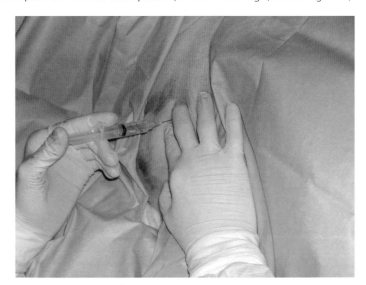

Plate 19 Local anaesthetic (1% Lidocaine) is injected. (See also Fig. 6.13).

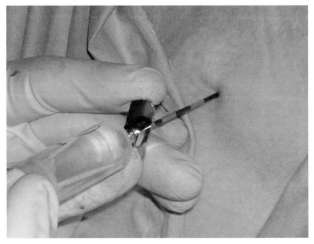

Plate 20 Insertion of a 16g Tuohy needle. (See also Fig. 6.14).

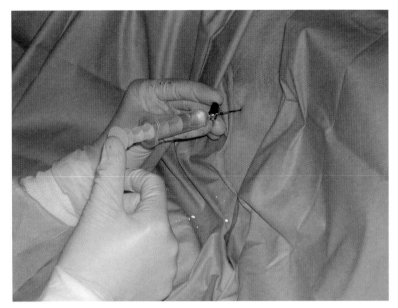

Plate 21 Testing for loss of resistance to saline. A sudden loss of resistance indicates that the epidural space has been entered. (See also Fig. 6.15).

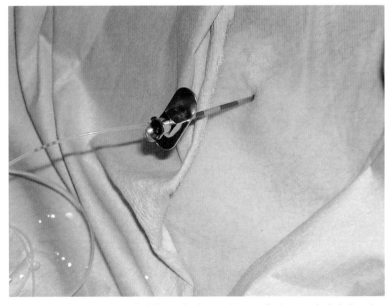

Plate 22 Epidural catheter is threaded through the Tuohy needle in a cephalad direction. (See also Fig. 6.16).

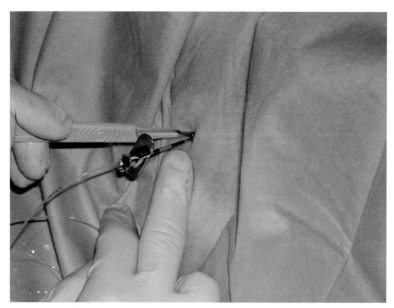

Plate 23 A small incision is made in the back adjacent to the Tuohy needle for tunnelling. (See also Fig. 6.17).

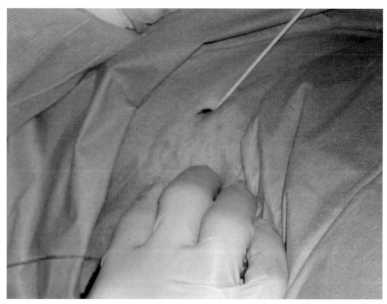

Plate 24 The tunneller (16g long Abbocath®-T, Hospira) is inserted subcutaneously from front to back. (See also Fig. 6.18).

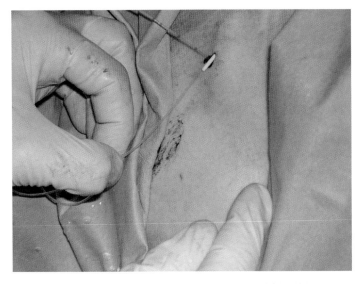

Plate 25 The epidural catheter is threaded through the tunneller from back to front. (See also Fig. 6.19).

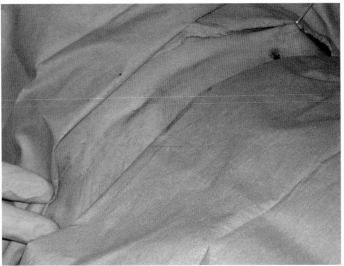

Plate 26 Two or three tunnellings are performed until the catheter reaches the anterior chest or abdominal wall. (See also Fig. 6.20).

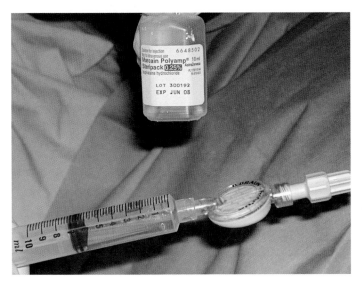

Plate 27 A filter is placed on the end of the epidural catheter and a test dose of 2 ml 0.25% bupivacaine is given. (See also Fig. 6.21).

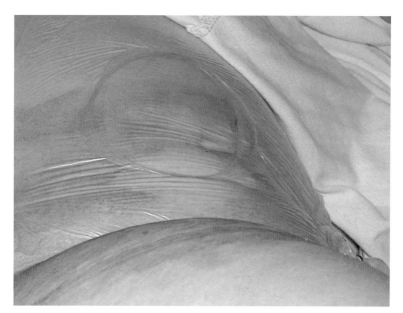

Plate 28 The epidural catheter is looped around and secured with Tegaderm transparent dressings. (See also Fig. 6.22).

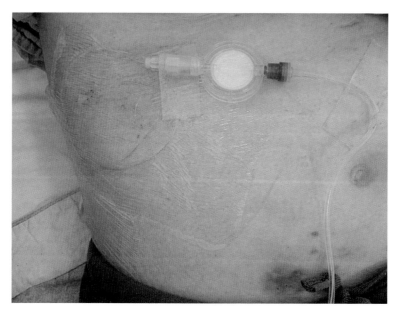

Plate 29 The tunnelled epidural catheter as it comes out at the skin (exit site) showing attached filter and transparent dressing. Patient at St Christopher's Hospice, by permission. (See also Fig. 7.1).

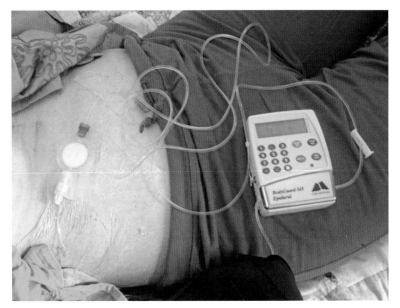

Plate 30 Illustration showing infusion pump and site. Patient at St Christopher's Hospice, by permission. (See also Fig. 7.2).

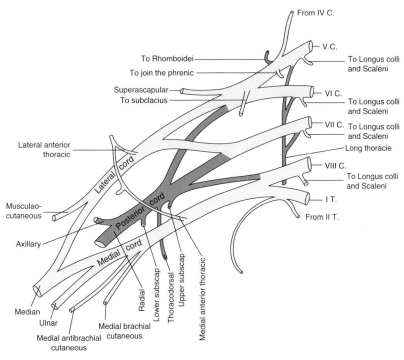

Plate 31 The brachial plexus. (See also Fig. 8.1).

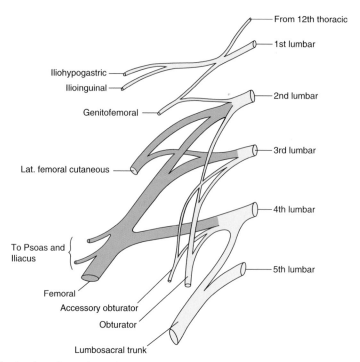

Plate 32 The lumbar plexus. (See also Fig. 8.2).

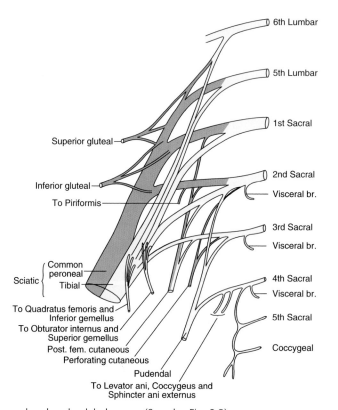

Plate 33 The sacral and pudendal plexuses. (See also Fig. 8.3).

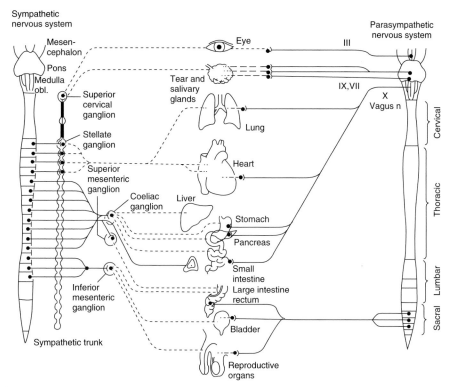

Plate 34 Outline diagram of the autonomic nervous system.
Reproduced from Janig, W. (1995). In Physiologie des menschen (Ed. R. F. Schmidt and G. Thews), 26th edn, pp. 340–69, Springer Verlag, Heidelberg, Berlin, with permission. (See also Fig. 9.1).

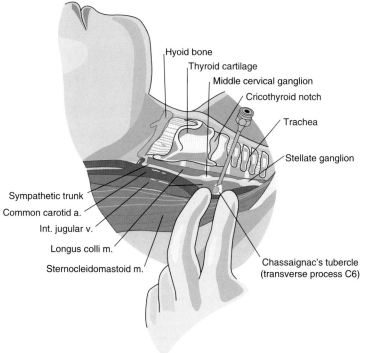

Plate 35 Stellate ganglion block—anterior approach. Reproduced from The Atlas of Pain management Injection techniques by Steven D Waldman (2007), Saunders 2nd edition, with permission from Elsevier. (See also Fig. 9.2).

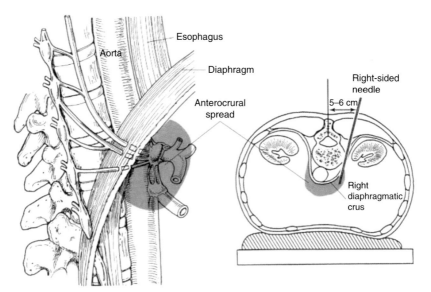

Plate 36 Coeliac plexus block, posterior approach, showing anterocrural spread. The greater, lesser and least splanchnic nerves are also demonstrated.
Reproduced from Brown: Atlas of Regional Anesthesia, 3rd ed., Copyright © 2006 Saunders, with permission from Elsevier. (See also Fig. 9.3).

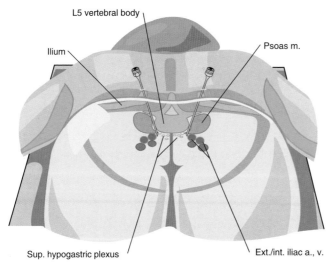

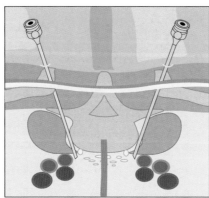

Plate 37 Superior hypogastric plexus block, showing two needle approach.
Reproduced from Waldman, Atlas of Interventional Pain Management. Elsevier. (See also Fig. 9.6).

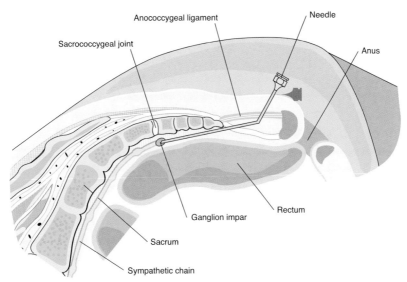

Plate 38 Ganglion of Impar block showing the anococcygeal approach.
Reproduced from Waldman, Atlas of Interventional Pain Management, Elsevier. (See also Fig. 9.7).

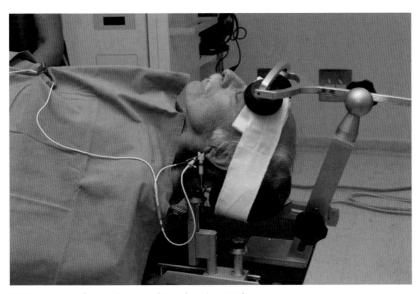

Plate 39 Positioning for cordotomy. (See also Fig. 10.2).

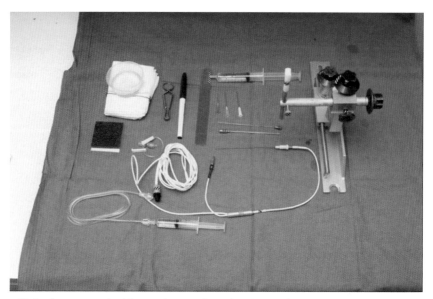

Plate 40 Equipment required for cordotomy. (See also Fig. 10.3).

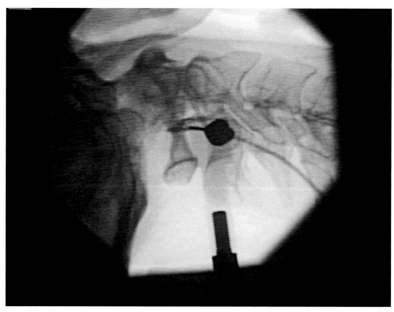

Plate 41 Injection of radio-opaque contrast at C1/2 to outline the dentate ligament. (See also Fig. 10.5).

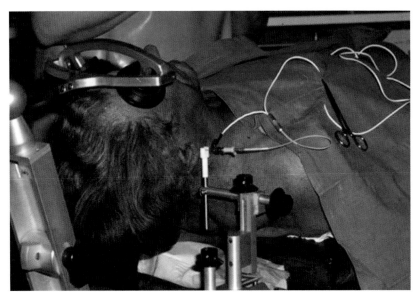

Plate 42 Localization of the spino-thalamic prior to making a radio-frequency lesion. (See also Fig. 10.6).

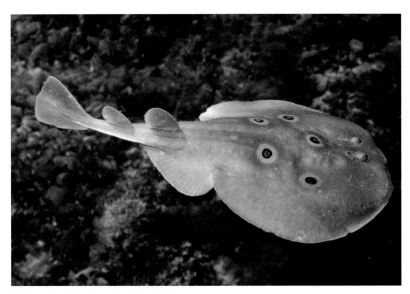

Plate 43 Torpedo fish. (See also Fig. 11.1).

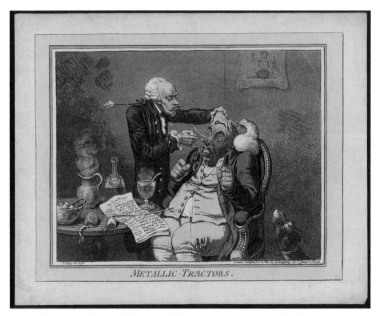

Plate 44 'Dr' Benjamin Perkins and the metallic tractor. Reproduced with permission courtesy of Historical Collections & Services, Claude Moore Health Sciences Library, University of Virginia. (See also Fig. 11.2).

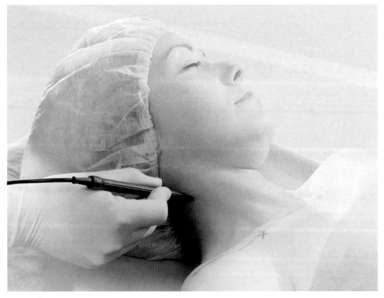

Plate 45 Braun® Stimulplex 'pen' peripheral nerve mapper/stimulator. © B. Braun Medical Ltd. Reproduced with permission. (See also Fig. 11.3).

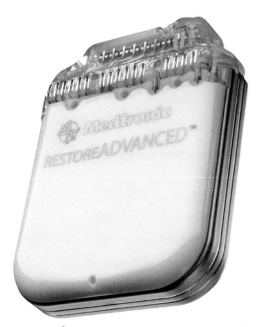

Plate 46 Restore Ultra Medtronic® Impulse Generator. Photo courtesy of Medtronic, Inc. (See also Fig. 11.4).

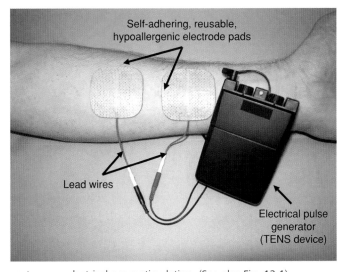

Plate 47 Transcutaneous electrical nerve stimulation. (See also Fig. 12.1).

with possible contributions from C4 or T2. The nerves making up the plexus lie in close association with the subclavian artery, running between the anterior and middle scalene muscles, over the first rib beneath the clavicle and into the axilla. The plexus gives rise to the musculocutaneous, median, ulnar, axillary and radial nerves (32). The point at which the plexus is blocked (i.e. the 'approach') will affect the clinical response, since the various approaches used will preferentially affect different parts of the plexus (33).

Brachial plexopathy, with associated shoulder, arm and hand pain, is most commonly encountered in cancer pain patients with metastatic breast and lung cancer, Pancoast tumour, radiation plexopathy and schwannoma. Benign causes include demyelination and thoracic outlet syndrome. The major question for the patient with plexopathy will be whether their symptoms are secondary to primary or recurrent disease, or to nerve damage following treatment, in particular neural damage following radiation and/or chemotherapy, which can have a delayed onset. The cause of the pain must be carefully considered when discussing the available therapeutic options, and if this is in doubt then MRI of the plexus is the investigation of first choice (34).

Refined imaging techniques can be used to accurately identify masses in the region of the plexus, which are highly predictive of tumour infiltration. MRI is exceptionally useful in differentiating recurrence from radiation damage. In one series of 50 breast cancer patients with plexopathy, imaging has been demonstrated to have a sensitivity and specificity of over 90% (35).

Assessment for brachial plexus block

The optimum approach to the plexus is crucially dependent on individual pathology, available resources and the skill of the operator (please see below for details of the techniques used). To be effective the block must be undertaken proximal to the level of the lesion. Careful clinical assessment is required to delineate whether arm/shoulder pain and any coexistent motor symptoms are being experienced in the distribution of the dermatones/myotomes, suggesting pathology at nerve root level, or in the sensory distribution of a single nerve, suggesting the presence of more peripheral pathology. Pain secondary to pathology located at nerve root level, particularly if it is liable to extend to within the cervical epidural space, which is associated with neck pain, is unlikely to respond well to brachial plexus block, especially if the more peripheral approaches are used.

Side effects secondary to brachial plexus block

The degree of motor deficit will be dependent on the part(s) of the plexus blocked and the concentration of the agents used. Before this block is contemplated it should be remembered that total block of the plexus will result in considerable sensory and motor deficit, which may require the provision of some support for the arm, and hand function may be compromised or lost.

The area of the limb that will be most affected is determined to some degree by the technique used. In the post-operative setting the interscalene and cervical paravertebral approach will provide analgesia in the shoulder and upper humeral region, and the infraclavicular and axillary approaches are used for pain occurring distal to the elbow (36). Ultrasound may be useful if optimum localization is to be achieved (6). Specific approaches that may offer the advantages of improved safety and less likelihood of catheter displacement have been described in cancer patients (37–39).

Systemic uptake of local anaesthetics has been demonstrated to be higher following the use of supraclavicular techniques than following the use of infraclavicular techniques (40). Systemic toxicity following accidental intravascular injection/systemic uptake of high doses of local anaesthetic is a particular problem associated with brachial plexus blocks, and is well described, even with ropivacaine (41). Appropriate precautions should be taken, and resuscitation facilities must be available if potentially toxic doses are used. Levobupivacaine has similar efficacy to that of bupivicaine when used in the post-operative setting via a supraclavicular approach, and less potential for inducing cardio-vascular toxicity (42).

Paresis of the phrenic nerve, and consequent impairment of diaphragmatic activity, is a possibility following brachial plexus block, particularly following the interscalene approach. Movement of the diaphragm can be easily demonstrated using ultrasound, which can be used both for pre- and post-block assessment. Any pre-existing pathology liable to compromise respiration is a relative contraindication to the use of the more central approaches to the plexus, particularly the interscalene, where even low doses of anaes-thetic can cause significant phrenic nerve dysfunction unless careful needle placement under ultrasound control is used (43). A prospective study of 100 patients has demon-strated that it is possible to provide continuous analgesia using a refined technique via the supraclavicular approach without inducing significant phrenic nerve paresis (44).

Bilateral brachial plexus block is undertaken relatively rarely due to the possibility of bilateral pneumothorax and/or bilateral phrenic nerve paresis. With accurate location of catheters, and appropriate delay between establishing a block on one side before estab-lishing it on the other, bilateral blocks have been safely undertaken in the peri-operative setting, but the interscalene approach is best avoided due to the possibility of bilateral phrenic nerve paresis (45).

Continuous infusions given via perineurally sited catheters are used both in the cancer-pain and post-operative settings. Elastomeric pumps are light and highly portable, and make outpatient management a realistic possibility, but the option of infection should be considered, and strict asepsis maintained whilst setting up the infusion (46).

Lumbar plexus block

The lumbo-sacral plexus

The lumbo-sacral plexus arises from the L1–S3 spinal roots and supplies sensory and motor inervation to the whole of lower limb and regions of the perineum. The anat-omy of the lumbar plexus is much more variable than that of the brachial plexus, with a greater or lesser contribution to the sacral plexus. The ventral divisions of the first four lumbar nerves (L1–L4) and contributions from the subcostal nerve (T12) usually make up the lumbar plexus. The ventral rami of the fourth lumbar nerves pass communicating branches to the sacral plexus. The lumbar plexus is formed lateral to the intervertebral foraminae and passes through psoas major, distributing motor branches directly to the muscle. The branches of the lumbar plexus include the ilio-hypogastric, ilio-inguinal, genito-femoral, lateral cutaneous, obturator and femoral nerves. Larger branches run obliquely down through the pelvic area to leave the pelvis under the inguinal ligament, with the exception of the obturator nerve, which exits the pelvis through the obturator foramen (47).

Lumbar plexus block

Because of its proximity to the vertebral bodies, transverse processes, para-aortic nodes and the posterior abdominal organs, the lumbar plexus can be involved in the spread of many intra-abdominal, pelvic and spinal primary and secondary tumours. As with investigation of brachial plexopathy, investigation of cancer patients presenting with low-back, pelvic and lower-limb pain is greatly assisted by refined CT and MRI techniques. This, combined with appropriate tissue sampling, will usually differentiate common benign causes of lower limb pain (e.g. disc prolapse) from malignant processes involving the lumbo-sacral plexus. However, both can initially present with similar patterns of referred pain, and can often coexist. In particular, care should be taken to fully investigate patients with radicular pain in the absence of demonstrated nerve compression within the spinal canal (48), and, as with the brachial plexus, it should be remembered that previous radiation can cause a plexopathy (49). Direct invasion of the plexus and psoas muscle may result in severe pain and muscle spasm—known as the 'malignant psoas syndrome'. The pain associated with this syndrome is often refractory to polymodal analgesic therapy, and may respond well to lumbar plexus block (50–52).

Neuraxial or lumbar plexus block?

A major advantage of lumbar plexus or lower limb nerve blocks over epidural and intrathecal infusions is the lack of autonomic block and preservation of function of the contralateral limb. These advantages may be particularly significant for patients who do not have a urinary catheter *in situ* and who wish to maintain mobility. Catheter fixation and variations in anatomy can present significant challenges and, if rapid and reliable analgesia is required for severe pain involving the whole limb, epidural or intrathecal infusion is a more familiar and reliable option. However, an analysis of randomized trials of epidural anaesthesia in comparison with peripheral nerve blockade delivered via a variety of approaches after major knee surgery has indicated that there is no difference in analgesic efficacy or post-operative morphine consumption, and the use of peripheral techniques may well be associated with increased patient satisfaction and an improved side effect profile (53).

Choice of technique from blocking the lumbar plexus

A number of approaches to both the plexus itself and to nerves supplying the lower limb (e.g. femoral, obturator and sciatic) have been described (see below). These are commonly used in isolation or combination for the control of acute traumatic and post-operative pain in the lower limb (54). Due to the variable anatomy and depth of the plexus, anatomical differences between males and females, and the need for more than one injection when some techniques are used, the possibility of systemic toxicity and block failure should be carefully considered. Spread of local anaesthetic into the epidural space can occur following some approaches to the lumbar plexus (55).

Catheters placed in the psoas compartment delivering 0.2% ropivacaine following a bolus of 0.4 ml/kg give safe and reliable analgesia following total hip arthroplasty, virtually removing the need for opioid analgesia (55). A more peripheral, and possibly easier and safer, approach can equally well be used for pain arising in the knee. Patient-controlled anaesthesia using bupivacaine (40 ml 0.25% followed by boluses of 10 ml 0.125%) delivered via psoas compartment or femoral catheters has been shown to be equally effective for knee surgery over a 48-h period (56). The use of techniques similar to those used in acute pain has been reported as effective in managing cancer pain, delivering good analgesia with few side effects, particularly when the facility for patient-controlled boluses is provided (52).

Anatomy and techniques

Brachial plexus

The anatomy of the brachial plexus

The brachial plexus gives rise to 17 different nerves, supplying the upper limb and shoulder girdle. Arising from five roots, C5–T1, fibres branch off to give rise to three trunks, which each divide into anterior and posterior parts to form three cords. These finally give rise to the five terminal nerves (see Table 8.1 and Fig. 8.1). The detailed anatomy is beyond the scope of this chapter but is readily available from anatomy reviews (57, 58) or regional blockade textbooks (59). Theoretically, single injections given proximal to the

Table 8.1 The brachial plexus

Parts of the plexus	
Roots (emerge from intervertebral foramina)	C5–T1
Trunks (emerge from between scalenus anterior and medius)	Superior (C5–6)
	Middle (C7)
	Inferior (C8–T1)
Divisions (occurs at lateral border of 1st rib)	Anterior (one from each trunk)
	Posterior (one from each trunk)
Cords (on entering axilla)	Lateral
	Medial
	Posterior
Terminal nerves	Musculocutaneous
	Median
	Ulnar
	Axillary
	Radial

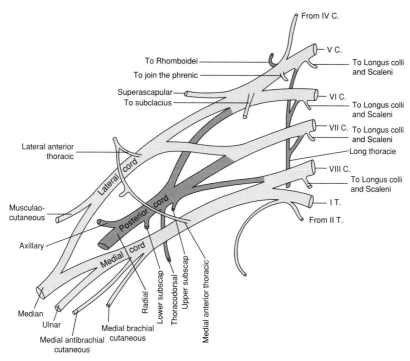

Fig. 8.1 The brachial plexus. Also appears in colour in the colour plate section, Plate 31.

axilla should block the whole plexus, since it is encased in a sheath from its origin to the axilla. This sheath arises from the prevertebral fascia, anterior scalenus and middle scalenus muscles, and joins distally with the fascia of the biceps and coracobrachialis muscles. It is well organized proximally, but much looser distally, and has also been shown to contain connective tissue septae. Clinical experience using ultrasound imaging for real-time nerve blockade would support these findings, as the extent of the spread of local anaesthetic can be highly variable. Furthermore, it is rare to find the musculocutaneous nerve within this sheath. Instead it is typically found in the sheath between biceps and coracobrachialis, and occasionally within the biceps muscle itself (57).

Interscalene Brachial plexus block—Winnie's approach

This is one of the more commonly described approaches and is widely practised using a nerve-stimulator technique, although blind placement may also be used.

Positioning

The patient is positioned supine with the head rotated laterally away from the side to be blocked.

Procedure

The level of the cricoid cartilage is identified and traced laterally to the posterior border of the sternocleidomastoid muscle. The interscalene groove can often be palpated, especially if accentuated by asking the patient to lift their head. The skin is infiltrated with local anaesthetic and the needle inserted in the direction of the sternal notch. A fascial 'pop' is often felt at 1–2 cm depth as it enters into the sheath of the brachial plexus. This can be confirmed using ultrasound, where a short-axis technique can be utilized. Paraesthesiae in the required territory can be elicited to confirm placement. Nerve stimulation will stimulate muscle contractions, which ideally should be shoulder abduction (C5 root) or elbow flexion (C5/6). Elevation of the scapula indicates that the needle is too posterior as it will be stimulating the dorsal scapular nerve, which is derived from the C5 root. Hiccupping indicates that the needle is too far anterior and is stimulating the phrenic nerve.

Injection

After careful aspiration for blood or CSF, 20 ml is usually sufficient to achieve adequate blockade of the plexus. Up to 40 ml is commonly described, as is the use of digital pressure to encourage spread either caudally or cranially. However, in the experience of these authors 20 ml is usually sufficient. Bupivacaine 0.25–0.5%, with or without steroid, may be used.

Complications

The following complications may be encountered:

◆ infection

◆ blockade of other nerves—recurrent laryngeal nerve (hoarseness), cervical sympathetic block (Horner's syndrome), phrenic nerve block (hemi-diaphragm paralysis)

◆ Inadvertent vascular injection—injection of even very small volumes of local anaesthetic into the vertebral artery will induce rapid onset of loss of consciousness and/or seizures

◆ inadvertent epidural/intrathecal injection

◆ pneumothorax/haemothorax/chylothorax.

Interscalene brachial plexus block—Meier's approach

This approach in essence aims to approach the brachial plexus at a reduced angle, running from proximal to distal, compared to the more tangential approach of Winnie.

Procedure

The procedure is much as for Winnie's approach, except for a more cephalad entry point at the level of the thyroid cartilage. The needle is aimed in the same direction as the course of the plexus, which corresponds to a line running from the posterior border of the sternocleidomastoid muscle at the level of the thyroid cartilage to the pulsation of the subclavian artery at the clavicle. As it is a less tangential approach, the fascial 'pop' is felt at a depth of about 35–50 mm.

Interscalene brachial plexus block—ultrasound-guided

An increasingly practiced technique, ultrasound guidance requires a high-frequency linear probe set to image to a depth of 2.5–3 cm. Additionally, a good sonographic technique is required to allow fixation of the probe to stabilize the image given the curvature of the neck and the use of slippery gel.

Positioning

The patient should be sitting at approximately 30–45°, with the head turned away from the side to be blocked. Pulling the pillow out away from the side to be blocked in such a way that there is no pillow protruding out from behind the head and neck is useful in improving access for the needle. The ultrasound machine can be placed on the contralateral side and the operator stands on the ipsilateral side. In this way the operator can clearly see the images without having to twist. Additionally the patient can also observe the procedure on the screen should they wish to do so.

Procedure

The anatomy is typically identified by observing the nerves posterior to the subclavian artery when the probe is lying in a parallel orientation just posterior to the clavicle. These nerves can then be traced proximally to the level of the cricoid cartilage, the operator being mindful to keep the probe tangential to the nerves when doing so. Alternatively the anatomy can be traced from anterior to posterior at the level of the cricoid cartilage. Local infiltration is performed at the point of planned needle insertion. A 50-mm 22G needle is most often used, using an in-plane approach from a posterior to anterior direction. An out-of-plane approach can be used if the anatomy is distorted by tumour infiltration, blocking the path of the needle along the in-plane tract. However, the posterior in-plane approach allows greater sparing of the more anterior phrenic nerve. Limiting volumes injected to 20 ml also helps this sparing, but the use of direct visualization allows better accuracy and placement of the medication around individual roots (C5, 6 and occasionally 7).

Supraclavicular brachial plexus block

Supraclavicular block theoretically allows better coverage with smaller volumes as this is where the plexus is most compact within the sheath. If the first rib and subclavian artery are easily palpable this approach can be undertaken relatively safely and reliably without the need for imaging or stimulation.

Position

The patient should be supine with head turned towards the contralateral side.

Procedure

The interscalene groove is located and traced caudally to where the skin flattens out. It is possible to feel the pulsations of the subclavian artery in some patients. The entry point is infiltrated with local anaesthetic and a 22G 50-mm needle is inserted into the groove. It should be directed caudally in a parasaggital plane, and aimed posterior to the artery. Medial trajectory is avoided in order to reduce the likelihood of pleural puncture. If ultrasound is used then the procedure is very similar to that used for the interscalene approach. The cranio-caudal distance between probe placement for interscalene and supraclavicular block is approximately 2–3 cm. The more caudal supraclavicular images reveal much closer proximity of the plexus to the artery and the pleura. In practice, a slightly more cephalad image is perhaps more acceptable as it allows greater separation between the brachial plexus and the subclavian artery. As with the interscalene block, the needle approach is in-plane. Deposition of solution, which lifts the plexus away from the artery on direct vision, has a tendency to give a faster onset and a better quality block.

Injection

The technique is the same as for the interscalene approach. Theoretically less volume is required.

Infraclavicular brachial plexus block

This blocks the brachial plexus where it has divided into the cords. It targets the more diffuse part of the plexus and can lead to patchy blockade depending upon the spread of the solution. Direct vision using ultrasound overcomes this. The chance of accidental pleural injury is very low using this approach, since at this point the plexus lies lateral to the thoracic cage. The infraclavicular region is a comfortable exit site for an indwelling or tunnelled brachial plexus catheter and it is less likely to be displaced because of movement.

Position

The patient should be supine. The head position should be neutral although it will have little effect on the anatomy.

Procedure

The insertion point is 2 cm below and 1 cm medial to the coracoid process. The insertion point is infiltrated with local anaesthetic, and a 22G 100-mm needle is inserted perpendicularly. The plexus is typically 5–7 cm deep. Up to 50 ml may be needed, but 30–40 ml usually suffices.

Infraclavicular brachial plexus block—ultrasound-guided

Position

Ensure the patient is positioned on the bed closer to the edge of the contralateral side, as arm abduction may be required.

Procedure

Images are first obtained by setting the depth to 6 cm initially, and placing a linear probe in the parasagittal plane inferior to the clavicle at its midpoint. Imaging more laterally will show the pectoralis minor muscle more readily, but also adds extra reassurance in that the lung lies medially. The axillary artery is then visualized, but due to the depth of the structures, clear imaging of the cords is not common. The short-axis approach can be performed with the arm by the side. The long-axis approach sometimes requires the arm to be abducted to avoid obstruction by the clavicle.

Utilising a 100-mm needle, local anaesthetic solution is deposited around the artery to allow complete block of the brachial plexus. Direct visualization allows a block to be undertaken with volumes as small as 20 mls.

Axillary brachial plexus block

This approach is suitable for providing analgesia at and distal to the level of the elbow. However, axillary block is often incomplete unless separate blockade of individual nerves is carried out. Typically the musculocutaneous nerve is not blocked as it often lies outside of the sheath that encases the rest of the nerves in the neurovascular bundle. The use of ultrasound gives much more predictable and consistent blocks as the individual nerves are identified and blocked. The axilla is more prone to infection than other sites used for blocking the plexus and hence this approach is not very suitable for inserting an indwelling catheter.

Position

The patient should be supine with the arm abducted to 90° and the elbow flexed to 90°.

Procedure

The axillary artery is palpated and the entry site infiltrated with local anaesthetic. The needle can then be inserted and manipulated to the desired position, depending which nerves need to be blocked. If stimulation is used an indication of the location of the needle can be obtained as follows:

- above the artery—closest to the median nerve (wrist/finger flexion and pronation)
- below the artery—closest to the ulnar nerve (thumb abduction, little/ring finger flexion)
- through the artery—closest to the radial nerve (extension of elbow, wrist and fingers)
- superior to the sheath and into the body of coracobrachialis—to look for the musculo-cutaneous nerve (elbow flexion).

Typically when blocking the ulnar, radial and median nerve, a 'pop' can be felt as the needle enters into the sheath. A total volume of 30–40 ml of solution is injected after careful aspiration for blood to allow adequate spread through the sheath.

Axillary brachial plexus block—ultrasound-guided

The use of ultrasound in axillary blockade indicates why an unguided block can easily fail. The structures are quite spread out within the sheath, and the musculocutaneous nerve is outside of it within coracobrachialis. In addition, the radial nerve 'hides' deep to the artery with the fascia of the triceps muscle immediately below the nerve. Direct vision using ultrasound allows accurate placement of injectate, which results in a reduction of volumes required. This is important if using steroid as it allows the concentration applied around each nerve to remain higher.

Position

The patient should be supine with arm abducted to 90°. The elbow can be straight in which case an arm board is required. Alternatively the elbow can be bent to 90° and in this situation the patient can lie close to the edge of the contralateral side of the bed with the pillow pulled through towards the side to be blocked, in order to offer support to the flexed arm.

Procedure

Utilising a 50-mm 22G needle, each nerve can be blocked individually. A long-axis approach from the cephalad side avoids placing the needle in the axilla. A total of 20 ml of solution is usually sufficient.

Neurolysis of the brachial plexus

There is a paucity of literature on the use of neurolytic solutions on the brachial plexus, and only occasional case reports are available (60, 61). Neurolysis of the brachial plexus should only be considered within the context of other available treatments for severe upper-limb pain (e.g. cervical epidural, cordotomy or dorsal root entry zone lesioning), particularly if the patient has some motor function in the arm. The potential for permanent motor block means that neurolysis of the brachial plexus should not be undertaken without very careful consideration. A 'test block' using local anaesthetic or the use of a catheter should be performed before neurolysis is considered. This allows the potential effects to be assessed and gives the patient time to consider available options. Even with careful dose adjustment of local anaesthetics given via a catheter, some patients find the resultant weakness and numbness more intolerable than the pain, and before neuroloysis is undertaken the implications of a permanent block should be fully understood.

Anatomy and techniques—lumbar plexus

Anatomy of the lumbar plexus

The lumbar plexus is formed by the anterior divisions of L1, 2 and 3 nerve roots, and a variable contribution from the L4 nerve roots. LI often receives a branch from T12. The plexus is situated in the posterior part of psoas major muscle, in front of the transverse processes of the lumbar vertebrae. LI, L2 and L3 supply the skin of the lower abdomen, groin, genitalia (genito-femoral nerve), inside of the thigh (obturator nerve) and antero-lateral aspect of the thigh (lateral cutaneous nerve and femoral nerve). The nerves pass obliquely downwards behind the psoas major. Normally a small part of the fourth nerve joins with the fifth to form the lumbosacral trunk, which makes a contribution to the sacral plexus. Anatomical variations described include situations where the third, third and fourth, or fifth nerves make contributions to both the lumbar and the sacral plexus (57) (see Figs 8.2 and 8.3).

Techniques for lumbar plexus block

It will be clear from the section above that any approach to the lumbar plexus will not provide analgesia to the entire lower limb, and is unpredictable in view of the extent of possible variations in the anatomy. If this is required, supplementary block of peripheral nerves will be needed in addition to lumbar plexus block. These are described in standard text books, where details of techniques for blocking individual nerve can be obtained (e.g. the obturator, saphenous, sciatic, peroneal and tibial nerves).

Two lower-limb blocks will be described here, since they are useful and relatively reliable and simple to undertake without the use of imaging—posterior lumbar plexus block

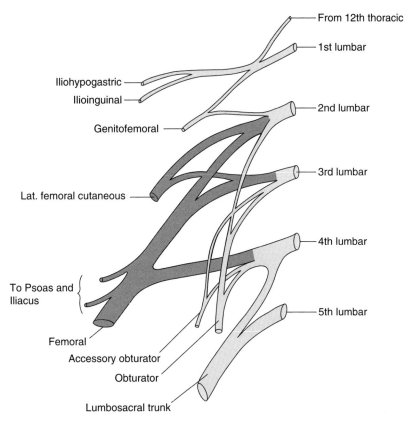

From 12th thoracic

1st lumbar

Iliohypogastric

Ilioinguinal

2nd lumbar

Genitofemoral

3rd lumbar

Lat. femoral cutaneous

4th lumbar

To Psoas and Iliacus

5th lumbar

Femoral

Accessory obturator

Obturator

Lumbosacral trunk

Fig. 8.2 The lumbar plexus. Also appears in colour in the colour plate section, Plate 32.

and femoral nerve block. An informative review of the available data regarding the efficacy of differing techniques as used in acute pain has been undertaken (62), and this will give some idea of the suitability of any one technique for an individual patient with cancer pain in the lower limb.

Posterior approach to the lumbar plexus

Continuous modifications to this technique are being described as techniques for localization improve (55, 63, 64), but in essence local anaesthetic is introduced into a fascial sheath that contains the plexus as it lies posterior to the psoas muscle and anterior to the transverse process of the lumbar vertebrae. Providing the main bony landmark (the transverse process of L3 or L4) can be correctly identified by needle contact this block can be easily undertaken without imaging or nerve stimulation facilities in patients with normal anatomy in the region. A continuous plexus block can provide excellent unilateral pain relief, particularly for unilateral malignant psoas syndrome, acetabular secondaries, or hip and groin pain.

Positioning

The patient is placed either prone with a pillow under the abdomen to correct the lumbar lordosis, or in the lateral (foetal) position with the side to be blocked uppermost.

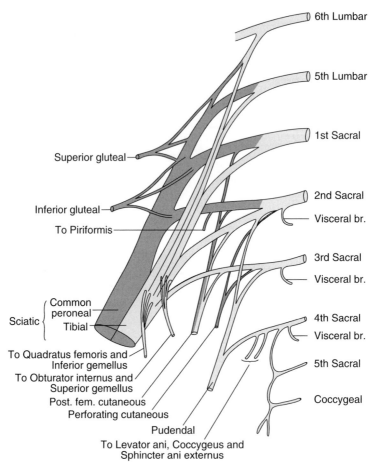

Fig. 8.3 The sacral and pudendal plexuses. Also appears in colour in the colour plate section, Plate 33.

Procedure

The spinous process of L3 or L4 is located by palpation and/or imaging and the skin anaesthetized at a point approximately 2 cm lateral to the midline, or directly over the transverse process if imaging is being used. The needle is introduced at this point at 90° to the skin and advanced until contact is made with the transverse process. If no bony contract is made the needle is re-angled in a cephalad/caudal direction until contact is made with the process. Care should be taken not to angle the needle medially as it may then enter the spinal canal. Ideally the needle point will be in contact with the flat bone of the transverse process at an angle of 90°. It will be clear that the transverse process has been contacted rather than the side of a vertebral body from the characteristic firm 'feel' of the contact. The depth of the L3 or L4 transverse process is very variable, being dependent on gender and body mass index, but is unlikely to be more than 8 cm from the skin. The needle is then 'walked off' the transverse process in a cephalad or caudal direction until it just slips past the bone into the posterior part of the psoas muscle. A 'loss of resistance' can usually be detected not more than 0.5–1 cm anterior to the posterior surface of the transverse process. If ultrasound/nerve stimulation techniques are not being used, and imaging is available, then positioning in the psoas sheath can be confirmed using 1–2 ml of a suitable X-ray contrast (e.g. Omnipaque) and screening in the anterior–posterior plane. The contrast will track towards the pelvis in the direction of the psoas muscle.

Injection

A single shot of bupivacaine 0.25% 10–20 ml with methylprednisolone (Depomedrone) 80 mg can be injected. A catheter may be inserted, and this can be tunnelled under the skin to a convenient position for the patient and attached to an external pump as for epidural or intrathecal infusions. Depending on the degree of spread required, an infusion rate of 5–10 ml/h of bupivacaine may be needed.

Complications

Some degree of weakness and / or numbness of the lower limb, and in particular weakness of hip flexion on the side of the block is to be expected. Epidural / paravertebral spread of the injectate may cause a degree of neurological deficit and rarely hypotention may occur. Haematoma and infection, including a psoas abscess may occur.

Femoral nerve block

Positioning

This block is undertaken with the patient supine. It may be helpful to place a pillow under the buttocks.

Procedure

The femoral artery on the affected side is located by palpation and a needle inserted lateral to the pulsation, over the femoral nerve where it passes under the inguinal ligament enclosed in the femoral sheath. The needle is directed in a cephalad direction and advanced slowly until parasthesia is elicited or correct placement identified using ultrasound (64) or stimulation. The nerve is quite superficial and will usually be found no more than 1–2 cm beneath the skin.

Injection

Care should be taken to avoid inter neural injection, the needle being withdrawn slightly before injection if eliciting parasthesia is being used for nerve localization. A single-shot injection of a relatively large volume of local anaesthetic can be used to provide rapid onset dense analgesia for control of pain following fractures (e.g. 40 ml 0.25% bupivacaine). Often a catheter is inserted to provide continuous analgesia (55). This technique has been successfully used for the management of cancer pain (65).

Complications

Some degree of lower limb weakness and numbness is to be expected. Haematoma may occur, particularly following damage to the femoral artery, and permanent parasthesia and neuropathic pain can following injury to the femoral nerve.

Neurolytic block in the lower limb

There is a limited place for neurolytic blocks of the lower limb, which should be undertaken with extreme caution. However, they do offer the advantage of continuous pain relief without the need for an indwelling neuraxial, paravertebral or lumbar plexus catheter and infusion (66), and the consequences of permanent motor block induced by these agents is not relevant to patients who already have no useful motor function in the limb or who have had amputations.

Intrathecal neurolytic blocks

Intrathecal chemical neurolytic solutions were first used in 1931 by Doglotti (67), who used alcohol injections for sciatica. Twenty-five years later Maher (68) used hyperbaric phenol intrathecally, saying it is 'easier to lay a carpet than to paper a ceiling', meaning that the spread of a hyperbaric solution (phenol) in the CSF is easier to control than a hypobaric one (alcohol). The emergence of neuraxial opioids and reversible methods of pain control, and fear of the unwanted side effects of intrathecal neurolysis, such as loss of bladder and bowel control and muscle weakness, has almost brought the technique to the point of extinction, but it should not be forgotten as a means of treating cancer pain, as explained in an interesting recent review article by Candido and Stevens (69).

In their article Candido and Stevens remind us that the physical separation of the dorsal and ventral nerve roots in the spinal canal theoretically allow disruption of the sensory fibres while preserving motor function (Fig. 8.4). The fine dorsal rootlets (fila radicularia, which supply the extremities), where the nerve roots attach to the spinal cord, are more susceptible than the nerve roots themselves to the action of neurolytic agents. The goal of therapy is to selectively destroy the nociceptive input to the spinal cord via a selective block of these rootlets and roots between the spinal cord and the dorsal root ganglion. The effect is not permanent, as axonal regeneration will occur. The challenge of the technique is to confine the spread of the injected substance to precisely the right nerve roots and rootlets to have the desired effect without blocking motor fibres. When using phenol, the area to be blocked is dependent; when using alcohol, the area to be blocked is uppermost. When the patient is in the lateral position a 45° tilt is used to direct the injectate towards the dorsal nerve roots (Fig. 8.5).

Neurolytic block is said to be more effective for visceral and somatic pain than for neuropathic pain, though no definitive studies have been performed to confirm this, and the pain should be known to be well localized and consistent before these blocks are considered. Other alternatives are tried first, and it is wise to perform a test dose with intrathecal local anaesthetic. The patient should understand that weakness of bowel and bladder sphincters and leg muscle weakness are potential side effects, and that there is no firm evidence to support the technique; there is historical and anecdotal evidence only. Intrathecal neurolysis is now usually confined to a limited block of the lower sacral nerve roots, using a hyperbaric solution. The patient is in the sitting position so that the solution is directed to the lowest sacral roots of the cauda equina.

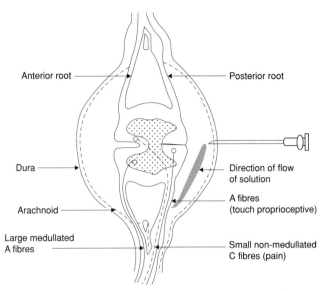

Fig. 8.4 Cross-section of spinal cord to show separation of dorsal (sensory) and ventral (motor) roots for intrathecal neurolysis.

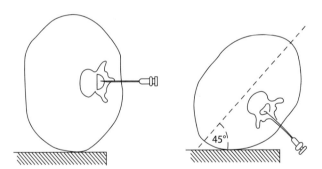

Fig. 8.5 Positioning for hyperbaric intrathecal injection.

Neurolytic agents

Phenol is hyperbaric and is manufactured as an aqueous solution or mixed with glycerol. As it is relatively insoluble in water, 7.5% is the strongest aqueous solution available. The usual strength used is 6% aqueous phenol or 5% phenol in glycerol. The latter is a viscous solution and hard to inject through a small-gauge needle. Warming phenol in glycerol prior to injection makes it much easier to inject. Clinically, phenol acts initially as a local anaesthetic, giving a feeling of warmth and numbness. The pain may return at 24 h, and it then produces chronic, non-selective denervation. The degree of neural destruction produced with be greater with higher concentrations. Phenol in glycerol is rapidly diluted in CSF, such that after 15 min the concentration is 0.1% of the original. Pain relief typically lasts for two months or more.

Alcohol is available in ampoules of 100% concentration. It is hypobaric with respect to CSF, and is very soluble, so the patient has to be positioned with the affected part uppermost. It spreads rapidly and high volumes may be required to have the desired effect, which makes a localized effect much more difficult to achieve. Forty per cent alcohol appears to be equivalent to 3% phenol, this is the minimum concentration required to produce neurolysis. Alcohol is irritant and causes burning dysaesthesias when injected. The duration of analgesia may be longer than that of phenol— over six months in one study (70). With alcohol, the axon may regenerate over its former course, in contrast to phenol, so that function does return, and complications are fewer.

Indications for intrathecal neurolytic block

Although intrathecal neurolysis has been used for localized nerve root pain, especially in the thoracic region, its use now is restricted to low sacral, rectal and perineal pain from cancer, especially where there is a colostomy and/or urinary diversion, where bladder function is already compromised or where the patient is already confined to bed.

Lumbar puncture is performed in the midline at L5/S1 with a 20G spinal needle (viscous phenol cannot easily be injected down a finer needle) with the patient in the sitting position. Aliquots (0.2ml) of warmed 5% phenol in glycerol are injected and the patient is asked to report any feelings of warmth and numbness. One millilitre is usually sufficient to anaesthetize the perineum, but up to 2 ml may be used. The patient remains sitting for 45 min after the block. This will produce a 'saddle block', which can be very effective for patients with intractable perineal pain not responding well to systemic analgesia (71). As with other neurolytic procedures it is advisable to undertake a 'test block' with local anaesthetic (i.e. an intrathecal block with heavy bupivicaine) to allow the patient the possibility of experiencing the effects of neurolysis before undertaking the definitive procedure.

Conclusions

Despite advances in the pharmacotherapy of cancer pain, neuroablative techniques and neuroaxial delivery of analgesics, a clear place for peripheral nerve blocks exists. In the field of acute pain management peripheral nerve blocks are being increasingly used to good effect: in expert hands they provide superb pain control with few side effects. As the described techniques for peripheral nerve block become better known, and more expertise is gained in nerve localization and infusion techniques as used in acute pain, it can be expected that this expertise can be made available to more patients with cancer pain. As always, careful patient assessment and a multidisciplinary approach to what are often very complex situations is the key to delivering the highest quality care possible to the limited group of patients that would be expected to benefit from peripheral nerve block.

Case study

A pain in the bottom

Fred's life was dedicated to the rhythm of the seasons and the local produce shows. This season he'd had an anterior resection for colon cancer and had missed a few important planting dates. We met in A&E one sunny August afternoon. He had come because the pain in his 'tail' was impossible, the drugs he was on made no sense to him and were not helping. His wife had had enough of it all.

We discussed the options—he was 100% against 'pills' of any description—they just did not work and just made him sick and sleepy, and there was no way he was having any more investigations or treatments. His priorities were pain relief, pain relief and pain relief. He had 'a red hot poker up the bottom', which was getting hotter by the day, and was most certainly *not* interested in any theories as to why. There was nothing to see on clinical examination, other than a normal looking rectum with what appeared to be completely normal skin with normal sensation around it. His colostomy worked fine and he'd declined a reversal. We had a detailed discussion as to the advisability and merits of an intrathecal block, first with local anaesthetic, then with phenol if he accepted the possibility of permanent side effects.

To his wife's delight he was admitted. The test block (heavy bupivicane) provided him with excellent analgesia, and we obliged his demands for the 'real block' the next day. Within an hour of the 0.5 ml phenol in glycerol being administered he promptly got up and discharged himself—his garden was waiting!

That evening he returned to A&E—this time with abdominal pain. Acute retention was the clear diagnosis, easily solved in time for him to get back up his ladder and picking his plums before nightfall. These had been carefully thinned in June and July and were now large, ripe, juicy and destined for a prize. He'd had 'a prostrate' a few seasons before, and knew all about catheters. They were very convenient, particularly for evenings in the pub with his mates after a hard day's digging.

Of course we booked him an outpatient appointment, and liaised carefully with the district nurses and his GP, but he told us he'd be back if/when he needed us—and that was the end of the matter.

Learning point

Consider the use of intrathecal phenol blocks for patients with localised neuropathic pain in the perineum which has not responded to other treatments.

References

1. Chambers WA (2008). Nerve blocks in palliative care. *Br J Anaesth* **101**(1), 95–100.
2. Joshi M, Chambers WA (2010). Pain relief in palliative care: a focus on interventional pain management. *Expert Rev Neurother* **10**(5), 747–56.
3. Tay W, Ho KY (2009). The role of interventional therapies in cancer pain management. *Ann Acad Med Singapore* **38**(11), 989–97.

4. Keller SM, Carp NZ, Levy MN, Rosen SM (1994). Chronic post thoracotomy pain. *J Cardiovasc Surg (Torino)* **35**(6 Suppl 1), 161–4.

5. Hans GH, Robert DN, van Maldeghem KN (2008). Treatment of an acute severe central neuropathic pain syndrome by topical application of lidocaine 5% patch: a case report. *Spinal Cord* **46**(4), 311–3.

6. Tran de QH, Munoz L, Russo G, Finlayson RJ (2008). Ultrasonography and stimulating perineural catheters for nerve blocks: a review of the evidence. *Can J Anaesth* **55**(7), 447–57.

7. Heavner JE (2007). Local anesthetics. *Curr Opin Anaesthesiol* **20**(4), 336–42.

8. Huschak G, Rüffert H, Wehner M, *et al.* (2009). Pharmacokinetics and clinical toxicity of prilocaine and ropivacaine following combination drug administration in brachial plexus anesthesia. *Int J Clin Pharmacol Ther* **47**(12), 733–43.

9. Leone S, Di Cianni S, Casati A, Fanelli G (2008). Pharmacology, toxicology, and clinical use of new long acting local anaesthetics, ropivacaine and levobupivacaine. *Acta Biomed* **79**(2), 92–105.

10. Weiniger CF, Golovanevski M, Sokolsky-Papkov M, Domb AJ (2010). Review of prolonged local anesthetic action. *Expert Opin Drug Deliv* **7**(6), 737–52.

11. Johansson A, Hao J, Sjölund B (1990). Local corticosteroid application blocks transmission in normal nociceptive C fibres. *Acta Anaesthesiol Scand* **34**(5), 335–8.

12. Jackson TP, Gaeta R (2008). Neurolytic blocks revisited. *Curr Pain Headache Rep* **12**(1), 7–13.

13. Cornish PB, Leaper CJ, Nelson G *et al.* (2007). Avoidance of phrenic nerve paresis during continuous supraclavicular regional anaesthesia. *Anaesthesia* **62**(4), 354–8.

14. Weinberg GL (2010). Treatment of local naesthetic toxicity (LAST). *Reg Anesth Pain Med* **35**(2), 188–93.

15. Zausig YA, Zink W, Keilm M *et al.* (2009). Lipid emulsion improves recovery from bupivacaine-induced cardiac arrest, but not from ropivacaine- or mepivacaine induced cardiac arrest. *Anaesth Analg* **109**(4), 1323–6.

16. Kopp SL, Wynd KP, Horlocker TT *et al.* (2009). Regional blockade in patients with a history of seizure disorder. *Anaesth Analg* **109**(1), 272–8.

17. Bleckner LL, Bina S, Kwon KH *et al.* (2010). Serum ropivavaine concentrations and systemic local anesthetic toxicity in trauma patients receiving long term continuous peripheral nerve block catheters. *Anaesth Analg* **110**(2), 630–4.

18. Dhir S, Ganapathy S, Linsay P, Athwal GS (2007). Case report: ropivacaine neurotoxicity at clinical doses in interscalene brachial plexus block. *Can J Anaesth* **54**(11), 912–6.

19. Vadivelu N, Screck M, Lopez J *et al.* (2008). Pain after mastectomy and breast reconstruction. *Am Surg* **74**(4), 285–96.

20. Defalque RJ (1982). Painful trigger points in surgical scars. *Anaesth Analg* **61**(6), 518–20.

21. Han SC, Harrison P (1997). Myofascila pain syndrome and trigger-point management. *Reg Anesth* **22**(1), 89–101.

22. Cummings TM, White AR (2001). Needling therapies in the management of myofascial trigger point pain: a systematic review. *Arch Phys Med Rehabil* **82**(7), 986–92.

23. Torres Lacomba M, Mayoral del Moral O, Coperias Zazo JL, Gerwin RD Goñí AZ *et al.* (2010). Incidence of myofascial pain syndrome in breast cancer surgery: a prospective study. *Clin J Pain* **26**(4), 320–5.

24. Tamimi MA, McCeney MH, Krutsch J (2009). A case series of pulsed frequency treatment of myofascial trigger points and scar neuromas. *Pain Med* **10**(6), 1140–3.

25. Wong FC, Lee TW, Yuen KK *et al.* (2007). Intercostal nerve blockade for cancer pain: effectiveness and selection of patient. *Hong Kong Med J* **13**(4), 266–70.

26. Dravid RM, Paul RE (2007). Interpleural block–Part 1. *Anaesthesia* **62**(10), 1039–49.

27. Dravid RM, Paul RE (2007). Interpleural block–Part 2. *Anaesthesia* **62**(11), 1143–53.

28. Demmy TL, Nwogu C, Solan P *et al.* (2009). Chest tube delivered bupivacaine improves pain and decreases opioid use after thoracoscopy. *Ann Thorac Surge* **87**(4), 1040–6.

29. Amesbury B, O'Riordan J, Dolin S (1999). The use of interpleural analgesia using bupivacaine for pain relief in advanced cancer. *Palliat Med* **13**(2), 153–8.

30. Mercadante S, Sapio M, Villari P (1995). Suprascapular nerve block by catheter for breakthrough shoulder cancer pain. *Reg Anesth* **20**(4), 343–6.

31. Petersen PL, Mathiesen O, Torup H, Dahl JB (2010). The transversus abdominis plan block: a valualble option for postoperative analgesia? A topical review. *Acta Anaesthesiol Scand* **54**(5), 529–33.

32. Thompson GE, Rorie DK (1983). Functional anatomy of the brachial plexus sheaths. *Anaesthesiology* **59**(2), 117–22.

33. De Tran QH, Clemente A, Doan J, Finlayson RJ (2007). Brachial plexus blocks: a review of approaches and techniques. *Can J Anaesth* **54**(6), 662–74.

34. Bowen BC, Pattany PM, Saraf-Lavi E, Maravilla KR (2004). The brachial plexus: normal anatomy, pathology and MR imaging. *Neuroimaging Clin N Am* **14**(1), 59–85.

35. Qavyum A, MacVicar AD, Padhani AR *et al.* (2000). Symptomatic brachial plexopathy following treatment for breast cancer:utility of MR imaging with surface-coil techniques. *Radiology* **214**(3), 837–42.

36. De Tran QH, Clemente A, Doan J, Finlayson RJ (2007). Brachial plexus blocks: a review of approaches and techniques. *Can J Anaesth* **54**(8), 662–74.

37. Vranken JH, van der Vegt MH, Zuurmond WW *et al.* (2001). Continuous brachial plexus block at the cervical level using a posterior approach in the management of neuropathic cancer pain. *Reg Anesth Pain Med* **26**(6), 572–5.

38. Vranken JH. Zuurmond WW, de Lang JJ (2000). Continuous brachial plexus block as a treatment for the Pancoast syndrome. *Clin J Pain.* **16**(4), 327–33.

39. Wang MY, Teitelbauum GP, Loskota WJ *et al.* (2000). Brachial plexus catheter reservoir for the treatment of upper-extremity cancer pain: technical case report. *Neurosurgery* **46**(4), 1009–12.

40. Rettig HC, Leron JG, Gielen MJ *et al.* (2007). The pharmacokinetics of ropivacaine after four different techniques of brachial plexus blockade. *Anaesthesia* **62**(10), 1008–14.

41. Satsumae T, Tanaka M, Saito S, Inomata S (2008). Convulsions after ropivacaine 300mg for brachial plexus block. *Br J Anaesth* **101**(6), 860–2.

42. Pedro JR. Mathias LA, Gozzani JL *et al.* (2009). supraclavicular brachial plexus block: a comparative clinical study between bupivacaine and levobupivacaine. *Rev Bras Anestesiol* **59**(6), 665–73.

43. Renes SH, Rettig HC, Gielen MJ *et al.* (2009). Ultrasound- guided low-dose interscalene brachial plexus block reduces the incidence of hemidiaphragmatic paresis. *Reg Anesth Pain Med* **34**(5), 498–502.

44. Cornish PB, Leaper CJ, Nelson G *et al.* (2007). Avoidance of phrenic nerve paresis during continuous supraclavicular regional anaesthesia. *Anaesthesia* **62**(4), 354–8.

45. Holborow J, Hocking G (2010). Regional anaesthesia for bilateral upper limb surgery: a review of challenges and solutions. *Anaesth Intensive Care* **38**(2), 250–8.

46. Capdevila X, Jaber S, Pesonen P *et al.* (2008). Acute neck cellulites and mediastinitis complicating a continuous interscalene block. *Anaeth Analg* **107**(4), 1419–21.

47. Di Benedetto P, Pinto G, Arcioni R *et al.* (2005). Anatomy and imaging of lumbar plexus. *Minervera Anestesiol* **71**(9), 549–54.

48. Planner AC, Donaghy M, Moore NR (2006). Causes of lumbosacral plexopathy. *Clin Radiol* **61**(12), 987–95.

49. Dropcho EJ (2010). Neurotoxicity of radiatioin therapy. *Neurol Clin* **28**(1), 217–34.

50. Agar M, Broadbent A, Chye R (2004). The management of malignant psoas syndrome: case reports and literature review. *J Pain Symptom Manage* **28**(3), 282–93.

51. Stevens MJ, Atkinson C, Broadbent AM (2010). The malignant psoas syndrome revisited: case report: mechanisms, and current therapeutic options. *J Palliat Med* **13**(2), 211–6.

52. Douglas I, Bush D (1999). The use of patient-controlled boluses of local anaesthetic via a psoas sheath catheter in the management of malignant pain. *Pain* **82**(1), 105–7.

53. Fowler SJ, Symons J, Sabato S, Myles PS (2008). Epidural analgesia compaired with peripheral nerve blockade after major knee surgery: a systematic review and meta-analysis of randomized trials. *Br J Aneasth* **100**(2), 154–64.

54. Hogan MV, Grant RE, Lee L (2009). Analgesia for total hip and knee arthroplasty: a review of lumbar plexus, femoral, and sciatic nerve blocks. *Am J Orthop (Belle Mead NJ)* **38**(8), E129–33.

55. Capdevila, X, Macaire P, Dadure C *et al.* (2002). Continuous psoas compartment block for postoperative analgesia after total hip arthroplasty: new landmarks, technical guidelines, and clinical evaluation. *Anesth Analg* **94**(6), 1606–13.

56. Ozalp G, Kaya M, Tuncel G *et al.* (2007). The analgesia efficacy of two different approaches to the lumbar plexus for patient-controlled analgesia after total knee replacement. *J Anesth* **21**(3), 409–12.

57. Grays Anatomy–on line version. From Gray's Anatomy, 6d The Lumbosacral Plexus http://www.freebookcentre.net/medical_books_download/Gray's-Anatomy.html

58. Orebaugh SL, Williams BA (2009). Brachial plexus anatomy: normal and variant. *Scientific World* **9**, 300–12.

59. Fingerman M, Benonis JG, Martin G (2009). A practical guide to commonly performed ultrasound-guided peripheral-nerve blocks. *Curr Opin Anaesthesiol* **22**(5), 600–7.

60. Kori SH (1995). Diagnosis and management of brachial plexus lesions in cancer patients. *Oncology* **9**(8), 756–60.

61. Lema MJ (2001). Invasive analgesia techniques for advanced cancer pain. *Surg Oncol Clin N Am* **10**(1), 127–36.

62. Tran D, Clemete A, Finlayson RJ (2007). A review of approaches and techniques for lower extremity nerve blocks. *Can J Anaesth* **54**(11), 922–34.

63. Awad IT, Duggan FM (2005). Posterior lumbar plexus block: anatomy, approaches and techniques. *Reg Anesth Pain Med* **30**(2), 143–9.

64. Marhofer P, Harrop-Griffiths W, Willschke H, Kirchmair L (2010). Fifteen years of ultrasound guidance in regional anaesthesia: Part 2–recent development in block techniques. *Br J Anaesth* **104**(6), 673–83.

65. Pacenta HL, Kaddoum RN, Pereiras LA *et al.* (2010). Continuous tunnelled femoral nerve block for palliative care of a patient with metastatic osteosarcoma. *Anaesth Intensive Care* **38**(3), 563–5.

66. Calava JM, Patt RB, Reddy S *et al.* (1996). Psoas sheath chemical neurolysis for management of intractable leg pain from metastatic liposarcoma. *Clin J Pain* **12**(1), 69–75.

67. Dogliotti AM (1931). Traitement des syndromes doloreux de la peripherie par l'alcoholisation subarachnoidienne des raciness posterieure à leur emergence de la moelle epineri. *Presse Medicale.* **39**, 1249–52.

68. Maher RM (1955). Relief of pain in incurable cancer. *Lancet* **268**(6853), 18–20.

69. Candido K, Stevens R (2003). Intrathecal neurolytic blocks for the relief of cancer pain. *Best Pract Res Clin Anaesthesiol* **17**(3), 407–28.

70. Parese DM (1958). Subarachnoid alcohol block in the management of pain of malignant disease. *Arch Surgery* **76**(3), 347–54.

71. Slatkin NE, Rhiner M (2003). Phenol saddle blocks for intractable pain at the end of life: report of four cases and literature review. *Am J Hosp Palliat Care* **20**(1), 62–6.

Chapter 9

Blocks of the autonomic nervous system

Richard Griffiths, Jon Norman, and Kevin Fai

This chapter describes the anatomy of the autonomic nervous system and explains its role in the processing of visceral pain from cancer, as far as it is currently understood. The following nerve blocks are considered in detail and their place in the management of cancer pain evaluated:

◆ stellate ganglion

◆ thoracic sympathetic chain

◆ coeliac plexus

◆ splanchnic nerves

◆ lumbar sympathetic chain

◆ superior hypogastric plexus

◆ ganglion of Impar

◆ vagus nerve

Introduction

The autonomic nervous system regulates non-voluntary functions. The sympathetic division lies along the length of the axial skeleton and its various plexi and ganglia are accessible to interruption using percutaneous or surgical techniques. Autonomic blocks may be considered when non-interventional techniques fail to give satisfactory pain relief and/or medication is causing unacceptable side effects (1–6). Blockade of the coeliac plexus is the most commonly performed block of the autonomic nervous system in cancer patients, and is used for controlling pain secondary to upper abdominal malignancy, particularly carcinoma of the pancreas. Lumbar sympathetic block may be performed for tenesmus and superior hypogastric plexus block for controlling pain relating to pelvic malignancies.

   When considering the place of these techniques the balance of potential benefits should be weighed against risks. Major vessels and viscera (including lungs heart and gastrointestinal tract) all lie in close proximity to the target for blockade or in the likely path of the needle used. Thus the potential for harm when performing autonomic blocks is considerable, particularly if neurolytic solutions are being injected. The incidence of such complications is hard to quantify, but if they are to be minimized these procedures should be carried out by a skilled clinician with a clear understanding of the risks in a facility equipt to deal with immediate and late complications.

Most importantly, the patient requires clear guidance as to the likely benefits and risks of the intended procedure and they or their advocate must be in a position to make an informed choice and give informed consent in accordance with General Medical Council guidance (5).

Anatomy and function of the autonomic nervous system

The autonomic nervous system is the part of the nervous system that regulates non-voluntary functions of the cardiorespiratory system, gastrointestinal tract and other body systems. It is divided into the sympathetic and parasympathetic systems which differ in their function, anatomy and pharmacology, as shown in Fig. 9.1.

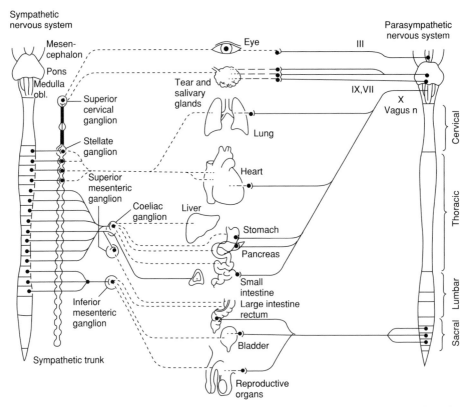

Fig. 9.1 Outline diagram of the autonomic nervous system. Reproduced from Janig, W. (1995). In Physiologie des menschen (Ed. R. F. Schmidt and G. Thews), 26th edn, pp. 340–69, Springer Verlag, Heidelberg, Berlin, with permission Also appears in colour in the colour plate section, Plate 34.

The sympathetic nervous system

The sympathetic chain is composed of two ganglionic trunks that progress inferiorly from the base of the brain, through the neck, thorax and abdomen, where they run in the retroperitoneal space over the antero-lateral aspect of the vertebral column. These two chains merge into a solitary structure anterior to the vertebral column at the approximate level of the sacro-coccygeal junction.

The sympathetic nervous system sends pre-ganglionic fibres from the mediolateral columns of the spinal cord into the ventral roots at T1–L2. They pass via the white rami communicans into the ganglionated sympathetic chain which comprises:

- three cervical ganglia
- one stellate ganglion
- eleven thoracic ganglia
- five lumbar ganglia
- four sacral ganglia
- one coccygeal ganglion (ganglion of Impar)

The sympathetic trunk lies at the anterolateral aspect of the vertebral bodies in the cervical region and descends in the neck behind the carotid sheath before entering the thoracic cavity. In the thorax it lies over the necks of the ribs close to the somatic nerve roots. It enters the abdomen behind the medial arcuate ligament of the diaphragm anterolateral to the bodies of the lumbar vertebrae. In the lumbar region it is separated from the somatic nerve roots by the psoas muscle and fascia. It then descends into the pelvis, lying anterior to the sacral ala. The two chains terminate on the anterior surface of the coccyx forming the ganglion of Impar (or Walther). Sympathetic innervation of the viscera is carried via the cardiac, coeliac and hypogastric plexuses.

The function of the sympathetic nervous system is complex and beyond the remit of this chapter. Broadly, it provides efferent transmission to the eye, heart, blood vessels, lungs, gut, adrenals, kidney and pelvic organs. Its effects are characterized by the phrase: 'fight or flight', i.e. pupil dilation, increased cardio-respiratory performance, decreased gut motility and decreased pelvic organ activity. Afferent transmission of pain and temperature are thought to contribute to the pathophysiology of some painful states, hence interruption may relieve pain (7).

Parasympathetic nervous system

The parasympathetic nervous system consists of myelinated pre-ganglionic efferent fibres from the nuclei of the cranial nerves three, seven, nine and ten, and the spinal nerves S2, S3 and S4. They pass directly to the target organs, namely the walls of the viscera, where they synapse with short non-myelinated post-ganglionic fibres. The vagus nerve carries approximately 75% of all parasympathetic fibres and it innervates the heart, lungs, liver and gastrointestinal viscera up to the splenic flexure. The pelvic parasympathetic nerves run directly as pelvic splanchnic nerves to the pelvic plexuses, and from there they run uninterrupted to the walls of the bladder, gut and sex organs.

The effects of parasympathetic stimulation include vasodilatation, increased gut motility and relaxation of sphincters.

Visceral pain

The characteristics of visceral and somatic pain differ (8, 9, 10). Visceral pain is diffuse, poorly localized and occurs as a response to a variety of different stimuli (e.g. distension of a hollow organ, ischaemia, traction on the mesentery, malignant invasion of nerve plexuses or endogenous chemical release). These characteristics are thought to be secondary to sparse efferent innervation spread over several spinal segments (including contralateral innervation) (9). Examples of acute visceral pain include urinary colic and acute myocardial ischaemia. Convergence of spinal afferent inputs may give rise to the phenomenon of referred pain, for example from the liver to the shoulder tip. Chronic visceral pain arising from abdominal malignancy can be particularly difficult to manage, and sympathetic blocks can be usefully employed in addition to medical management to relieve pain and nausea (8, 9, 10).

It is important that the nature of pain is correctly diagnosed and that its assumed origin correlates with scan findings and knowledge of the disease. Somatic and visceral pains often coexist and somatic pain will not be alleviated by an autonomic block. In these circumstances a neuraxial block will offer better pain relief. The importance of accurate diagnosis of the pain type and sources cannot be overstated (See Chapter 3).

Several mechanisms have been proposed for how sympathetic interruption can reduce pain (10).

1. Interruption of visceral sensory afferents. Sympathetic efferents accompany visceral sensory afferents. Blockade of the sympathetic ganglia interrupts these pathways and may reduce pain from the viscera.

2. Reduction in sympathetic tone resulting in vasodilatation and increased perfusion. This has the potential to reduce the pain of tissue ischaemia caused by vascular insufficiency.

3. Reduction in pain maintained by the sympathetic nervous system (sympathetically mediated pain). Following nerve or tissue injury pain may be maintained by sympathetic efferent activity and by circulating catecholamines.

General indications for sympathetic blockade

Several conditions may benefit from interruption of the sympathetic nervous system (3, 11, 12, 13).

Visceral pain

Pain caused by abdominal or pelvic malignancy may be alleviated by neurolytic sympathetic blockade, which has also been advocated for pain in the urinary system (loin-pain haematuria syndrome) and chronic pelvic pain. Additionally, patients with intractable angina may benefit from stellate ganglion blockade.

Peripheral vascular disease

Sympathetic nerve blocks may benefit those with end stage occlusive arterial disease, predominately in the lower limbs.

Hyperhidrosis, complex regional pain syndrome and chronic neuropathic pain.

Sympathetic blockade leads to anhidrosis (lack of sweating). Percutaneous chemical lumbar sympathectomy and endoscopic transthoracic sympathectomy have been used for the treatment of excessive sweating of the feet and hands respectively, but can induce compensatory sweating in other parts of the body and are now rarely indicated for these conditions. BoTox injections are now the treatments of choice for excessive sweating. Stellate ganglion block and lumbar sympathectomy have been traditionally used to treat reflex sympathetic dystrophy (RSD), now commonly known as complex regional pain syndrome (CPRS) (11). However, the aetiology of CRPS is complex, the pain and associated symptoms are unlikely to be sympathetically maintained, and these blocks are now rarely used for this indication. Sympathetic nervous system dysfunction has been implicated in neuropathic pain, although this may have been overemphasized.

General Contraindications to Sympathetic Blockade

Coagulopathy, the presence of local infection or tumour in the intended path of the needle track, relevant anatomical abnormalities, hypovolemia and unavailability of adequate resuscitation facilities are usually contraindications to these procedures (3, 12). The close proximity of the sympathetic trunk to major blood vessels, e.g. the aorta during coeliac plexus blockade, make it particularly important that sympathetic blockade is not carried out in the presence of abnormal blood clotting,. Imaging may be necessary to determine the position of the tumour prior to a procedure. Alternative entry points, e.g. an anterior or a posterior approach to the coeliac plexus, may circumvent the need to pass a needle through a tumour and risk spreading malignant cells to previously unaffected areas. Abnormalities in the anatomy of the spinal column (e.g. scoliosis) or in the local vasculature (e.g. of the carotid sheath) may make access to the target area less reliable, and increase the likelihood of damage to adjacent structures. Patients who are hypovolemic, or have limited cardiovascular reserve, are particularly susceptible to hypotension secondary to loss of sympathetic vasomotor tone, making it essential that these blocks are only carried out in environments where skilled assistance and resuscitation facilities are available (3, 12).

Injectates and lesioning

Many descriptions of sympathetic nerve blockade involve a diagnostic block using local anaesthetic, which if successful is then followed by a therapeutic (neurolytic) block using alcohol or phenol (3, 12, 13, 14). Steroids have been used, and radiofrequency lesioning of the sympathetic trunk has been described as an alternative to chemical neurolysis (15).

Chemical neurolysis using alcohol or phenol

Alcohol (commonly 50%) causes Wallerian degeneration of nerves in a non-specific manner. Regeneration of the nerve usually occurs within three or four months, although there is a risk of developing post-neurolysis deafferentation neuralgia, which may occur less commonly than when using phenol (16).

Phenol (typically 5–12% formulated in water) destroys sensory and motor nerves by protein denaturation. It causes neuritis on contact with somatic nerves (though less so than alcohol) and can cause soft tissue ulceration if injected subcutaneously (16).

Radiofrequency lesioning

Radiofrequency lesioning involves the use of electricity to generate heat. A well-circumscribed lesion is formed around the tip of the probe (which does not itself heat up) in the shape of a matchstick head with a diameter of 2–4 mm. Radiofrequency lesions cause Wallerian degeneration, and in all nerve fibres delayed axonal regeneration follows. The precise pathophysiology is not yet clear, although regeneration of axons occurs over a matter of months. Deafferentation pain has been described following radiofrequency lesioning of somatic nerves (15).

Complications of sympathetic blocks

The general complications may be stratified into those caused by the needle insertion (e.g. local bruising, pain at injection site, injury to blood vessels and viscera, transmission of infection or tumour along a needle tract) and those caused by the injectate (e.g. neuritis, tissue necrosis, induction of anaesthesia dolorosa [pain in an area of numbness], motor paralysis, cardiovascular, urological and sexual dysfunction) (16). Each block has possible specific complications related to the anatomical site, and these are described separately in the relevant sections of this chapter.

Stellate ganglion block
Anatomy

The stellate ganglion takes its name from the Latin word for star. It is formed from the fusion of the inferior cervical ganglion and the first thoracic ganglion in 80% of the population. In the remaining 20% they exist as individual entities. The preganglionic fibres originate from the anterolateral horn of the spinal cord at a thoracic level. Head and neck fibres originate from T1 and T2 before synapsing in the cervical ganglia. Postganglionic fibres travel with the carotid artery, cervical plexus and upper cervical roots. Upper-limb fibres originate from T2–8 and synapse in the inferior cervical and upper two thoracic ganglia. The postganglionic fibres join either the brachial plexus or the subclavian perivascular plexus.

The stellate ganglion lies anterior to the neck of the first rib, in a fascial space between the prevertebral muscles posteriorly and the carotid sheath anteriorly. The dome of the pleura lies anterior to its lower part and the vertebral artery lies anterior to its upper part, although there are variations in the anatomy in relation to the cervical spine (17).

Indications

Stellate ganglion block has been used for a range of painful conditions including carcinomatous infiltration of the brachial plexus, carcinoma of the head, neck, upper chest and breast, complex regional pain syndrome, acute herpes zoster and intractable angina (12).

Specific contraindications and complications

Recent myocardial infarction, contralateral pneumothorax or pneumonectomy, and the presence of glaucoma increase the risks of undertaking this procedure. Specific complications include an increase in intraocular pressure, and inadvertent intravascular, epidural or intrathecal injection of local anaesthetic and/or neurolytic solution. There is a risk of inducing seizure activity and induction of loss of consciousness even if very small volumes of local anaesthetic are injected into the vertebral artery, and epidural or intrathecal injection at this level can cause total paralysis and cardiovascular collapse. Blockade of other nerves in close proximity to the site injected can cause hoarseness (recurrent laryngeal nerve), diaphragmatic paralysis (phrenic nerve) and Horner's syndrome (middle and superior cervical ganglion). Injury to the vagus nerve, brachial plexus, lung, thoracic duct and oesophagus have been described (12).

Techniques

C6 anterior (paratracheal) approach

This is the most commonly described technique. It is often performed blind, but accuracy can be supplemented by the use of fluoroscopic guidance.

Positioning and procedure The patient lies supine with their head a neutral position. The jaw should be slightly open to prevent swallowing or talking, as these movements may displace the needle tip. The tip of the 6th lateral transverse process (Chaussaignac's tubercle) is located by palpation at the level of the cricoid cartilage and the skin infiltrated with local anaesthetic (Fig. 9.2). The carotid sheath and sternocleidomastoid are then displaced laterally and a needle inserted perpendicularly until it contacts the transverse process (typically at 2–3 cm). Undertaking fluoroscopy prior to inserting the needle 2 cm allows the needle trajectory to be ascertained. Classically periosteal injection is avoided by withdrawing the needle 2–3 mm before injecting. If fluoroscopy indicates that the needle tip is on the more medial aspect of the transverse process, then withdrawing up to 5 mm may avoid injection into the longus coli muscle which limits caudad spread. Anatomical variations in the size and location of Chaussaignac's tubercle suggest that targeting the more medial portion of the C6 transverse process increases safety (17). If contrast is used this should spread under the prevertebral fascia in a cephalo-caudad fashion.

Injection After careful aspiration to exclude blood or CSF, in the experience of these authors, injection of 5 ml of bupivacaine 0.25% is usually sufficient to produce a satisfactory block, although up to 15 ml has been described. Cadaveric studies show 10 ml injected at the C6 level can spread as high as C2 and as low as T4 (18). Clinical studies

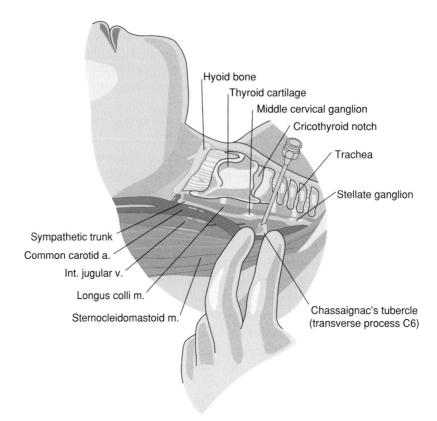

Hyoid bone
Thyroid cartilage
Middle cervical ganglion
Cricothyroid notch
Trachea
Stellate ganglion
Chassaignac's tubercle
(transverse process C6)
Sympathetic trunk
Common carotid a.
Int. jugular v.
Longus colli m.
Sternocleidomastoid m.

Fig. 9.2 Stellate ganglion block—anterior approach. Reproduced from The Atlas of Pain management Injection techniques by Steven D Waldman (2007), Saunders 2nd edition, with permission from Elsevier. Also appears in colour in the colour plate section, Plate 35.

indicate that 5 ml of solution caused spread from C3–T4 using a blind technique (19) and from C3–T2 using an ultrasound-guided technique (20). Cephalad spread to the superior cervical ganglion (C3) or above, leads to Horner's syndrome, with caudad spread below T1 causing vasodilation of the upper limb (19).

Neurolytic techniques involve the use of phenol 6% (3–5 ml) or absolute alcohol (3–4 ml) injected incrementally to effect. Neurolytic injections should ideally be delivered at the level of the stellate ganglion itself. However, given the other important structures in the vicinity, these authors would advocate a radiofrequency-based therapy, which allows sensory and motor testing prior to lesioning and should produce a more predictable result.

C7 anterior approach

This is undertaken in a similar manner to that outlined above, but the needle is inserted, using a blind technique, one finger's breadth caudad to Chassaignac's tubercle. This carries a higher risk of pneumothorax, but allows lower volumes to be utilized. Ackerman and Racz (21) compared 50 blocks at the C6 level using 10 ml of 0.5% bupivacaine versus 50 blocks using 5 ml at the C7 level. The success rates were 82% at C6 and 100% at C7.

Posterior approach

Theoretically neurolytic agents delivered via a lower approach are less likely to cause a permanent Horner's syndrome.

Positioning and procedure The patient lies prone, with the spine in a neutral position. A point 4 cm lateral to the spinous process of T1 or T2 is located and local anaesthetic infiltrated. A 22G 10-cm needle is advanced 3–4 cm perpendicular to the skin to contact the transverse process. If no bone is contacted at 4cm then the needle is either too lateral or passing between the adjacent transverse processes, and appropriate correction is made, with fluoroscopic assistance if needed. Once the transverse process is contacted, the needle is withdraw slightly and re-angled to allow it to pass below the transverse process and advanced to the anterolateral border of the vertebral body, using a similar technique to that employed during lumbar sympathetic blockade. Typically the vertebral body is contacted approximately 3 cm deeper than the transverse process and the final needle tip position will lie approximately 8–9 cm from the entry point (22).

Injection After careful aspiration, 5–7 ml of solution can then be injected. The lower approach allows smaller volumes to be used, although pneumothorax, aortic injury and blockade of the recurrent laryngeal nerve are more likely.

Ultrasound-guided lateral approach

A more contemporary approach is to place the needle under direct vision, utilizing ultrasound. As the stellate ganglion is a relatively superficial structure this approach is feasible. It was initially described in 1995 by Kapral *et al.* (23), who used it to guide the needle towards the transverse process of C6. Since then, there have been two more descriptions of an ultrasound-guided lateral approach (20, 24), both of which aim to place the local anaesthetic below the prevertebral fascia at the posterolateral component of the longus coli muscle. Gofeld *et al.* (20) describe an in-plane lateral approach, which theoretically is much safer than the blind approaches as the needle only has to traverse sternocleidomastoid and scalenus anterior before piercing the prevertebral fascia. Constant direct visualization of the needle tip reduces inadvertent damage to adjacent structures and medication is seen going into the correct tissue plane. These authors injected 0.2 ml of methylene blue into cadavers using ultrasound and found the cervical sympathetic chain at C6 was bathed in dye, thus confirming the accuracy of this technique.

Positioning and procedure—Gofeld The patient is placed in the lateral decubitus position with the side to be blocked uppermost and the head supported to keep the cervical spine straight. The anatomy is identified using a high-frequency linear probe placed at the level of the cricoid cartilage, giving a short-axis view of the C6 vertebra. The prevertebral fascia can be seen as a hyperechogenic white line between the transverse process and the vertebral body. Between the fascia and the vertebra lies the longus coli and longus capitis muscles.The entry point posterior to the probe is infiltrated with local anaesthetic and a 22G short bevelled needle advanced in-plane into the subfascial plane.

Confirmation of needle position can be achieved with normal saline prior to injecting 5 ml of local anaesthetic (20).

Thoracic Sympathetic Block

Anatomy

The exact location of the sympathetic chain at each spinal level is highly variable and, even in the same cadaver, only 16% of individuals have the same anatomy bilaterally (25). The actual position of the ganglia can vary in the antero-posterior plane by up to around 20 mm (26), explaining the variations in textbook descriptions of where to position the needle relative to the vertebral body in the lateral view. In general, however, the upper thoracic ganglia lie more posteriorly than the lower thoracic ganglia. The relations of the sympathetic ganglia include the vertebral body medially, the rib, intercostal muscles and somatic nerve posteriorly, and the pleura anterolaterally.

Indications and use

Thoracic sympathetic blockade has been used to aid a variety of conditions affecting the upper limb and the trunk. However, the proximity of the somatic nerves to the sympathetic trunk has meant that percutaneous techniques have been largely superseded by endoscopic ablation under direct vision. Furthermore, stellate ganglion block can be utilized without the same level of risk in the management of conditions of the upper limb and thoracic wall and for intractable angina. It has been documented that spread from a stellate ganglion block can go as inferiorly as the fourth thoracic ganglion (27). This encompasses the important 'gateway' where preganglionic fibres arising from thoracic levels synapse onto postganglionic fibres. Splanchnic nerve blockade encompasses fibres originating from the lower thoracic levels. Cancer pain is rarely purely sympathetically mediated so that tunnelled epidurals or intrathecal techniques are more often used than sympathetic block for controlling chest and upper abdominal pain secondary to malignancy. Furthermore, ability to cover all thoracic segments using stellate ganglion and splanchnic blockade means that thoracic sympathetic block is rarely performed.

Specific contraindications and complications

Relative contraindications include contralateral pneumothorax or pneumonectomy and thoracic aortic aneurysm.

Complications

Pneumothorax is the main concern and can be made less likely by limiting the needle entry point to a less lateral approach; Erdine (28) recommends staying within 4 cm of the spinous process. Intercostal blockade can be avoided by placement of the needle anteriorly, with careful sensory and motor testing during radiofrequency lesioning. Inadvertant intravascular, epidural, sub-dural or intrathecal injection have been described. Horner's syndrome is associated with cephalad spread of solutions, and is less likely if low volumes are injected.

Technique

Positioning and procedure

The patient should be lying prone with the arms overhanging the edge of the table to manoeuvre the scapulae laterally. Placement of a pillow below the chest can help this further. Alternatively the patient can be sitting upright which may facilitate more accurate imaging. The level to be blocked is identified and an entry point (typically 3–5 cm lateral to the spinous process) is selected and infiltrated with local anaesthetic. A fluoroscopically guided gun-barrel technique can be used to mark this, with the C-arm approximately 20% oblique to the ipsilateral side. A 10-cm 22G needle is then advanced towards the vertebral body to make contact with it. If the transverse process is encountered, the needle can be re-angled to pass cephalad or caudad to it . The final needle-tip position should lie at least at the mid-point of the vertebral body in the lateral view, although several descriptions recomend that the needle tip be placed 2–3 mm posterior to the anterior edge of the vertebral body. Given the variations in anatomy it is prudent to place the needle tip anterior to the midpoint of the vertebral body in order to reduce likelihood of blockade of the emerging somatic nerve. Contrast should spread along the thoracic vertebral column.

Injection

Following careful aspiration, 6–8 ml of solution is injected for a diagnostic block. Typically these authors would use 0.25% bupivacaine containing 40–80 mg methylprednisolone. If neurolytic solutions are to be used then the volume should be restricted to 2-3 ml due to the high likelihood of spread onto the somatic nerve. Gabrhelik *et al.* (29) compared radiofrequency thermocoagulation at both T2 and T3 versus single lesioning at T2 plus 0.5 ml of 6% phenol for the treatment of Raynaud's phenomenon. No statistical difference was demonstrated in outcomes or quality of life, and the authors also claim a lower rate of complications for the first technique, lending support to the general principle suggesting that sensori-motor testing and radiofrequency-based treatment allows better targeting of lesions.

Coeliac plexus and splanchnic nerve block

Coeliac plexus block is perhaps the best established of any autonomic block for cancer pain, having first been described 90 years ago by Labat (30). Since then many techniques have been reported (12).

Anatomy

The splanchnic nerves comprise the greater, lesser and least splanchnic nerves which arise from branches of the sympathetic trunk within the thorax. The nerves contain preganglionic sympathetic and visceral afferent fibres. The anatomy of these nerves varies considerably between individuals. The greater splanchnic nerves arise from T5–T10, the lesser from T9–T12 and the least from T11–T12. The greater splanchnic nerves descend obliquely on the anterolateral aspect of the thoracic vertebral bodies (at 10 and 2 o'clock

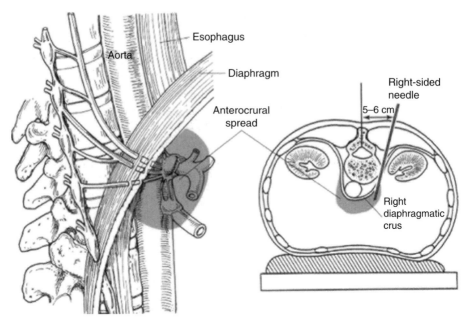

Fig. 9.3 Coeliac plexus block, posterior approach, showing anterocrural spread. The greater, lesser and least splanchnic nerves are also demonstrated

on an axial section). The nerves perforate the diaphragm and enter the coeliac ganglia of the same side, where they synapse, providing the largest contribution to the coeliac plexus. The lesser splanchnic nerve lies posterolateral to the greater nerve in close proximity to the vertebral bodies and contributes to superior mesenteric and coeliac ganglia. The least splanchnic nerve gives a small contribution to the coeliac ganglia. The coeliac plexus comprises several diffuse ganglia and nerve fibers that lie anterolateral to the aorta approximaly 1.5 cm anterior to the T12 and L1 vertebral bodies 0.6–0.9 cm caudal to the origin of the coeliac artery. The number, size and position of the coeliac ganglia vary considerably, with those on the left being situated more caudal than those on the right by a distance of up to 1½ vertebral bodies. The plexus represents the major sympathetic supply to the upper abdomen, supplying the bowel from distal oesophagus to transverse colon, including the stomach, liver, pancreas and spleen. Parasympathetic fibers also pass through the coeliac plexus. (See Fig. 9.3).

Indications and efficacy

Coeliac plexus or splanchnic nerve block have been used successfully for cancer-associated pain originating from the pancreas, liver and stomach, and occasionally from the large bowel and kidneys (31). It is usually recommended for use in cancer pain only, as potential serious complications and regeneration of the plexus make its use in non-cancer pain conditions inadvisable, although it is still sometimes undertaken for chronic pancreatic pain. Splanchnic nerve blockade may avoid some of these complications, and is also usually possible in late disease where anatomical distortion from tumour mass, metastases or ascites can make coeliac block technically impossible.

Coeliac plexus block has been the subject of several large case series, a few controlled trials, and one meta-analysis, which together offer a better evidence base than is available for any other neuroablative procedures. The immediate success rate approaches 90% for pancreatic cancer, as assessed by reduction in pain and possibly opioid consumption. Treatment failure may be due to technical difficulties, the presence of other non-visceral pain or prolonged survival. Duration of effectivness may be longer than six months, or up till death in 70% of patients. In these studies over 60% of patients had carcinoma of the pancreas, and published series for other upper gastrointestinal cancers are less numerous, but appear to show similar good response rates (31). Whilst the procedure may be repeated, a successful block often lasts until the end of life.

Pulished literature indicates a remarkable consistency in the efficacy of this block, regardless of the technique used. Older studies were subjected to meta-analysis by Eisenberg involving 1145 patients, and indicate a 70% to 90%.response rate (32). Polati et al. suggested that although 25% were pain free after a neurolytic block alone, most patients require continued opioid and/or anti-inflammatory analgesia, albeit at reduced dose and with an improvement in pain scores which lasted between 4 weeks and 5 months or until death (33). When considering these results it needs to be remembered that coeliac or visceral pain is not necessarily the only pain suffered by this patient group.

There is no clear consensus as to which one of the many techniques described for coaeliac plexus block is the most effective or safe. Ischia compared three techniques in a prospective randomized trial: the classic retrocrural approach, the transaortic approach and chemical splanchnectomy (34). There were no differences in outcome and no major complications. Nearly 50 % of patients had complete pain relief initially, which was more likely to occur if the block was performed within two months of the onset of pain. Relapse was related very closely to prolonged survival. Orthostatic hypotension occurred less often in patients who underwent a transaortic approach. Özyalçın et al. compared chemical transaortic and splanchnic blockade using alcohol (35). In this small (40 patients), randomized prospective study, improved analgesia and quality of life along with reduced opioid consumption were observed in the group treated with splanchnic blockade. The splanchnic group survived an average of 23 days longer than the transaortic group. Persistent diarrhoea occurred in 25% of the coeliac plexus block group, but in none of the splanchnic group. Marra et al. presented a series of 150 cases of CT-guided coeliac and/or splanchnic blocks using an anterior approach (36). The authors concluded that splanchnic or combined blocks were superior to coeliac block alone.

In advanced pancreatic cancer, coeliac plexus blocks can be technically impossible. The spread of dye and drug can be comprised by the anatomical distortion, even with anterior approaches, thus reducing efficacy (37). Splanchnic denervation can be considered in these cases, and this approach also theoretically lowers the risk of haematoma in patients with coagulation abnormalities. Gunaratnam et al. reported, in a series of 58 patients, a 78% response rate to endoscopically guided coeliac plexus block using an anterior approach (38). The benefits were maintained at six months, making the results comparable with more established techniques. They and other authors have theorized that advantages may include direct vision of tumour, allowing accurate staging and a reduced rate of neurological complications.

There is discussion over whether blocks should be offered early or only in late-stage disease. Oliveira *et al.* (39) concluded in a small trial that coeliac blocks were more effective in early disease. The same was shown by Rykowski and Hilgier (40), who found that coeliac blocks were less effective in relieving pain when the tumour was located in the body and tail of the pancreas rather than the head. Those with carcinoma of the head of the pancreas had far less tumour load and longer survival than the comparator group. The authors used a single-injection technique, which may not have been very appropriate for those with advanced disease. In the UK it is true to say that most patients are only referred for consideration of neuroablative techniques in the later stages of their illness.

Survival and quality of life improvements have been investigated, as well as pain control. Wong demonstrated that percutaneous spanchnic block resulted in improvements in pain scores up till death as compared to active conventional therapy, but there was no reduction in opioid consumption, improvement in survival or quality of life, and no reduction in side effects (41). The results mirror those of Kawamata *et al.* (42). Stefaniak *et al.* (43) compared a traditional coeliac plexus block with videothoracoscopic splanchnectomy (VSPL). Whilst both groups had significantly reduced pain, the VSPL group had significantly greater pain relief. However, quality of life was only improved for the coeliac plexus group. Open splanchnic nerve ablation has been the subject of one significant double-blind trial containing 137 patients (44). Here, a lesion was achieved peroperatively in patients with unresectable pancreatic cancer using 50% alcohol with a saline control group. The treatment significantly reduced pain for six months, reduced the likelihood of pain developing and, in those with pre-operative pain, a statistically significant improvement in survival. A few case series exist for percutaneous denervation, the largest showing an excellent or good response in 75% of patients (45).

Contraindications and complications

Absolute contraindications to coeliac plexus and splanchnic nerve blocks include coagulopathy and inadequate imaging and resuscitation facilities. Relative contraindications include cardiac failure, and inability to maintain the necessary position for duration of procedure. The latter may be overcome using approaches to plexus appropriate to the individual patients' situation and provision of sedation.

Immediate short term complications include acute localized upper abdominal pain, hypotension and diarrhoea (12). These are common and should be expected and managed appropriately. Needle trauma or the use of neurolytic solutions may cause damage to blood vessels, kidney, ureters, phrenic nerve and lung (45, 46) and inadvertent epidural, intrathecal or intradiscal injection is possible. Long term failure of ejaculation and sexual dysfunction may occur (47). Anterior approaches are associated with an increased risk of infection, abscess and fistula formation (48).

Permanent paraplegia has been reported with posterior approaches (1 per 683 blocks, or 0.15%) (49). In four cases studied, three patients suffered associated disturbance of bladder and or bowel sphincter function. Such sphincter dysfunction was not reported in isolation. It is postulated that the cause may be cord ischaemia secondary to acute hypotension or damage to the artery of Adamkiewicz, or to the neurolytic solution tracking back into the spinal canal.

Techniques

Many different techniques for blocking the coeliac plexus have been described, including posterior approaches above or below the crura, either avoiding the aorta or going through it. An anterior approach was first described 20 years ago, and is performed under ultrasound or CT guidance. Anatomical variations make it possible that any of these techniques may block the splanchnic nerves, ganglia and plexus when fluoroscopy or CT guidance is used. Splanchnic nerve block can be performed percutaneously using either a neurolytic drug or a radiofrequency generator. The block may also be achieved using a thorascopic surgical approach under one-lung general anaesthesia.

Despite large case series and some controlled trials there is no clear consensus on whether to use a 1- or 2-needle technique, an anterior or posterior approach, or whether a diagnostic block with local anaesthetic should be undertaken before attempting neurolysis. Most patients will get short term benefit from a diagnostic block, so some authorities argue that these are unhelpful in predicting outcome from neurolysis. The inconvenience and discomfort of undergoing two procedures within a short time needs to be balanced against potential safety aspects, particularly in view of the risks of major neurological sequelae.

Posterior anterocrural approach

This is the most commonly described technique (12) and in the UK is still the most frequently practised and so will be described in greater detail. It requires bilateral injections. For patients unable to lie prone a single left-sided injection may work with the patient lying on their right, although this is less reliable than bilateral blocks.

Positioning and procedure This is performed in an operating theatre environment with expert assistance, good i.v. access, monitoring, resuscitation equipment and X-ray screening available. The patient lies prone, with a pillow placed under the abdomen to reduce lumbar lordosis. Sedation is usually necessary, especially if there is discomfort from lying prone, but meticulous technique should mean that consciousness can be maintained, at least while gaining correct needle placement, and heavy sedation used during the injection of neurolytic substance, which can be profoundly painful.

The caudal aspects of the spinous processes of T12 and L1 are located and local anaesthetic infiltrated below the 12 th rib approximately 7–8cm lateral to the caudal aspect of L1 bilaterally at the points of the isosceles triangle which has its apex at T12. There are anatomical variations in the position of the 12th rib which need to be considered. The points chosen are usually level with the inferior third of the L1 vertebral body on the antero-posterior (AP) view. Using fluoroscopy with AP and lateral (and gun-barrel views when available), a tract is infiltrated towards the antero-lateral aspect of the body of L1 using local anaesthetic. A 20 or 22 gauge 150-mm needle is then advanced down this track, aiming to strike the centre of L1 vertebral body whilst avoiding the transverse process. Further local anaesthetic infiltration is made before advancing the needle off the vertebral body anteriorly. This may be achieved by redirection of the needle or by 'walking off' the vertebral body. Using a lateral view on fluoroscopy, each needle is advanced in turn very slowly, feeling for arterial pulsation, and checking regularly for any fluid in the needle using careful aspiration (blood, CSF and urine are all possible). Small volumes of radio-opaque dye injected as the needle is advanced will help guide the operator in finding the end points, which will be around 1 cm anterior to vertebral body on the left and up to 2 cm on the right, thereby avoiding the aorta. The final needle depth will depend on the needle angle and the patients anatomy, but is usually in the region of 10–13 cm from the skin entry site.

Injection Contrast injection (eg Omnipaque 300) should appear as a butterfly pattern on the AP view (Fig. 9.4) and run in a smooth pattern up and down the anterior surface of the vertebral bodies in a wedged-shaped pattern on the lateral view (Fig. 9.5). There should be no spread into the psoas sheath or nerve roots laterally, or epidural and intrathecal spaces posteriorly. Vascular spread should be checked for and excluded with great care.

Due to the diffuse nature of the plexus, a volume of 15–20 ml of neurolytic solution is injected each side. This makes alcohol, in concentrations ranging from 50% to absolute alcohol, the neurolytic agent of choice. The alcohol should be injected slowly, which often causes severe but short-lived pain. To minimize this problem, 0.25% bupivacaine 10 ml either side or 20 ml using a single needle may be injected first. Alternatively local anaesthetic may be mixed with either the contrast or neurolytic solution to achieve the same effect. Sedation may be used or increased for the injection, but heavy sedation in patients often already on high doses of potent systemic analgesia can be unpredictable. Careful monitoring following injection is required as hypotension occurs in up to 60 % of patients and this often requires active management with fluids and vasoconstrictors.

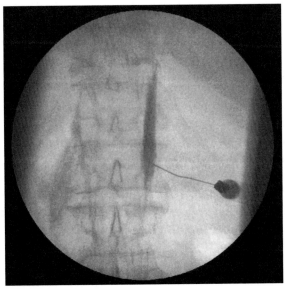

Fig. 9.4 Coeliac plexus block, anteroposterior imaging showing spread of radio-opaque contrast.

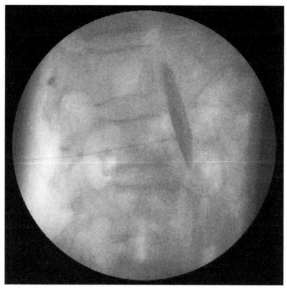

Fig. 9.5 Coeliac plexus block, lateral imaging showing spread of radio-opaque contrast.

Posterior retrocrural approach

A similar approach to that out lined above is used, but at the T12 level. Here the end point is less than 1 cm in front of the vertebral body and posterior to the diaphragm. This approach carries the risk of inducing bilateral pneumothoraces.

Transaortic approach

Some practitioners favour the transaortic approach (34). Here a single-needle is advanced from the left side, as above, past the upper third of the first lumbar vertebral body. Here when arterial pulsation is felt, the needle is advanced through the aorta with the end point being anterior to it. A characteristic pop is described when the needle breeches the aortic wall. Clearly, great care must be taken to exclude intra-arterial injection. The end point for the needle is 3–4 cm anterior to body of vertebrae on the lateral view and between the left lateral edge of body and spinous process on the AP view. Contrast should cross to the centre/centre left of the L1 body on antero-posterior view and the standard neurolytic injection is 30 ml of absolute alcohol.

Advocates for the transaortic approach argue that the single-needle technique gives closer placement and allows a lower volume of neurolytic solution to be used; others argue that this technique carries a greater risk of vascular damage, bleeding or inadvertent intravascular injection.

Transdiscal approach

The end point for the needle is posterior to the aorta, having passed through the T12–L1 disc from a paramedian approach (15–20° from the midline) using a loss-of-resistance technique.

Anterior approaches

The anterior approach has been used since the 1980s in some centres. The block is performed under ultrasound or, more commonly, CT guidance. Advantages include the use of the more comfortable supine position, a single-needle technique and, theoretically, a reduced risk of paraplegia. The needle may pass through the stomach, small intestine or liver; the large intestine is best avoided. Prior clotting studies are essential. Complications may include peritonitis, abscess or fistula formation and haemorrhage. An endoscopic technique has also been described; here the needle is guided through the stomach, again via an anterior approach.

Splanchnic nerve neurolysis

Splanchnic nerve blocks are less well established than coeliac plexus blocks in the management of upper gastrointestinal cancer pain. However, in patients with significant anatomical distortion around the coeliac plexus they become the block of choice. The block is similar to the posterior retrocrural approach for coeliac plexus ablation or chemical splanichectomy using alcohol or radiofrequency neurolysis. Percutaneous blockade interrupts the greater and lesser splanchnic nerves at the level of the 11th and 12th vertebral bodies. Splanchnic nerve blockade may be performed either percutaneously or surgically, using an open or laparoscope technique. Bilateral blocks are usually required.

Positioning and procedure

The patient is positioned prone with a pillow under the abdomen to reduce lumbar lordosis. Sedation is often necessary, but meticulous technique should mean that this only need be light, at least while gaining correct needle placement and for sensory testing prior to radiofrequency ablation. It is important to identify the diaphragm and stay medial to it. The insertion points may need to be altered accordingly. Generally insertion points are 4–6 cm from the midline level with middle of the lower third of the 11th and 12th vertebral bodies at the costal angle. A correctly placed needle will lie across the border of the upper and middle third of the T11 or T12 vertebral body. On the lateral view the needle tip should be 0.5 cm posterior to the anterior edge of the vertebral body, closely approximated to the body on the AP view such that the needle tip appears to lie slightly medial to the lateral edge of the vertebral body. Contrast should not project lateral to the margins of the vertebral bodies and should spread in a thick band over the lower two or three thoracic vertebrae.

For neurolysis, each side is injected with 6–8 ml of absolute alcohol. For the radiofrequency technique sensory (50/100 Hz) and motor (2 Hz) stimulation is mandatory to exclude accidental thoracic root lesioning. The patient may describe poorly localized anterior upper abdominal discomfort. A long lesion across the anterior half of the lateral surface of the vertebral body will be necessary to maximize the chance of a complete lesion. For this, a needle with a 15-mm active tip is required if it is to be done as a single lesion. Not all RF machines are powerful enough for this, and in this situation two lesions with a 10-mm active needle should be performed sequentially and adjacently, with the needle advanced 7–8 mm.

Conventional radiofrequency with the probe heated to around 80°C for 90 s will be necessary to create a lesion in a large nerve. Some practitioners lesion up to three times for 60 seconds.

Lumbar sympathetic block

Anatomy

The lumbar sympathetic chain descends from the thoracic chain and passes into the retro-peritoneal space under the crura of the diaphragm. It continues inferiorly on the anterola-teral aspect of the spine. Its position with respect to the anterior border of the vertebral bodies varies in a U-shaped distribution, with the chain being closest (0.5 cm) to anterior border at the level of L3, and up to 3 cm more posterior to it at the L2 and L4 levels (50). Laterally it is located 1.8–3 cm from the midline of the vertebral body, with L3 again being the least lateral. The number, size and shape of the of ganglia can vary, averaging 2.2 ganglia per chain between L1 and L5. The locations of the ganglia are also unpredictable, but are most frequently located around the disc regions of L2/3 and L3/4.

Relations to the sympathetic chain include the fascia of the psoas muscle laterally and the vertebral body posteriorly. Medially, it is bounded by the vertebral body and immediately anteriorly lies the parietal peritoneum. Anterior to this lies the inferior vena cava on the right and the aorta more anteromedially on the left side. The genitofemoral nerve lies laterally within the psoas sheath, and emerges from it anteriorly below the level of L3 (51). This anatomical relationship explains the not infrequent possibility of genitofemoral nerve blockade or neuralgia post-neurolysis. More posterolaterally lie the ureter and kidney. The L3 level is usually used for a single-level block since this shows the least variation in anatomical location at this level (50). Block above this increases the risk of renal puncture, and blockade below it increases the risk of accidental genitofemoral nerve damage, since this nerve typically emerges from the psoas sheath below the level of L3 (51).

Indications

Lumbar sympathetic block has been used for a wide range of conditions, which fall into the two large categories of vascular conditions and pain conditions. Pain conditions where lumbar sympathetic block can be used include: carcinomatous infiltration or compression of the nerves of the lower limb, rectal tenesmus (52), renal tract pain (high block at L1), complex regional pain syndrome and pain related to vascular insufficiency (12). Evidence is lacking, but bilateral lumbar sympathetic block may have a role in the relief of rectal tenesmus, which can be a very difficult symptom to treat and one that is highly distressing. A diagnostic block with local anaesthetic and steroid would be simple to perform under imaging and would carry little risk (52).

Contraindications and complications

Anatomical abnormalities that may make undertaking this block potentially hazardous need to be evaluated on a case by case basis. Complications are more likely after bilateral block due to the increased risk of needle trauma and bilateral sympathetic denervation. Specific complications include inadvertent puncture of the kidney causing haematuria, neuralgia secondary to inadvertent block/lesioning of somatic nerve (typically genitofemoral, which occurs in 5 % of patients), diarrhoea, ischaemic colitis, hypotension, failure of ejaculation, impotence and compensatory sweating. There are no reports of permanent nerve damage from neurolytic lumbar sympathetic block, although there are case reports of protracted groin pain.

Technique

The lateral approach is the technique most often described.

Positioning and procedure The patient is placed prone or in the lateral decubitus position. The former gives a more stable position. The level to be blocked is identified using fluoroscopy and the position of the transverse process identified. The skin and deeper tissues are infiltrated with local anaesthetic at an entry point 15 cm lateral to the spinous process. Alternatively, tilting the C-arm 60° from the midline plane can be used to help determine the point of entry utilising a gun-barrel technique,

A 20–22G 15-cm long needle is inserted at an angle of approximately 60° from the midline plane and advanced until contact is made with the lateral aspect of the vertebral body. It is then 'slid along' the vertebral body, emerging through the anterior fascia covering the psoas muscle, until the needle tip comes to lie on the anterolateral aspect of the vertebral body. AP views should show the needle tip just medial to the lateral border of the vertebral body, and the lateral view should show it to be either at or just a few millimetres behind its anterior border.

Contrast (0.5–1 ml) can be injected to confirm needle position. This should spread in a cephalo–caudad direction outlining the contours of the vertebral bodies and discs on the lateral view, without lateral spread on the AP view. Sprague and Ramamurthy describe a technique whereby 0.5 ml of contrast is deliberately injected within the substance of the psoas to show its characteristic striations (53). The needle is then advanced under continuous fluoroscopy until tenting of the psoas fascia is demonstrated. A further 0.5 ml of contrast injected subfascially reveals an obvious radio-opaque line delineating the fascia, which is penetrated, and further contract injected to demonstrate correct needle placement.

Injection Following careful aspiration, 10 ml of bupivacaine 0.25–0.5% with 40–80 mg of methylprednisolone can be injected with the aim of achieving short term therapeutic effect. Neurolytic blocks utilize aqueous phenol 6% or absolute alcohol. Phenol is more often used as there is a theoretical lower risk of neuralgia when compared to alcohol. Contrast can be mixed in to observe the extent of spread. Typically 5 ml is sufficient for adequate spread, although volumes up to 15 ml have been used. Flushing the needle with saline before removing it prevents neurolytic solution coming into contact with the skin and other structure in the needle track.

Radiofrequency ablation Sensory stimulation at 50 Hz should create vague back discomfort, ideally at a threshold lower than 0.5 V. Groin sensations indicates lateral placement of the needle, which should be repositioned medially. Motor stimulation at 2 Hz up to 2 V should not cause movement of the lower extremity. Lesioning should be completed by applying temperatures of 80°C for 90 s, with or without prior injection of 0.5–1 ml of lignocaine. The use of RF has the distinct advantage of allowing pre-lesioning testing and delivering a more discrete and more controlled lesion, therefore inadvertent involvement of the genitofemoral or somatic nerve should be less likely. Conversely the duration of therapeutic effect is better with neurolytics. Rocco describes 15 of 20 patients deriving very temporary or no benefit at all after radiofrequency lesioning (54). The difference in effect is presumably because injectates spread over a wider area than a localised RF lesion.

Superior hypogastric plexus block

Blockade of the superior hypogastric plexus is well documented. It has been used for visceral pain arising from pelvic organs, namely bladder, uterus, cervix and rectum. Varying techniques have been described for patients with pain from a variety of malignant and non-malignant conditions. However, the technique has a limited evidence base and supporting evidence for effectiveness is founded predominately on case reports and unblinded cohort studies. Blockade of the inferior hypogastric plexus is not commonly described due to its inaccessible location.

Anatomy

Post-ganglionic fibres from the lumbar sympathetic chain combine with those from the parasympathetic fibres from the S2, S3 and S4 ganglia to form the superior hypogastric plexus. It is in continuity with the lumbar sympathetic chains and innervates the pelvic viscera via the hypogastric nerves (a purely sympathetic nerve). The plexus comprises a diffuse network of ganglia that lie retroperitoneally, anterior to the fifth lumbar vertebra. The ureters lie close to the anterolateral aspect of L5 and are close to the plexus laterally, as are the iliac vessels. The superior hypogastric plexus supplies both sympathetic and parasympathetic innervation to the bladder, uterus, cervix, vagina and rectum.

The inferior hypogastric plexuses, both right and left, are predominantly formed from post-ganglionic, parasympathetic and sympathetic efferents at the S2, S3 and S4 levels, and are closely related to the viscera of the pelvis. As such, they cannot be routinely isolated and blocked.

Indications and efficacy

Blockade of the superior hypogastric plexus may be helpful for visceral pain arising from cancer of any of the pelvic organs, or so-called 'frozen pelvis'. Visceral pain is diffuse and difficult to localize accurately. A patient will often describe it as a deep, internalized, boring pain that never goes and is extremely unpleasant. Visceral pain is often associated with other pain syndromes, especially in advanced cancer of the pelvic organs, which may cause noiciceptive, neuropathic, bone and inflammatory pain spread throughout the pelvis and pelvic wall.

Non-cancer conditions in which blockade of the superior hypogastric plexus has been described, using local anaesthetic with or without steroid, include endometriosis, chronic pelvic pain, interstitial cystitis, severe penile pain and chronic prostatitis.

In 1990, Plancarte and colleagues describe performing superior hypogastric plexus blocks on 28 patients with pelvic malignancy (55). The majority (20) were female patients with poorly controlled pain secondary to advanced cervical cancer despite pharmacotherapy, radiotherapy and chemotherapy. They describe a mean reduction in pain of 70%.

Plancarte *et al.* published a cohort of 227 patients who had 'poor pain control' secondary to advanced malignancy (gynaecological, colorectal or genito-femoral cancer) over a three-year period (56). They received diagnostic superior hypogastric plexus blocks using 0.25% bupivicaine and, if successful, a neurolytic block was performed the following day using 10% phenol. Effective pain relief (defined as a decrease in VAS to below four on a zero-to-ten scale) was reported in 72% of patients that received a neurolytic block (51% of those enrolled). No complications were detected during a follow-up period of three months.

Leon Casasola and colleagues describe neurolytic bilateral superior hypogastric plexus blockade in 26 patients with pelvic cancer from a variety of primary tumour types (57). Sixty-nine per cent of patients gained satisfactory pain relief following one or two blocks using 10% phenol (success defined as a decrease in VAS to below four on a zero-to-ten scale).

Erdine and colleagues report a case series of transdiscal neurolytic superior hypogastric plexus blocks on 20 patients with a variety of malignancies of the pelvic viscera (58). Twelve patients had significant pain relief post procedure, but this was maintained for only one month. No significant difference in pain scores was observed from one to six months post procedure. In 25% of patients no pain relief was reported.

From the above it can be concluded that blockade of the superior hypogastric plexus can provide significant analgesia for patients with pain in the pelvis that is visceral in origin. However, the evidence for its effectiveness is provided by a small number of patients in trials of limited quality. No studies exist comparing the effectiveness of epidural or intrathecal analgesia versus blockade of the superior hypogastric plexus for patients with severe pelvic pain.

Plancarte *et al.* reported no neurological complications in a series of 227 cases (55). Possible specific complications include haemorrhage (due to the close proximity of the iliac vessels), intravertebral disc infection or rupture (during transdiscal approach), impotence (and sexual dysfunction), ureteric injury, accidental epidural, subdural or subarachnoid injection and somatic nerve injury.

Techniques
Postero-lateral approach

The postero-lateral approach to the superior hypogastric plexus has been described using fluoroscopy as the imaging modality (54, 55). A similar technique under CT-guidance is also described (59, 60). With the patient in the prone position and under strict asepsis the approximate position of the L4–L5 interspace is found from palpating the posterior superior iliac crests. This can be confirmed using imaging. Approximately 5–7 cm from the mid-line and under local anaesthesia, 150-mm needles are advanced bilaterally, aiming to place the needle tips on the anterolateral aspect of the junction of the L5 and S1 interspace. If the transverse process or nerve root is encountered the needle is redirected caudad or cephalad. Angulation of the needle into the correct position cannot always be achieved because of the proximity of the ilium. Lateral views should confirm the needle tip just beyond the antero-lateral margin at L5/S1. Aspiration of blood here is possible due to the close proximity of the common iliac vessels. Non-ionic water-soluble contrast solution is injected to confirm positioning. If correctly positioned this should, on an antero-posterior view, show spread confined to the midline. On lateral images contrast should be seen anterior to the L5–S1 interspace in a smooth contour, confined within the retroperitoneal space. For diagnostic blockade of the superior hypogastric plexus, 6–8 ml of 0.25% bupivacaine can be injected via both needles. For a therapeutic neurolytic block the injection of, 6–8 ml aqueous 10% phenol has been described. The anatomy and needle insertion for superior hypogastric block is shown in Fig. 9.6.

Transdiscal approach

Access to the superior hypogastric plexus can also be achieved via the intervertebral disc. This approach may be an alternative means of accessing the plexus if the classic postero-lateral approach is not possible. This approach has the added risks of discal infection and injury. The technique has been described using fluoroscopic (61, 62) and CT imaging (63).

Positioning and procedure The patient is placed in the prone position and the L5–S1 interspace is identified. Under local anaesthetic infiltration, a 150-mm 22G needle is inserted 5–7 cm from the midline and advanced towards the L5–S1 disc via the inferior aspect of the facet joint. Under imaging, the position of the needle is confirmed within the disc and advanced until it leaves the anterior disc. This can be confirmed using a loss-of-resistance syringe. Position of the needle tip is confirmed using radio-opaque contrast. Its spread should be seen in the cephalo-caudad plane and not within the disc. A diagnostic or neurolytic block can be performed as described above. During neurolytic block, to avoid intra-discal injection of phenol it is recommended that a small volume (0.5 ml) of air is injected around the superior hypogastric plexus before withdrawing the needle into the disc and injecting a small volume of intra-discal antibiotic (cephalsporin). This is addition to intravenous antibiotic cover.

Anterior approach

Blocking the superior hypogastric plexus via the anterior approach is less frequently described. Due to the risks of visceral perforation and presumed risk of infection, its use is limited to patients where blockade of the superior hypogastric plexus is deemed advantageous but access to it is compromised by altered anatomy by the presence of tumour mass. This technique has been described under fluoroscopic guidance (64) and CT guidance (65, 66)

Positioning and procedure The patient is placed in the supine position and local anaesthetic is infiltrated 3–5 cm below the umbilicus. A single or double needle technique can be performed. A 6-cm 22G needle is then advanced perpendicularly until contact with

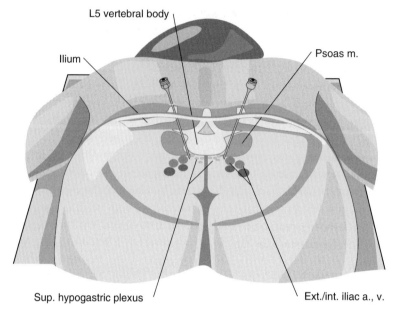

L5 vertebral body

Ilium

Psoas m.

Sup. hypogastric plexus

Ext./int. iliac a., v.

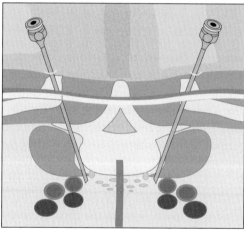

Fig. 9.6 Superior hypogastric plexus block, showing two needle approach from Waldman, Atlas of Interventional Pain Management. Elsevier. Also appears in colour in the colour plate section, Plate 37.

bone is felt. Fluoroscopy should confirm the needle tip lying anterior to the body of the L5 vertebrae. A quantity of 20–30 ml of 0.25% bupivicaine is suggested for a diagnostic block, using a single-needle technique. When using a two-needle technique, 6–8 ml of 0.25% bupivicaine per needle is recommended. Therapeutic neurolysis is described using a two-needle technique. Here the above technique is performed and 6–10 ml of aqueous phenol is injected each side of the L5 vertebral body.

Cariati and colleagues perform the anterior-approach superior hypogastric plexus block under CT guidance for patients with pelvic malignancy (65). After confirming correct needle position they injected a solution of absolute alcohol, bupivicaine and contrast medium. They describe the spread of contrast medium seen around the iliac vessels.

Ganglion of Impar block

Pain from the perineum, rectum and anus may be relieved by interruption of the sympathetic chain as afferent fibres accompany sympathetic efferent nerves. Blockade of the terminal part of the sympathetic chain—the Ganglion of Impar—is well documented and varying techniques have been described. However, there is a limited evidence base and supporting evidence is founded predominately on case reports and unblinded cohort studies. The ganglion of Impar block has been described for pain of malignant and non-malignant (including coccydynia) conditions originating in the pelvis.

Anatomy

The ganglion of Impar marks the termination of the sympathetic chain as it merges into a solitary structure lying anteriorly to the sacrococcygeal junction. Post-ganglionic fibres innervate the perineum, distal rectum, vulva, distal vagina and urethra via the grey rami communicantes. Location of the ganglion of Impar can vary (67), such that it can lie caudally to the mid-coccyx. This emphasizes the need for imaging to ensure correct needle placement.

Indications and efficacy

Blockade of the ganglion of Impar is indicated for visceral pain from the rectum, or possibly the vagina and distal urethra. It has been used for both cancer pain, tenesmus and non-cancer conditions such as proctalgia fugax, endometriosis and pain following radiation therapy. Injection of local anaesthetic and steroid is commonly used for diagnostic procedures. Neurolytic blocks can also be performed with relative safely.

Evidence for the use of this block in cancer patients is weak, and comes from individual case reports and case series only. Plancarte *et al.* studied 16 patients with advanced pelvic malignancy (68). All had poorly controlled pain despite pharmaceutical and surgical measures. Following a neurolytic block the authors reported that half the patients had a 100% reduction in pain, although details of pain assessment and length of follow-up are lacking.

Agarwal-Kozlowski and colleagues describe a case series of 43 patients with perineal pain from a variety of causes (69). They report a reduction in pain scores from 8.2 to 2.2 (on an 11-point scale) at follow-up four months later.

Basagan and colleges performed ganglion of Impar blockade through the sacral-coccygeal junction in nine patients who had localized perineal pain of visceral origin (70). They report significantly reduced pain scores and opioid requirement in eight patients who were followed up for up to two months. Studies comparing the effectiveness of the ganglion of Impar block with other interventional techniques (superior hypogastric block or intrathecal neurolytic block) for severe pain in the perineum do not exist, but the evidence points to it being a relatively safe procedure.

Complications are seldom reported in the case series reviewed. A review in 2007 reported no complications from blockade of the ganglion of Impar (71). Theoretically specific complications may include rectal puncture, pre-sacral abscess, and sacral nerve root damage.

Techniques

There are four approaches described for blockade of the ganglion of Impar. These are via the sacro-coccygeal ligament, via the anococcygeal ligament, using a lateral approach, and in the lithotomy position. X-ray screening (fluoroscopy), CT scanning and ultrasound have all been used for imaging.

Approach via the sacro-coccygeal ligament

The trans-sacrococcygeal approach involves inserting a 22G needle directly through the sacro-coccygeal ligament under fluoroscopy (72). The needle tip should lie just anterior to bone, as the posterior wall of the rectum lies anteriorly. Its position is confirmed using non-ionic water-soluble radio-opaque contrast.

Approach via the ano-coccygeal ligament

Plancarte originally described a pre-sacral block technique for perianeal pain associated with cancer. This technique became the standard for blocking the ganglion of Impar (68) and is shown in Fig. 9.7.

The patient is placed in the lateral position and a bent needle is inserted anterior to the coccygeal tip, through the anococcygeal ligament, and directed under fluoroscopy guidance so the tip lies just anterior to the saccrococcygeal junction. Attention should be

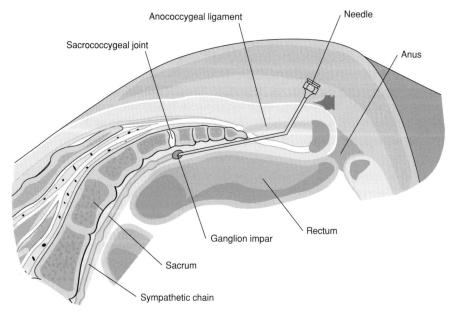

Fig. 9.7 Ganglion of Impar block showing the anococcygeal approach from Waldman, Atlas of Interventional Pain Management, Elsevier. Also appears in colour in the colour plate section, Plate 38.

drawn to the proximity of the anus and the posterior rectal wall. The position was confirmed using contrast medium and 4 ml of 1% lignocaine injected (diagnostic purposes). For neurolysis, 4–6 ml of 10% phenol dissolved in radiographic contrast is described. Bent or curved needles may be required to perform the procedure safely (73, 74).

Lateral approach

CT-guided ganglionic blockade allows a different approach (69, 75, 76). The lateral approach to the ganglion of Impar is performed with the patient in the prone position. Entry points are made approximately 10 cm from the midline (bilaterally), at the level of the sacrococcygeal junction. After local anaesthesia infiltration, a needle is inserted to the region of the ganglion (anterior to the sacro coccygeal junction). Both diagnostic injections (using 1.0% ropivicaine) and therapeutic blocks (using alcohol) are performed.

A bilateral lateral approach has been described under CT guidance in a patient with advanced vulval cancer. The authors speculate that CT guidance may avoid the potential for rectal perforation, which is possible using the anococcygeal approach (76).

Lithotomy position

An alternative approach is to place the patient in the lithotomy position (77). Direct access to the ganglion of Impar is possible due to the avoidance of the curvature of the coccyx. The technique requires imaging (fluoroscopy is described) and a finger placed into the rectum for guidance.

Ultrasound guidance

A recent case report describes the blockade of the ganglion of Impar under ultrasound guidance (78). The needle was inserted under direct guidance via the anococcygeal ligament. Spread of the diagnostic solution (4 ml of 0.5% bupivicaine) was observed in real time. Therapeutic neurolysis was performed with the above technique using 4 ml of 50% ethanol.

Radiofrequency denervation

Radiofrequency denervation of the ganglion of Impar has been described (79, 80).

Vagus nerve block

The vagus nerve is part of the parasympathetic nervous system. Blockade of the vagus nerve has been reported, although the literature reveals little in the way of case reports or cohort studies to support its use (81). The review by Waldman gives a thorough description of the technique and suggests its indications are for vagal neuralgia or ill-defined pain in the head and thorax, but there are few studies to support its use (12). However, as it forms part of the autonomic nervous system it is included here.

Anatomy

The vagus nerve forms the major part of the parasympathetic nervous system. It leaves the skull through the jugular foramen and descends through the neck within the carotid sheath between the carotid artery and internal jugular vein. It enters the thorax behind the root of the lung to form the pulmonary plexus and the oesophageal plexus with the contralateral vagus nerve. The vagus nerve plays an unresolved role in the afferent conduction of visceral pain.

Indications and efficacy

The indications for blockade of the vagus nerve are vagal neuralgia or in patients with cancer pain involving the structures of the neck and thorax. Vagal neuralgia is described as ill-defined 'shock-like' sensations in the laryngeal and thyroidal areas. It has been described as paroxysms of pain lasting a few seconds to minutes, precipitated by swallowing, coughing or sneezing (81). Blockade of the vagus nerve has been reported for pain in the distribution of the vagus nerve or ill-defined pain in the head and neck due to cancer. Despite increasing knowledge of the role of vagal afferents in the transmission of visceral pain, little published research supports the use of vagal nerve blockade. The blind technique described below has the potential to cause considerable problems. Inadvertent intravascular or intrathecal injection of local anaesthetic or phenol has the potential to cause morbidity and mortality. As such, careful aspiration is essential, observing carefully for blood or CSF. Specific complications include dysphonia or difficulty in coughing, tongue weakness and reflex tachycardia. A technique involving stimulation of the vagus nerve for pain in the head and face has been described, although evidence regarding its efficacy and safety is lacking (82). However, blockade of the vagus nerve remains in the armamentarium of interventional pain clinicians when dealing with difficult pain management problems of the cancer patient.

Technique

Blockade of the vagus nerve has been described using a blind technique (12).

Position and procedure

The patient is placed in the supine position. and an imaginary line between the angle of the mandible and the mastoid process is visualized. After local anaesthetic is injected a 22G needle is advanced perpendicular to the skin and in contact with the styloid process. The needle is withdrawn and walked off posteriorly and advanced approximately 0.5 cm.

Here the position of the vagus nerve is expected to lie deep to the posterior border of the styloid process.

Injection

The injectate can be both diagnostic (bupivicaine and methyprednisolone) and therapeutic (neurolyic agents including phenol). For a diagnostic block 5 ml 0.5% lignocaine is used. For a therapeutic block 80 mg methyprednisolone has been used and small quantities of alcohol or phenol can be used to obtain a destructive block.

Ultrasound guided technique

The use of ultrasound in guiding the needle position and observation of injectate spread has many advantages and its role in this technique is very attractive. Ultrasound-guided injection of the stellate ganglion is described and it is feasible that injection of the vagus nerve in the neck could be achieved using similar principles.

Neurostimulation

As an extension of the use of vagal nerve stimulation for epilepsy, a technique for stimulating the vagus nerve for treatment of refractory pain has been described (83). No clinical report or evidence is forthcoming, however.

Conclusion

Coeliac plexus and splanchnic nerve block are the most widely practised and effective of all autonomic blocks for visceral pain. When performed at an early stage in disease progression these techniques can offer good pain relief, a reduction in opioid side effects and improved quality of life. However, serious complications are described, benefit and risk have to be carefully weighed up and explained in every individual case, and patients are often referred too late.

There appears to be no difference in effectiveness between the different approaches and it is unknown if improved imaging and CT guidance lower the incidence of complications.

References

1. World Health Organization (1986). Cancer Pain Relief. WHO Publications Centre, Albany, NY.

2. Scottish Intercollegiate Guidelines Network (2008). Control of Pain in Adults with Cancer: A National Clinical Guideline (Number 106). Scottish Intercollegiate Guidelines Network. Available from: www.sign.ac.uk/pdf/SIGN106.pdf.

3. Justins D (2002). Pain and autonomic nerve block. In: Wildsmith J, Armitage E, McClure J (eds). Principles and Practice of Regional Anaesthesia, 3rd edn, pp. 291–306. Churchill Livingstone, Edinburgh.

4. Miguel R (2000). Interventional treatment for cancer pain: The fourth step in the World Health Organisation analgesic ladder? Cancer Control 7(2), 149–56.

5. Good Medical Practice. General Medical Council. Available from: www.gmc-uk.org/static/documents/content/GMC_GMP_0911.pdf.

6. Reisfield G, Wilson G (2004). Blocks of the sympathetic axis for visceral pain. J Palliative Medicine 7(1), 76–77.

7. Bonica J (1968). Autonomic innervation of the viscera in relation to nerve block. Anesthesiology 29(4), 793–813.

8. Giamberardino M (2005).Visceral Pain Pain Clinical Updates Vol 13(6). International Association for the Study of Pain. Available from: www.iasp-pain.org.

9. Charlton J (2005). Visceral pain. In: Core Curriculum for Professional Education in Pain. IASP Press, Seattle.

10. International Association for the Study of Pain (2008). Mechanisms of Cancer Pain. In: Global year against cancer pain fact sheet. Available from: www.iasp-pain.org.

11. Schott GD (1998). Interrupting the sympathetic outflow in causalgia and reflex sympathetic dystrophy: a futile procedure for many patients. BMJ 316(7134), 792–3.

12. Waldman SD (2004). Atlas of Interventional Pain Management, 2nd edn. Saunders, Elsevier, Philadelphia.

13. Leon-Casasola O (2005). Neurolysis of the sympathetic axis for cancer pain management. Techniques in Regional Anaesthesia and pain management. 9(3), 161–66.

14. Williams J (2003). Nerve blocks–chemical and physical neurolytic agents. In: Rice A, Warfield C, Justins D, Eccleston C (eds). Clinical Pain Management: Chronic Pain. Arnold, London.

15. Gauci C (2008). Sympathetic nervous system radiofrequency/pulsed radiofrequency. *Manual of RF Techniques*, 2nd edn, pp 138–40. Flivopress, Amsterdam.

16. Alshab A, Goldner J, Panchal S (2007). Complications of sympathetic blocks for visceral pain. Techn Region Anaesth **11**(3), 152–56.

17. Janick JE, Hoeft MA, Ajar AH *et al.* (2008). Variable osteology of the sixth cervical vertebra in relation to stellate ganglion block. Region Anesth Pain M, **33**(2), 102–108.

18. Honma M, Murakami G *et al.* (2000). Spread of injectate during C6 stellate ganglion block and fascial arrangement in the prevertebral region: an experimental study using donated cadavers. Region Anesth Pain M **25**(6), 573–83.

19. Ackerman WE, Ahmad M (1999). Effects of stellate ganglion block: A result of ganglion blockade or vertical spread of local anaesthetic. Poster discussion VII. Region Anesth Pain M **24**(3), 65.

20. Gofeld M, Bhatia A *et al.* (2009). Development and validation of a new technique for ultrasound guided stellate ganglion block. Region Anesth Pain M **34**(5), 475–79.

21. Ackerman WE, Racz GB (1995). A comparison of two techniques for stellate ganglion blockade. ASRA Annual Meeting. Anesth Pain Med **20**(2), 147.

22. Walls WKJ (1955). The anatomical approach in stellate ganglion injection. British Journal of Anaesthesia **27**(12), 616.

23. Kapral S, Krafft P, Gosch M, *et al.* (1995). Ultrasound imaging for stellate ganglion block: direct visualization of puncture site and local anaesthetic spread. A pilot study. Region Anesth **20**(4), 323–28.

24. Shibata Y, Fujiwara Y, Komatsu T (2007). A new approach of ultrasound-guided stellate ganglion block. Anesth Analg **105**(2), 550–51.

25. Zhang B, Zhuang L *et al.* (2009). Anatomical variations of the upper thoracic sympathetic chain. Clin Anat **22**(5), 595–600.

26. Yarzebski JL, Wilkinson HA (1987). T2 and T3 sympathetic ganglia in the adult human: a cadaver and clinical-radiographic study and its clinical application. Neurosurgery **21**(3), 339–42.

27. Ackerman WE, Ahmad M (1999). Effects of stellate ganglion block: a result of ganglion blockade or vertical spread of local anaesthetic. Poster discussion vii. Region Anesth Pain M **24**(3), 65.

28. Raj PP, Lou L, Erdine S *et al.* (2008). Interventional pain management. In: L Lou, S Erdine, PS Staats (eds). *Image guided procedures*, 2nd edn. WB Saunders, Philadelphia, p259.

29. Gabrhelik T, Michalek P *et al.* (2009). Percutaneous upper thoracic radiofrequency sympathectomy in Raynaud phenomenon. a comparison of T2/T3 procedure versus T2 lesion with phenol application. Region Anaesth Pain Manage **34**(5), 425–29.

30. Ischia S, Polati E, Finco G *et al.* (1998). Labat Lecture: the role of the neurolytic celiac plexus block in pancreatic cancer pain management: do we have the answers? Reg Anesth Pain Med **23**(6), 611–4.

31. Yamamuro M, Kusaka K, Kato M, Takahashi M. (2000). Celiac plexus block in cancer pain management. Tohoku J Exp Med **192**(1), 1–18.

32. Eisenberg E, Carr DB, Chalmers TC. (1995). Neurolytic celiac plexus block for treatment of cancer pain: a meta-analysis. Anesth Analg. **80**(2), 290–5.

33. Polati E, Finco G, Gottin L *et al.* (1998). Prospective randomized double-blind trial of neurolytic coeliac plexus block in patients with pancreatic cancer. Br J Surg **85**(2), 199–201.

34. Ischia S, Ischia A, Polati E, Finco G (1992). Three posterior percutaneous celiac plexus block techniques a prospective, randomized study in 61 patients with pancreatic cancer pain. Anesthesiology **76**(4), 534–40.

35. Özyalçın NS, Talu GK, Çamlıca H, Erdine S. (2004). Efficacy of coeliac plexus and splanchnic nerve blockades in body and tail located pancreatic cancer pain. Eur J Pain **8**(6), 539–45.

36. Marra V, Debernardi F, Frigerio A *et al.* (1999). Neurolytic block of the celiac plexus and splanchnic nerves with computed tomography. The experience in 150 cases and an optimization of the technique. Radiol Med **98**(3), 183–8.

37. De Cicco M, Matovic M, Bortolussi R *et al.* (2001). Celiac plexus block: injectate spread and pain relief in patients with regional anatomic distortions. Anesthesiology **94**(4), 561–5.

38. Gunaratnam NT, Aruna V. Sarma, Ian D *et al.* (2001). A prospective study of EUS-guided celiac plexus neurolysis for pancreatic cancer pain. Gastroint Endoscopy **54**(3), 316–24.

39. Oliveira R, Reis M, Prado W. (2004). The effects of early or late neurolytic sympathetic plexus block on the management of abdominal or pelvic cancer pain. Pain **110**(1), 400–408.

40. Rykowski JJ, Hilgier M. (2000). Efficacy of neurolytic celiac plexus block in varying locations of pancreatic cancer: influence on pain relief. Anesthesiology **92**(2), 347–54.

41. Wong GY, Schroeder DR, Carns PE *et al.* (2004). Effect of neurolytic celiac plexus block on pain relief, quality of life, and survival in patients with unresectable pancreatic cancer: a randomized controlled trial. JAMA **291**(9), 1092–99.

42. Kawamata M, Ishitani K, Ishikawa K *et al.* (1996). Comparison between celiac plexus block and morphine treatment on quality of life in patients with pancreatic cancer pain. Pain **64**(3), 597–602.

43. Stefaniak T, Basinski A, Vingerhoets A *et al.* (2005). A comparison of two invasive techniques in the management of intractable pain due to inoperable pancreatic cancer: neurolytic celiac plexus block and videothoracoscopic splanchnicectomy. Eur J Surg Oncol **31**(7), 768–73.

44. Lillemoe, KD, Cameron JL, Kaufman HS *et al.* (1993). Chemical splanchnicectomy in patients with unresectable pancreatic cancer a prospective randomized trial. Ann Surgery **217**(5), 447–57.

45. Brown DL, Bulley CK, Quiel EL (1987). Neurolytic celiac plexus block for pancreatic cancer pain. Anesth Analg **66**(9), 869–73.

46. Rosenthal J (1998). Diaphragmatic paralysis complicating alcohol splanchnic nerve block. Anaesth Analg **86**(4), 845–6.

47. Black A, Dwyer B (1973). Coeliac plexus block. Anaesth Intensive Care **1**(4), 315–8.

48. Romanelli DF, Beckman CF, Heiss FW (1993). Celiac plexus block: efficacy and safety of the anterior approach. Am J Roentgenol **160**(3), 497–500.

49. Davies DD (1993). Incidence of major complications of neurolytic coeliac plexus block. J R Soc Med **86**(5), 264–6.

50. Rocco A, Palombi D, Raeke D. (1995). Anatomy of the lumbar sympathetic chain. Region Anaesth Pain M **20**(1), 13–19.

51. Sayson S, Ramamurthy S, Hoffman J (1997). Incidence of genitofemoral nerve block during lumbar sympathetic block. Region Anaesth Pain M **20**(6), 569–74.

52. Bristow A, Foster J (1998). Lumbar sympathectomy in the management of rectal tenesmoid pain. Ann Royal Coll Surg **70**(1), 38–39.

53. Sprague R, Ramamurthy S (1990). Identification of the anterior psoas sheath as a landmark for lumbar sympathetic block. Region Anaesth Pain M **15**(5), 253–55.

54. Rocco A (1995). Radiofrequency lumbar sympatholysis. The evolution of a technique for managing sympathetically mediated pain. Region Anaesth Pain M **20**(1), 3–12.

55. Plancarte R, Amescua C, Patt R, Aldrete J (1990). Superior hypogastric plexus block for pelvic cancer pain. Anaesthesiology **73**(2), 236–39.

56. Plancarte R, Leon-Casasola O, El-Helaly, Allende, L (1997). Neurolytic superior hypogastric plexus block for chronic pelvic pain associated with cancer. *Reg Anaesth* **22**(6), 562–8.

57. Leon-Casasola O, Kent, Lema (1991). Neurolytic superior hypogastric plexus block for chronic pelvic pain associated with cancer. Pain **54**(2), 145–51.

58. Erdine S, Yucel A, Celik M (2003). Transdiscal approach for hypogastric plexus block. Reg Anaesth Pain Med **28**(4), 304–308.

59. Waldman S, Wilson W, Krops R (1991). Superior hypogastric plexus block using a single needle and computerise tomography guidance: description of a modified technique. Reg Anaesth **16**(5), 286–87.

60. Wechsler R, Maurer P, Halpern E, Frank E (1995). Superior hypogastric plexus block for chronic pelvic pain in the presence of endometriosis: CT techniques and results. Radiology **196**(1), 103–106.

61. Turker G, Basagan-Mogol E, Gurbet A *et al.* (2005). A new technique for superior hypogastric plexus block: the posteromedian transdiscal approach. Tohoku J. Exp Med **206**(3), 277–81.

62. Raj P, Lou L, Erdine S *et al.* (2008). Pelvic sympathetic blocks. In: Erdine S, Ozyalcin S (eds). Interventional Pain Management: Image Guided Procedures.

63. Dooley J, Beadles C, Kok-Yeun H *et al.* (2008). Computed tomography-guided bilateral transdiscal superior hypogastric plexus neurolysis. *Pain Medicine* **9**(3), 345–7.

64. Kanazi GE, Perkins FM, Thakur R, Dotson E (1999). New technique for superior hypogastric plexus block. Reg Anesth Pain Med **24**(5), 473–6.

65. Cariati M, De Martini G, Pretolesi F, Roy M (2002). CT-guided superior hypogastric plexus block. *J Comput Assist Tomogr* **26**(3), 428–431.

66. Michalek P, Dutka J (2005). Computed tomography-guided anterior approach to the superior hypogastric plexus for noncancer pelvic pain: a report of two cases. Clin J Pain **21**(6), 553–56.

67. Oh C, Chung I, Yooh D (2004). Clinical implications of topographic anatomy of the ganglion of Impar. Anaesthesiology **101**(1), 249–250.

68. Plancarte R, Amescua C, Patt R, Allende S (1990). Presacral blockade of the ganglion of Walther (ganglion Impar). *Anaesthesiology* **73**(3A), A751.

69. Agarwal-Kozlowski K, Lorke D, Habermann CR *et al.* (2009). CT-guided blocks and neuroablation of the ganglion Impar (Walther) in perineal pain. Clin J Pain **25**(7), 570–576.

70. Basagan ME, Turker G, Kelebek GN, et al. (2004). Blockade of ganglion Impar through sacrococcygeal junction for cancer-related pain. Agri **16**(4), 48–53.

71. Alshab AK, Goldner JD, Panchal SJ (2007). Complications of sympathetic blocks for visceral pain. Tech Reg Anaesth Pain Manage **11**(3); 152–56.

72. Wemm K, Sabershy L (1995). Modified approach to block the ganglion Impar (ganglion of Walther). Reg Anaesthesia **20**, 544–45.

73. De Medicis E, de Leon-Casasola O (2001). Ganglion of Impar block: Critical evaluation. Tech Reg Anaesth Pain Manage **5**(3), 120–122.

74. Nebab E, Florence I (1997). An alternative needle geometry for interruption of the ganglion of Impar. Anaesthesiology **86**(5), 1213–1214.

75. Wilsey C, Ashford N, Dolin S (2002). Presacral neurolytic block for relief of pain from pelvic cancer: description and use of a CT-guided lateral approach. *Palliat Med* **16**(5), 441–444.

76. Ho K-Y, Nagi P, Gray L, Huh B (2006). An alternative approach to Ganglion Impar neurolysis under computed tomography guidance for recurrent vulva cancer. Anaesthesiology **105**, 861–2.

77. Xue, Lema, de Leon-Casasola (1999). Ganglion Impar block. In: Benzon H, Rajas S, Borsook D (eds). Essentials of Pain Medicine and Regional Anaesthesia. Churchill Livingstone, Philadelphia.

78. Gupta D, Jain R, Mishra S *et al.* (2008). Ultrasonography reinvents the originally described technique for ganglion Impar neurolysis in perianeal cancer pain. Anaesth Anal **107**(4), 1390–92.

79. Gauci C (2008). Sympathetic nervous system radiofrequency/pulsed radiofrequency. In: Manual of RF Techniques, 2nd edn. Flivopress, Amsterdam.

80. Reig E, Abejon D, del Pozo C *et al.* (2005). Thermocoagulation of the ganglion Impar or ganglion of Walther: description of a modified approach. Pain Practice **5**(2), 103–110.

81. Chawla J, Falconer M (1967). Glossopharyngeal and vagal neuralgia. BMJ **3**(5564), 529–31.

82. Rutecki P, Wernicke J, Reese T (1992). Treatment of pain by vagal afferent stimulation. United States, Patent 533051.

83. Kirchner A, Birklein F, Stefan H, Handwerker HO (2000). Left vagus nerve stimulation suppresses experimentally produced pain. Neurology **55**(8), 1167–71.

Chapter 10

Cordotomy

Mike Williams and Derek Pounder

Cordotomy is destruction by division or ablation of the lateral spinothalamic tract of the spinal cord to relieve pain.

This chapter includes a description of the basic neuroanatomy, a detailed description of the technique, information about complications, selection of suitable cases, and description of outcomes of percutaneous cervical cordotomy

Cordotomy used to be performed by neurosurgeons by open laminectomy under general anaesthesia. This was done in the cervical or thoracic region to cut the lateral spinothalamic tract on the opposite side of the body from the pain. Cordotomy also abolishes the sensation of touch and temperature in addition to pain. The spinothalamic tract lies in the anterolateral part of the spinal cord close to the respiratory and motor tracts (Fig. 10.1). Technical precision is obviously of paramount importance, and this will deter all but the dedicated practitioner from performing cordotomy. The open procedure carries all the risks of surgery in a patient with advancing malignant disease, and has largely been discontinued in the UK. However, open operation on the thoracic spinal cord avoids the risk to respiration and the upper limb when pain is below the waist.

Since Sweet's work in the 1960s and 1970s on open cordotomy (1), Samson Lipton in Liverpool, UK, has pioneered percutaneous cervical cordotomy for unilateral pain from cancer, most importantly mesothelioma. It is a technique that can offer excellent pain relief, with marked reduction in or cessation of opioid and other drugs, and enhancement of quality of life, in a group of patients with one of the most unpleasant and painful tumours. We are fortunate that skilled and dedicated practitioners still exist in UK to provide cordotomy as an option in the management of pain from mesothelioma.

Percutaneous cervical cordotomy (PCC) is now performed using the precise placement of a percutaneous radiofrequency (RF) ablative lesion. Mullen first described a technique of PCC using a radioactive-tipped needle to cause a necrotic lesion within the cord (2, 3). Subsequently both Mullen and Rosomoff described similar techniques, which used an electrical current through a needle to cause a lesion (3, 4). The development of the percutaneous technique allowed patients with often significant co-morbidities to avoid high-risk open operative procedures. Since the early 1960s there have been advances in both X-ray and RF ablative technology. These advances include X-ray fluoroscopy, the measurement of impedance and a greater control of the lesioning process, all leading to greater safety and efficacy.

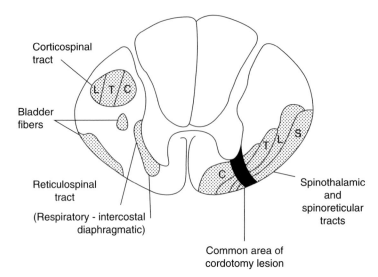

Fig. 10.1 Cross section of the spinal cord at at the high cervical level.

Neuroanatomy

The nociceptive pain pathway involves the transmission of action potentials along nerve fibres from the periphery to the brain. This pathway consists of three neurones.

The primary afferent neurone transmits the action potential from the peripheral nociceptors where they are generated to the dorsal horn laminae of the spinal cord. There they synapse with the second order neurones that traverse the midline and form the spinothalamic tract, which ascends on the contralateral side in the antero-lateral segment of the spinal cord, terminating in the thalamus. Tertiary fibres then project from the thalamus to areas of the brain to enable perception, localization and memory of, and reaction to, the pain. Interruption of the spinothalamic tract will therefore halt this transmission. A precise lesion within the spinothalamic tract high in the neck can produce analgesia to deep pin-prick and hypoalgesia in one half of the body from the shoulder down to the foot on the contralateral side. PCC is undertaken between the first and second cervical vertebrae because at this level the spinal cord is not completely surrounded by bone and so is directly approachable percutaneously with a radio-frequency (RF) ablative needle from the lateral side. It is carried out on the opposite side to that of the perceived pain, as the second order neurones cross the midline after they synapse with the primary nociceptive neurones. As the proximal second order neurones join the spinothalamic tract from the periphery, they displace the distal neurones within the tract in a postero-lateral direction. Within the cervical region the spinothalamic tract is more organized and forms a homunculus with the lower sensory dermatomes (sacral and lumbar) represented posteriorly, nearer the dentate ligament. The proximal sensory dermatome (thoracic and cervical) fibres are found anteriorly. In close proximity to the spinothalamic tract anteriorly lie neurones that control respiration, and posteriorly below the dentate ligament are the corticospinal tracts of motor function. Knowledge of the nerves within the spinal cord is important in localizing the position of the RF needle prior to a lesion being made, as well as understanding any possible complications (Fig. 10.1). Lahuerta *et al.* reported that the best analgesic results were associated with a lesion 5 mm deep in the anterior-lateral segment of the spinal cord involving destruction of 20% of the cord (5).

Patient selection

Cordotomy should be considered in patients with unrelieved severe unilateral pain from cancer who have tried medical management of their pain, including complex regimes using neuropathic pain agents, topical agents and other agents such as steroids, or who suffer unacceptable side effects from analgesic medications. Indications for consideration of PCC include costopleural syndrome (unilateral chest wall pain) caused by malignant mesothelioma of the lung. In some centres where cordotomy is practised frequently, cordotomy is offered as soon as the patient requires strong opioid analgesics for this condition (e.g. Portsmouth Hospitals NHS Trust). PCC may also be effective for unilateral pain from any tumour infiltration and for peripheral bone metastases (5–8). It may also be effective for unilateral neuropathic pain from nerve plexus infiltration, such as pancoast syndrome (6). There are also reports of its successful use for bilateral malignant pain and axial bone metastasis (8, 9), but this is not common practice.

Careful discussion should take place with the patient, relatives, carers and healthcare professionals regarding the risks and benefits of the procedure.

There are only three centres in the UK regularly performing PCC. We have found in Portsmouth that patients may be referred at too late a stage in their disease for the full benefits of the procedure to be realized (10).

Technique

The stages of cordotomy are:

- explanation/consent
- patient positioning
- needle positioning
- myelography
- spinal cord puncture
- stimulation/localization of tracts
- lesion generation
- post-cordotomy care.

The technique described below is that used in Portsmouth (Queen Alexandra Hospital, Portsmouth Hospitals NHS Trust, UK).

A single-needle technique is used, similar to that first described by Mullen and Rosomoff (2). This involves using a single all-metal spinal needle through which one may inject contrast media to delineate the dentate ligament and to act as introducer for the RF ablation electrode needle. We are aware of practitioners who use a two-needle technique for the separate functions (8). The procedure may be divided into stages, which are outlined below.

RF lesioning relies on an alternating electrical current at high frequency, which is generated by the lesion generator and causes a heat lesion. This lesion is produced by an alternating electric field at the tip of the RF needle, which causes ions in the tissue to move back and forth at a high rate, causing frictional heating. The heat is therefore produced in the tissue and not by the warming of the electrode. The field concentration is greatest at the tip and the lesion is localized around this point. The size of the lesion is dependent on the diameter of the electrode and the length of uninsulated exposed tip.

Preparation

Prior to the procedure the patient is given a full explanation of the procedure. This is reinforced by a patient information leaflet and fully informed consent is obtained. The procedure of PCC in expert hands takes approximately 40–70 minutes. To facilitate the procedure, which may be uncomfortable and stressful to the patient, titrated aliquots of analgesic and sedative medications are given. *It is imperative that communication be fully maintained with the patient throughout the procedure to allow precise localization of the spinothalamic tract prior to RF thermoablation.* Small doses of fentanyl are used (25-μg aliquots), up to a total dose of 150 μg. Small doses of midazolam are rarely required. Low dose remifentanil or propofol infusions may also be used. An experienced radiographer, fully familiar with the technique, and an experienced nurse, whose role is to reassure and comfort the patient throughout the procedure and to assess limb power during lesioning, are always in attendance.

Patient positioning

Positioning of the patient is very important. The patient must be positioned supine on a radiolucent operating table and must maintain position for the duration of the procedure. The patient's head is placed in a supportive head frame to facilitate this (see Fig. 10.2). X-ray image intensification is used to enable antero-posterior (AP) and lateral images of the cervical spine to be taken. Intravenous access is established with an infusion of Hartmanns or normal saline solutions. Pulse rate and oxygen saturation are monitored using a pulse oximeter. The equipment is shown in Fig. 10.3.

Needle positioning
Lateral X-ray

Lateral X-ray screening is performed to identify the lateral C1/C2 intervertebral foramen on the side opposite (contralateral) to that of the perceived pain (see neuroanatomy). It is important to obtain clear lateral images with no evidence of parallax distorting the foramen. A metal, radio-opaque marker can be used to identify the point on the skin overlying the junction of the anterior one third and posterior two thirds of the foramen.

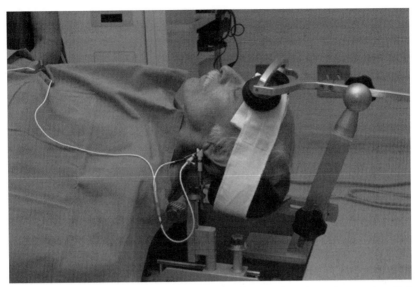

Fig. 10.2 Positioning for cordotomy. Also appears in colour in the colour plate section, Plate 39.

This point usually overlies the dentate ligament and should be marked with a sterile skin marker. Some C arm image intensifiers have a laser-targeting system, which allows an easier way of marking this point. Up to 10 ml of 1% lidocaine is infiltrated subcutaneously beneath the mark and more deeply in a horizontal direction using a standard intra-muscular injection needle. The syringe should be aspirated before injection to avoid

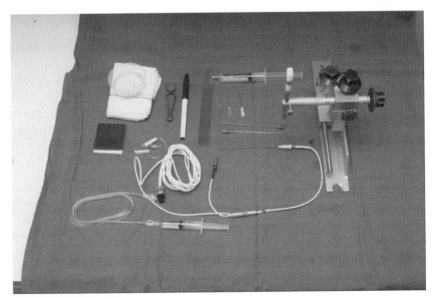

Fig. 10.3 Equipment required for cordotomy. Also appears in colour in the colour plate section, Plate 40.

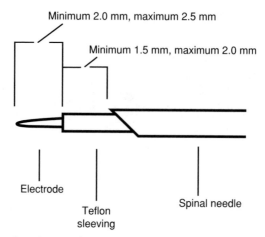

Minimum 2.0 mm, maximum 2.5 mm

Minimum 1.5 mm, maximum 2.0 mm

Electrode

Teflon
sleeving

Spinal needle

Fig. 10.4 Positioning of cordotomy electrode within spinal needle.

inadvertent intravenous injection of local anaesthetic. Five minutes is allowed for the local anaesthetic to take effect.

During this time the operator can adjust the RF cordotomy electrode so that it protrudes 4.5–5.0 mm from the tip of a 20G spinal needle. The hub of the electrode should be locked at this position (Fig. 10.4). This adjustment will ensure that the penetration of the electrode into the cord is limited to this depth.

The 20G metal spinal needle is then inserted subcutaneously in a horizontal direction toward the C1/C2 foramen as previously marked out. The needle is advanced until it is about 5 cm deep and targeting the foramen as outlined above. At this point, the electrode support apparatus is secured in position on the head frame and the shaft of the spinal needle placed in the V-shaped support.

Adjustments are made to the electrode support apparatus to ensure the spinal needle is targeted accurately. The X-ray intensifier is now positioned over the patient's face to acquire an AP view of the C1/C2 vertebrae of the cervical spine. Adjustments are made so that a clear view of the odontoid peg, with the needle approaching laterally through the lateral recess, can be seen on X-ray through the patient's mouth. The lateral border of the odontoid peg forms a good reference point for the beginning of the subarachnoid space.

Anteroposterior x-ray of the cervical spine

Further small amounts of local anaesthetic are given as the needle is advanced into the epidural space. Eventually the needle is guided through the dura mater and arachnoid mater into the cerebro-spinal fluid (CSF). Often, a distinct resistance is encountered when the needle penetrates the dura and care must be exercised to control the depth of penetration. Free flow of CSF must be observed from the needle hub when the stilette is removed. Further AP views of the C1/2 vertebra are taken to ensure the spinal needle tip has not passed the midline, i.e. that the spinal cord has not been traversed and that CSF fluid is not draining from the opposite side of the cord.

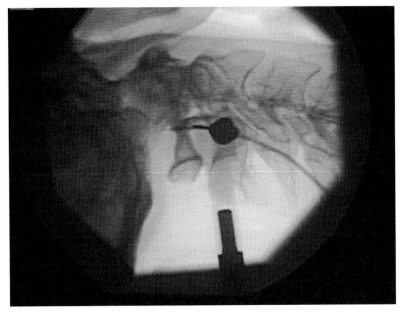

Fig. 10.5 Injection of radio-opaque contrast at C1/2 to outline the dentate ligament. Also appears in colour in the colour plate section, Plate 41.

Myelography

Lateral X-ray myelography

Lateral X-ray myelography is now required to identify the spinal cord and the supporting dentate ligament (Fig. 10.5). This fine frond-like ligament is formed from a fold in the arachnoid and is a good marker for identifying the antero-lateral tract, which lies just anterior to this ligament. Contrast media is injected into the CSF under continual screening and the sequence ideally recorded. Omnipaque 300 has been our choice of contrast medium since the late 1980s. It is water soluble and leaves sufficient short-term stain for the anterior cord and dentate ligament to be easily seen. If the dentate ligament and anterior cord are not easily seen, then it is most likely that entry into the CSF has been posterior to the dentate ligament and the needle will have to be repositioned more anteriorly until myelography indicates the needle tip to be anterior to this ligament. Usually about 2–4 ml of the contrast medium is required to give good pictures. There are descriptions of operators using an air myelogram, which involves the injection of up to 5 ml of air into the CSF to delineate the anterior border of the spinal cord. Previously, lipid soluble contrast medium agitated with air was used, and this lingered for longer on the structures, but we find that we get good visualization of the cord structures with relation to the needle tip using digital subtraction X-ray imaging and the ability to review our recorded screening image by image.

It is very important that the needle be targeted anterior to the dentate ligament, as any needle targeted posterior to it may direct the cordotomy electrode into the descending cortico-spinal tract, which carries the motor fibres from the brain. An inadvertent lesion within this tract would produce ipsilateral motor weakness and/or paralysis.

Once the spinal cord and dentate ligament have been clearly identified and the operator is satisfied that the needle is anterior to the ligament, then it is reasonable to proceed to the next stage of placing the electrode into the spinal cord.

Spinal cord puncture

The needle will have been accurately positioned with myelography, and fine adjustments made with the electrode support apparatus so that the electrode will enter the cord just above the dentate ligament. Impedance measurements are made to confirm that the electrode is completely sheathed within spinal cord tissue. To achieve this end, the lesion generator must be set to the impedance mode. Once free flow of CSF is observed from the needle hub, the RF electrode may then be fed down the needle shaft. As soon as the electrode tip enters the CSF the impedance will approximately measure 100–250 Ω. As the electrode comes into contact with the spinal cord the impedance will increase to 400–500 Ω and as the electrode punctures the cord and the tip becomes fully sheathed in the cord, then the impedance will measure in excess of 1000 Ω, commonly 1020–1040 Ω.

The Neurotherm® JK25T lesion generator that we currently use includes an auditory as well as a digital display of these impedance figures, which makes it easier to observe the electrode while puncturing the cord rather than having to look back at a digital display. The spinal cord, surprisingly, is quite tough to puncture and it often requires a firm, sharp degree of pressure to spike the electrode into the cord. A definite 'give' can often be felt, accompanied by a sudden increase in the impedance measurement. Sometimes the electrode can 'glance off' the cord and slide over the top. This can be confirmed by AP X-ray screening. In these situations, the needle-targeting angle has to be adjusted and further attempts at spinal cord puncture made. Occasionally, it may not be possible to enter the cord, especially where the anterior third of the cord is very shallow and narrow, resulting in the procedure being abandoned.

Stimulation/localization of tracts

Once the spinal cord has been punctured by the RF electrode needle, it is necessary to identify its location within the tracts. It is this stage of the procedure that requires the patient to be fully communicative. The lesion generator must now be set to stimulate. Initially, motor stimulation at 2 Hz is employed and the voltage level is progressively increased until visible muscle twitching in the ipsilateral neck muscles at 2 Hz is visualized. Where voltage levels of 0.3–0.5 V are producing satisfactory twitching of the scalene/ upper trapezius muscles, then it is highly likely that the electrode is located centrally in the spinothalamic tract. Twitching at lower voltage levels usually means that the electrode is placed anterior to the tract and is closer to the C2 anterior horn cells. Any other muscle group twitching, especially in the leg, means that the electrode is posterior to the spino-thalamic tract and is close to, or is lying within, the descending motor cortico-spinal tract. *Lesioning with the electrode in this position is absolutely contraindicated* as muscle weakness

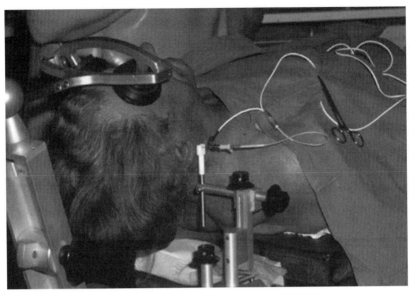

Fig. 10.6 Localization of the spino-thalamic prior to making a radio-frequency lesion. Also appears in colour in the colour plate section, Plate 42.

or hemiplegia would result. Repositioning of the electrode is required until satisfactory motor stimulation is achieved.

In all cases, it is important to increase the voltage until some identifiable muscle group is adequately stimulated, as too low a voltage level might miss an electrode placed in the motor tract (Fig. 10.6).

Sensory stimulation is then performed at 100 Hz. Progressive increase in voltage should be made until the patient reports the development of sensations. Ideally he/she should report a warm or cold sensation like running water, or a tingling sensation on the contra-lateral (painful) side. If this sensation is felt in the hand and arm then the electrode is placed centrally in the spinothalamic tract and a lesion made here will almost certainly produce excellent contralateral pain relief. If the stimulation is located in the lower contra-lateral limb, then the electrode is located more posteriorly than in the previous position but it is likely that lesioning here will still produce good pain relief.

Sometimes facial stimulation (can be bilateral) may be felt at 100 Hz and this usually means that the electrode is too anterior in the tract. Tetany of the neck muscle with stimulation can also indicate an electrode that is too anteriorly placed. In all cases, satis-factory right/left discrimination must be achieved before any lesions can be made.

Lesion generation

The lesion generator is now set to the RF lesion setting. A test lesion should be made at 70°C for 20 s. During the lesioning the patient should be asked to raise and lower the ipsilateral lower limb in a controlled fashion and to squeeze the assisting nurse's hand with the ipsilateral hand. This allows continuous checking of the motor power whilst the cord is being damaged. *At any sign of weakness the lesion should be immediately stopped.* After the lesion is completed the patient is tested for pinprick analgesia on the contralateral side. Lesions should be repeated at increasing temperature and duration until pin prick analgesia is clearly established. The authors would usually undertake a further lesion at 70°C for 20 s followed by another at 80°C for 20 s, repeated until satisfactory analgesia is achieved. Finally a lesion at 85°C for 40 s is often made to consolidate the lesion.

Post-cordotomy care

The patient is kept on bed rest until the next morning. Successful cordotomy resulting in good analgesia requires immediate reduction of opioid medications, otherwise toxicity in the form of drowsiness may ensue as pain is no longer present. However, too rapid a reduction can cause symptoms of acute opioid withdrawal. Routinely we halve the opioid dosing post procedure and monitor the patient overnight. These observations include standard observations of pulse, blood pressure, temperature, pain and sedation scores. The following morning the patient has a nurse-led review to identify any post-procedure complications prior to discharge. Further reductions in opioid dosing may then be supervised in the community. Patients are contacted a week later for a nurse telephone review.

Complications of cordotomy
Dysaethesiae

Interrupting the spinothalamic tract will cause a reduction in pain sensation to the contralateral side of the body. This may be total or partial depending on the extent of the lesion. Patients are warned that their perception of extremes of hot and cold will also be affected on the contralateral side of the PCC. This is important if patients are used to testing temperature with that side of the body, i.e. testing the temperature of a cup of hot fluid or bath water. Patients may also suffer deafferentation pain with neuropathic symptoms, including numbness, burning, hypo/hyperalgesia and allodynia in the hypoalgesic area. In the majority these sensations are either mild or transient; very occasionally a patient may find these sensations distressing.

Failure of procedure

Failure has often been quoted as being due to anatomical anomalies, e.g. flat anterior segments of the cord. Some may also be due to technical difficulties related to rotation of the cord due to patient positioning, making localizing of a definitive point to lesion difficult (6). This is compounded by the patient being required to maintain a constant, often uncomfortable, position for a prolonged period during the procedure. The use of sedation/analgesia has to be modified to enable lucid communication with the patient for the accurate localization of the lesion. A time limit for the attempted intervention may be set to 1.5 h, with failure rate of approximately 8%. A second attempt can be offered a week later, which in some may be successful. Sanders, in his series of 80 patients (including bilateral PCC (BPCC) patients), had a failure rate of 3.2% (8).

Mirror pain

Mirror pain is a pain that may appear soon after the procedure on the opposite side to that of the original pain and ipsilateral to the side of PCC. It is often similar both in character and location to the original presenting pain (11, 12). This pain is thought to be due to transmission bypassing the thermocoagulation lesion via interneurones that were previously inhibited by descending inhibitory neurones. Reported incidences of this complication vary from 6 to 72%. Ischia showed an incidence of 72% in patients having PCC for thoracic pain but only 32% for patients with pancoast tumour (6). Schrottner also revealed a differential between those having a PCC for lung cancer and those for breast cancer: 54 and 32%, respectively (13). In many of the series mirror pain was the main cause of recurrent pain and appeared related to the degree of analgesia attained and not the severity of the original pain. Fortunately in the majority the pain is weaker than the original pain and more easily controlled with conventional analgesic medication (6).

Motor weakness

The corticospinal motor tracts are located posterior to the spinothalamic tract and the dentate ligament. If the lesion extends into this area muscle weakness/hemiplegia may ensue on the ipsilateral side to that of the procedure. If the complication does arise then the leg is affected more than the arm. In our series of 52 patients, four suffered from lower limb weakness (7.6%). None was severe enough to prevent mobilization (10). Lahuerta *et al.* reported an incidence of 69% with lower limb weakness and 18% with concurrent upper limb weakness. Fortunately the majority were transient and resolved over a few days to weeks as oedema from the RF lesion subsided. Only 2% were left with weakness after one month (5).

Mortality

Mortality ranges from 1 to 27%. Pounder *et al.* reported a mortality rate of 6% (10) in a series of 52 cordotomies. It was noted that this occurred at the start of their practice, and it was also noted that a high proportion of the patients were frail and in the terminal stages of their disease process. We did recommend that patients be referred earlier in their illness when strong opioids are started. Subsequent to the reported series there has been only one death attributable to PCC in over 600 cases.

Respiratory insufficiency

Respiratory insuffiency has been well described in cases of cervical cordotomy and is the main reason for deterioration (3, 6). Lahuerta described 12 patients who died after cordotomy. The majority died during the night within 48 h of their cordotomy, and also had pre-existing respiratory pathology (5).

The mechanism for respiratory deterioration is unclear. It may be caused by effects on the efferent motor neurones, which innervate the phrenic and intercostal muscles. These fibres form the reticulospinal tract and lie in close proximity to the spinothalamic tracts in the anterior-lateral area of the ventral horn (see Fig. 10.1). Hitchcock revealed that surgical cordotomy lesions to a depth of 2–4 mm in the anterior-lateral surface of the cord in the high cervical area (C1–2) produced significant acute reductions in tidal volume measurements (14). This was greatest with lesions in the area of the anterior horn and the emerging roots. During the first post-operative day the vital capacity (VC) was reduced by 45%, independent of premorbid respiratory function. However, thereafter recovery was dependent on the pre-operative respiratory status. Unfortunately in some there may be a continued deterioration and mortality from respiratory insufficiency. Lahuerta *et al.* further confirmed the area of the lateral ventral horn to be affected, examining cadaver specimens of the spinal cord at the C2 cervical level from patients who had died of respiratory complications after PCC (15). The Portsmouth group showed that spirometry function (FEV1/FVC) and pulse oximetry are not significantly affected after cordotomy. We also showed that lung-function testing did not predict outcome for the cordotomy (16). This may indicate that it may not be the components of respiratory function that are the major cause of deterioration but the control of breathing.

Ondine's curse has been described in cases post cordotomy (17). This is a phenomenon whereby a patient while awake and aroused has normal respiratory drive, which is lost when the patient is asleep and has reduced arousal. Control of respiration is influenced by autonomic and voluntary mechanism. The autonomic control is from the respiratory centre via the reticulospinal tracts. The voluntary function is from corticospinal tracts and is able to override the autonomic function when the individual is in an aroused conscious state. During sleep this voluntary function is absent and breathing is then predominantly controlled by the autonomic tracts. A situation may arise where the autonomic reticulospinal tracts are interrupted and the voluntary corticospinal tracts remain intact. In an aroused conscious state the patient will breathe normally, but when they fall asleep there will be no autonomic respiratory drive and death ensues unless the patient is roused. There may be considerable bilateral/cross-over innervation for respiratory control, which may explain the increased risk seen with BPCC (17).

Regardless of the mechanism, the risk of respiratory deterioration appears to be related to high cervical analgesia, and those with pre-existing respiratory disease and BPCC. However, we believe that pre-existing respiratory disease in those with advanced cancer should not preclude patients from the possible benefits of cordotomy.

Miscellaneous

Urinary problems are described post cordotomy. Pounder *et al.* did not encounter any problems in over 600 cases. Lahuerta *et al.* reported a 20% incidence, but function was restored within a few days (5).

Horner's syndrome is a common occurrence and of little consequence, resolving over weeks.

Headache, or more specifically pain behind the ear in the C2 dermatome, is a frequent occurrence during RF lesioning and usually subsides rapidly after the procedure. It is controlled by simple analgesics.

Effectiveness

Mesothelioma

PCC appears to be effective in patients with pain from mesothelioma. Pounder *et al.* have reported reduction in pain, such that 83% of patients' opioid requirements could be halved, while 38% were able to stop their opiate medication completely (10). These results are consistent with that of other investigators (8, 18). However, there may be a reduction of efficacy over time. In the same study it was reported that 18 out of 52 patients required an increase in opioids within a median time of nine weeks (0.7–26 weeks). Others have reported a 50% reduction in efficacy over one year (7). Schrottner revealed, in his series of 78 patients, that 15% of patients had uncontrolled recurrence of pain. Interestingly, he also reported that the level of hypoalgesia to deep pin-prick remained stable in 91% of his patients with recurrent pain (13). Ischia reported in his series that there was a low incidence of recurrent pain on the side contralateral to the lesion (6). These observations would suggest that the majority of pain recurrence may not be due to direct failure of the technique (19). The mechanisms of pain recurrence may not be clearly reported when case series in the literature are reviewed.

The possible causes of recurrent pain are tumour spread across the midline or outside the area of hypoalgesia, metastasis to distant areas outside the area of hypoalgesia, reduction in the level of the hypoalgesic area (possibly due to resolution of oedema in the cord in the early stages after the cordotomy) or the development of deafferentation pain.

Deafferentation pain may be described as the development of mirror pain soon after PCC or neuropathic pain in the area of hypoalgesia. Although there may be a high rate of pain recurrence, in the majority recurrent pain is less strong than the original pain and more easily controlled by conventional analgesics (11).

Other tumours

The use of PCC for pancoast tumours and apical lung metastasis may be a less successful procedure. The pain from these tumours often involves the arm, but may extend to the shoulder and neck. To achieve hypoalgesia in these cephalad areas requires the lesion of the spinothalamic tract to include high cervical segments (C3–4). This involves either the placement of the lesion anterior within the homunculus of the spinothalamic tract or a greater area of lesioning, which may involve the neurones that control respiration and therefore a risk of respiratory complications if these fibres are damaged. The effectiveness of PCC for these conditions has often been quoted as poor. However, Ischia believes that poor results are due to incorrect technical operation; in his series comparing pancoast syndrome and chest wall (thoracic) pain, he found less recurrence of pain in the pancoast group (6).

Bilateral pain

Bilateral PCC has been described for bilateral cancer pain (8, 20). More favourable results have been attained when pelvic and lower extremity hypoalgesia is required as opposed to upper extremity and thoracic analgesia. However, complications have been reported as being greater than for unilateral PCC. In a series of 22 BPCC patients, Koulousakis reported six deaths from respiratory failure (27.2%) (21). All six had a level of sensory loss that was high on at least one side (C2 or C3). He quoted prognosis as being more favourable in those with no post-operative paresis, less than six coagulations of the cord during lesioning and where the interval between cordotomies was greater than one month.

Non-cancer pain

PCC appears to be more effective for the control of cancer pain as opposed to non-cancer pain. However, this may be due to the shortened life expectancy in cancer patients who would have had a recurrence of pain had they lived longer (5, 7).

Conclusion

This chapter explains how interrupting the contralateral spinothalamic tract can relieve intractable pain localized to one half of the body. The technique of percutaneous cervical cordotomy, as practised at Portsmouth Hospitals NHS Trust, has been explained in detail. It is recognized that there may be variations in technique in other centres. Although technically demanding, the described technique has relatively few complications as it is undertaken while the patient is awake, enabling the immediate effects of the lesion to be monitored closely during the procedure. Percutaneous cordotomy has been used very successfully at Portsmouth, especially for costopleural pain of malignant mesothelioma, in terms of both pain relief and quality of life. Epidemiology suggests that the incidence of this disease will peak over the next 15 years. It is unfortunate that Portsmouth Hospitals NHS Trust is one of only a few centres in the UK that performs this worthwhile procedure.

Case study

Mr B, a 68-year-old male, presented with increasing shortness of breath and right-sided chest pain to another hospital. His chest X-ray revealed a large pleural effusion, which was drained with symptomatic relief. Cytology and chest CT suggested a mesothelioma. He proceeded to a pleural biopsy, which confirmed the diagnosis. He had radiotherapy to the biopsy site and systemic chemotherapy. He had been exposed to asbestos as an apprentice marine engineer in the local dockyards as a youth.

Three months later he was referred to Portsmouth with increasing right-sided chest wall pain. He was taking MST 20 mg bd, meloxicam 15 mg od and paracetamol 1 g qds as oral analgesia. He scored his pain as 8/10 on a visual analogue scale. The pain was located around the right shoulder and upper chest wall, mainly posteriorly. He described it as a severe ache with episodes of very sharp pain within the same area. Positioning was difficult due to exacerbation of pain on pressure and movement, to the extent that his sleep was disturbed and sitting against anything was painful. He was becoming increasingly drowsy and lethargic on an increasing dose of opioid medication.

A left percutaneous cervical cordotomy was performed. Sensory testing at 100 Hz produced pain into the right hand and we undertook radiofrequency lesioning. This gave immediate reduction in pain of 80%. His MST was halved to 10 mg bd. At one week he was happy with the result and reported 90% pain relief, good sleep and travel by car was now bearable. At six months he reported 85% pain relief. He now takes only paracetamol as necessary for a discomfort he gets in his chest. He is keen to reassure us this is not a 'pain' and is very satisfied with the outcome.

Learning point

Cordotomy should be considered early in patients with mesothelioma.

References

1. Sweet WH, Poletti CE (1994). Operations in the brain stem and spinal canal, with an appendix on open cordotomy. In: Wall PD, Melzack R (eds). *Textbook of Pain,* 3rd edn. Churchill Livingstone, Edinburgh.

2. Mullan S, Harper PV, Hekmatpanah J *et al.* (1963). Percutaneous interruption of spinal-pain tracts by means of a strontium90 needle. *J Neurosurg* **20**, 931–9.

3. Mullan S, Hekmatpanah J, Dobben G, Beckman F (1965). Percutaneous, intramedullary cordotomy utilizing the unipolar anodal electrolytic lesion. *J Neurosurg* **22**(6), 548–53.

4. Rosomoff HL, Brown CJ, Sheptak P (1965). Percutaneous radiofrequency cervical cordotomy: technique. *J Neurosurg* **23**(6), 639–44.

5. Lahuerta J, Bowsher D, Lipton S, Buxton, PH (1994). Percutaneous cervical cordotomy: a review of 181 operations on 146 patients with a study on the location of 'pain fibers' in the C-2 spinal cord segment of 29 cases. *J Neurosurg* **80**(6), 975–85.

6. Ischia S, Ischia A, Luzzani A *et al.* (1985). Results up to death in the treatment of persistent cervico-thoracic (Pancoast) and thoracic malignant pain by unilateral percutaneous cervical cordotomy. *Pain* **21**(4), 339–55.

7. Cowie RA, Hitchcock ER (1982). The late results of antero-lateral cordotomy for pain relief. *Acta Neurochir (Wien)* **64**(1–2), 39–50.

8. Sanders M, Zuurmond W (1995). Safety of unilateral and bilateral percutaneous cervical cordotomy in 80 terminally ill cancer patients. *J Clin Oncol* **13**(6), 1509–12.

9. Ischia S, Luzzani A, Ischia A, Pacini L (1984). Role of unilateral percutaneous cervical cordotomy in the treatment of neoplastic vertebral pain. *Pain* **19**(2), 123–31.

10. Jackson MB, Pounder D, Price C *et al.* (1999). Percutaneous cervical cordotomy for the control of pain in patients with pleural mesothelioma. *Thorax* **54**(3), 238–41.

11. Nagaro T, Adachi N, Tabo E *et al.* (2001). New pain following cordotomy: clinical features, mechanisms, and clinical importance. *J Neurosurg* **95**(3), 425–31.

12. Nagaro T, Amakawa K, Kimura S, Arai T (1993). Reference of pain following percutaneous cervical cordotomy. *Pain* **53**(2), 205–11.

13. Schrottner O (1991). Results of percutaneous cordotomy in lung and breast cancer. A comparative study with strong support for a multidimensional nature of pain. *The Pain Clinic* **4**(4), 217–22.

14. Hitchcock E, Leece B (1967). Somatotopic representation of the respiratory pathways in the cervical cord of man. *J Neurosurg* **27**(4), 320–9.

15. Lahuerta J, Buxton P, Lipton S, Bowsher D (1992). The location and function of respiratory fibres in the second cervical spinal cord segment: respiratory dysfunction syndrome after cervical cordotomy. *J Neurol Neurosurg Psychiatry* **55**(12), 1142–5.

16. Price C, Pounder D, Jackson M *et al.* (2003). Respiratory function after unilateral percutaneous cervical cordotomy. *J Pain Symptom Manage* **25**(5), 459–63.

17. Tranmer BI, Tucker WS, Bilbao JM (1987). Sleep apnea following percutaneous cervical cordotomy. *Can J Neurol Sci* **14**(3), 262–7.

18. Nagaro T, Amakawa K, Yamauchi Y *et al.* (1994). Percutaneous cervical cordotomy and subarachnoid phenol block using fluoroscopy in pain control of costopleural syndrome. *Pain* **58**(3), 325–30.

19. Mooij JJ, Bosch DA, Beks JW (1984). The cause of failure in high cervical percutaneous cordotomy: an analysis. *Acta Neurochir (Wien)* **72**(1–2), 1–14.

20. Yegul I, Erhan E (2003). Bilateral CT-guided percutaneous cordotomy for cancer pain relief. *Clin Radiol* **58**(11), 886–9.

21. Koulousakis A, Nittner K (1982). Bilateral C1-2 cordotomies. *Can complications be avoided? Appl Neurophysiol* **45**(4–5), 500–3.

Chapter 11

The use of peripheral nerve and spinal cord neuromodulation in cancer pain

Nicholas Padfield

There has been an enormous change in the management of cancer in the last few decades. Patients are now surviving for years after their initial diagnosis due to advancements in treatments. However, this increased longevity has been achieved at a cost. Cancer treatments can cause direct neuronal damage, resulting in neuropathic pain (1, 2). Raynaud's phenomenon has been associated in one study of 20–30% cases of germ cell tumours treated with cisplatin, vinblastine and bleomycin (3, 4). Radiotherapy, whilst being constantly refined, may cause significant scarring and fibrosis, which leads to chronic problems in patients, who are now surviving for years after their treatment instead of the short time witnessed in earlier years. Brachial and lumbar plexopathies can develop early on following radiotherapy and can be difficult to differentiate clinically from tumour extension into the epidural space. They are frequently associated with autonomic involvement and dysfunction. Delayed onset progressive radiotherapy-induced plexopathy may follow a slow but relentless course with periods of plateauing (5). These unpleasant consequences of cancer treatments lead to intractable pain states, with pain that is very difficult to manage by medical and pharmacological methods.

Spinal cord stimulation has been shown to be preferentially effective for neuropathic pain (6–8) rather than nociceptive pain. As our understanding of the pathophysiology of chronic pain broadens, it becomes clear that modification of peripheral mechanisms alone will not address the complex challenges of central sensitization that occur as a result of prolonged nociceptor activity. Spinal cord stimulation appears to have effects both centrally and peripherally, which should match, in theory, the central and peripheral nature of neuropathic pain (9–11).

Under-treatment of cancer pain continues to be common and often remains undiagnosed, resulting in suboptimal management of the patient (12, 13).

The employment of neuromodulation techniques has been gathering momentum as the appropriate selection of treatable conditions, specific targets and equipment are all being refined. The experience in the exciting and rapidly developing field of neuromodulation is one of at last giving hope in situations originally deemed hopeless. However, it is invasive and expensive, and has its own set of drawbacks. Success will depend not only on rigorous patient selection but also multidisciplinary assessment to ensure a realistic outcome, based on a sound knowledge base of the limitations of the technique whilst giving the patient appropriately detailed individual information.

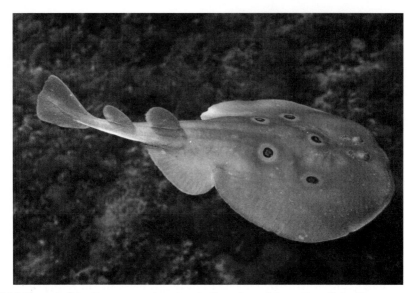

Fig. 11.1 Torpedo fish. Also appears in colour in the colour plate section, Plate 43.

The history of neuromodulation

The earliest recorded human effort at neurostimulation appears to have been that of the Mesopotamian healer Scribonius Largus, who used electrical currents to produce transient pain relief. By either the direct application of electrical torpedo fish (eels, of the type shown in Fig. 11.1) to the human body or by placing painful extremities into a pool of water containing torpedo fish. The resulting electrical shocks stunned the nervous system, allowing an immediate and residual numbness in the extremity.

In this application electrical torpedo fish were the very first means of achieving transcutaneous electrical nerve stimulation (TENS) for therapeutic purposes. This form of treatment was particularly popular for the treatment of gouty arthritis.

From these early efforts, the creation, storage and delivery of electrical energy then became the challenge. From the works of Volta, Faraday and others, batteries were soon developed. In the USA in the 1750s, pioneers such as Benjamin Franklin began to experiment with these new electrical devices and explore their nature. Unfortunately the time was ripe for the appearance of various notorious quack 'doctors' such as James Graham and Benjamin Perkins. They purported to achieve miracle cures, from impotence, back ache and rhinophyma, and practised on a gullible public in eighteenth century London. The illustration in Fig. 11.2 is a caricature of electricity applied by a 'metallic tractor' to the nose of a patient with rhinophyma.

A significant scientific discovery came from Michael Faraday, Professor of Chemistry at the Royal Military Academy in Woolwich, whose 'law', announced in 1833, pointed out that an electric current can produce a magnetic field (and that the reverse was also true). This started the scientific basis for the medical application of electricity. Faraday's observation was the key to the development of the inductor, which then served as the

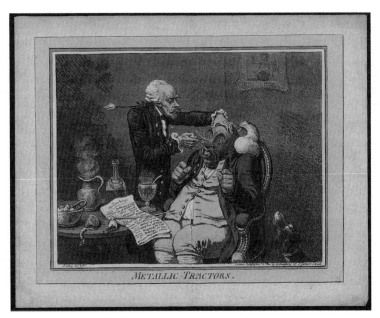

Fig. 11.2 'Dr' Benjamin Perkins and the metallic tractor. Reproduced with permission courtesy of Historical Collections & Services, Claude Moore Health Sciences Library, University of Virginia. Also appears in colour in the colour plate section, Plate 44.

basis for neurostimulation. This in turn led to the wire-wound transformer, which permits voltage control and the modern control of electricity in motors.

In 1863, Gaiffe, in Paris, had constructed a transcutaneous electrical nerve-stimulating device remarkably similar to those in use today. This device was the true precursor of the modern TENS unit, featuring removable batteries, an inductor, lead wires and skin electrodes. Its only limitation was its low electrical output under load (about 3 mA as opposed to modern TENS units with 90 mA outputs).

Unfortunately, the ever-gullible public were still to be prey to exaggerated claims. An advertisement from the 1882 Boston Globe states:

> One of the Most Marvellous (sic) Inventions of the Century!
> All cases of Rheumatism, Diseases of the Liver, Stomach and Kidneys, Lung Complaints, Paralysis, Lost Vitality, Nervous Disability, Female Complaints . . . are cured with the Electrifier.

The first commercially available device that would look like a modern TENS machine was the 'Electreat'. This device was patented by Charles Willie Kent in 1919 and manufactured in Peoria, Illinois. It has been estimated that as many as 250,000 of the Electreats were sold over the following 25 years. The device operated on two 'D' cell batteries and a mechanical inductor. A roller was built in at the top to be applied to the skin, and plug-in sponge pad electrodes were supplied. The Electreat was one of the very first high-output battery-operated TENS units manufactured. However, the claims for its efficacy were widely exaggerated. In fact, following passage of the Food, Drug and Cosmetic Act in 1938, Kent was the first individual prosecuted by the US government for making unsubstantiated medical claims and the Electreat company was then forced to limit their claims to pain relief alone. The Electreat was one of the first high-output battery-operated TENS units out of all the quack devices to survive into the twentieth century. Drawbacks include limited control of stimulation and inability to be worn.

The family of neurosurgeon C. Norman Shealy (who was the first surgeon to actually implant neuroaugmentive devices in humans) had used the Electreat in the past. Based on his personal experience he approached Medtronic, in Minneapolis, and encouraged them to begin to develop solid-state TENS devices. Pain relief is produced when electrodes connected to the unit are used to deliver electrical impulses through the skin, thus blocking the pain signal.

The evolution of TENS devices led to more compact units with better patient-safety provisions. At the same time there was an associated evolution in the technology of skin electrodes. Despite these advances, both TENS units and skin electrodes remained fairly primitive in design in regard to their future potential, as did the design of implanted neuroaugmentive devices. By the 1970s, in Minneapolis, Minnesota, a number of medical device manufacturing companies (i.e. Medtronic, Stimulation Technologies, Inc., etc.) started to take a serious look at TENS technology and began, for the first time, to apply solid-state technology to these therapeutic applications.

The new discipline of implanted electronic devices designed to influence the function of the nervous system for therapeutic purposes began in the 1960s. We have to thank the efforts of a small group of pioneers at Temple University in Philadelphia and C. Norman Shealy in Boston for this development (7).

The first reported implantation of a spinal-cord stimulating system by Shealy was, in fact, for a patient suffering with cancer.

The physiological basis of action of neuromodulation

In neuropathic pain the hyperexcitability shown by the wide dynamic range cells in the dorsal horns appears to be related to increased basal release of excitatory amino acids, such as glutamate, and to a dysfunction of the local GABA system (14). Animal work indicates that spinal cord stimulation reduces this hyperexcitability and induces release of GABA in the dorsal horn neurons, with a resultant reduction in the level of glutamate. In fact, there is likely to be a cascade of neuroactive substances, including adenosine, and multiple mechanisms are activated (15). For a review see Myerson and Linderoth (9).

A growing body of evidence indicates that the microglia in the dorsal horn of the spinal cord play a causal role in neuropathic pain behaviours resulting from peripheral nerve injury and specific neuron–microglia–neuron signalling has been discovered (15). Suppressing this signalling may therefore represent the basis for new forms of therapy in chronic pain following nerve injury.

With the advent of functional magnetic resonance imaging and microrecording techniques it has become possible to trace the activity of different populations of dorsal horn neurones. Different stimulation frequency and intensity will activate different areas within the brain, particularly the periventricular grey matter, a known target for electrically induced analgesia.

There also appears to be a complex interrelation between segmental (antidromic activation) and supraspinal mechanisms, an area which has been studied by the Karolinska research group. The major suppressive part of the Spinal Cord Stimulation (SCS) effects appears to be accomplished at a spinal segmental level (16). However, there is also evidence from rats that stimulation above a cord transection can produce analgesia. It is postulated that this is produced by activation in the pretectal nucleus (17). Activation of a supraspinal loop resulting in attenuation in a rat model has recently been demonstrated (18).

Practitioners of external neuromodulation and peripheral nerve stimulation know that low-frequency stimulation will often produce complete relief from pain, but that an increase in frequency will change the experience from one of analgesia to one of intense pain. There is evidence of the interaction between C fibres and a distinct population of dorsal horn neurones in the amplification of pain-related information (14). It has thus recently become possible to demonstrate the actions of peripheral nerve stimulation electrophysiologically and to link this to observed clinical phenomena. Patients with implanted spinal cord stimulators will also be quite particular about their preferred stimulation frequency, as well as intensity, as they experience a change in the nature of the electrically induced pararesthesiae.

Available neuromodulation systems

External neuromodulation

This is the least invasive form of neuromodulation. When there is a clear superficial trigger area this form of neuromodulation should be tried. A ball electrode is applied to the skin surface at the trigger point and a frequency of 2 Hz is applied; the output is increased until the patient indicates it is at the optimum level. If effective, the pain will diminish, even disappear, within a matter of seconds. Trial and error will determine how long to continue the stimulation. In our experience we would not continue to stimulate for longer than 10 minutes per site. Frequently the patient will indicate they have had enough before the 10 minutes is up.

In Fig. 11.3—a commercial image—the 'pen' is being used to map the brachial plexus. However, the pen can be used to stimulate other target peripheral nerves without the need for injection. If analgesia is achieved the patient has the option of loaning/purchasing their own apparatus.

Peripheral nerve stimulation

Peripheral nerve stimulation (PNS) is probably the most focused form of neuromodulation in that the stimulation directly targets the nerves that conduct pain impulses from the periphery to the CNS. Stimulation of large myelinated A-beta touch and pressure fibres sends non-painful touch signals to the brain and it is theorized that this prevents perception of pain by interfering with pain signal transmission.

There are several pain phenomena that should be understood. Nociceptive neuralgia refers to nerve pain from mechanical or tactile nerve irritation and ectopic neuralgia refers to nerve pain from a spontaneous abnormal nerve discharge without mechanical stimulation. Although the nociceptive type may respond to nerve transection and/or translocation, the ectopic form usually will not.

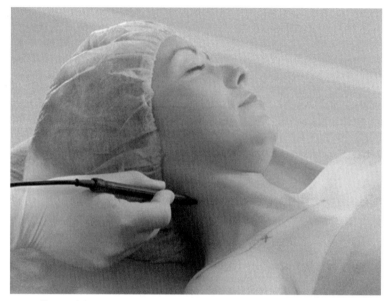

Fig. 11.3 Braun® Stimulplex 'pen' peripheral nerve mapper/stimulator. © B. Braun Medical Ltd. Reproduced with permission. Also appears in colour in the colour plate section, Plate 45.

Another important pain phenomenon is deafferentation, which refers to pain in the distribution of a nerve that has been transected. Disruption of afferent sensory input from the transected nerve may result in hypersensitivity caused by changes induced in adjacent sensory nerves. At times, these adjacent nerves may carry pain signals from the zone of deafferentation, even in the absence of light-touch sensation. This particular deafferentation sequela is termed by some as 'anesthesia dolorosa'.

The deafferentation phenomenon is theorized to occur at the spinal cord level, where the transected nerve pain signals are augmented, causing hypersensitivity. PNS is often effective for deafferentation pain and anesthesia dolorosa.

The choice of site will be detailed later in the chapter. The electrodes can be sited by percutaneous insertion through a specially designed needle or they can be applied in proximity to the peripheral nerve or nerve trunk at open operation. The choice of leads continues to expand, depending on the method of placement. There are micro- and standard leads, which carry four or eight cylindrical contacts for percutaneous insertion and placement.

Risks and benefits of peripheral nerve stimulation

Risks Side effects are uncommon, but do occur and it is important to be aware of these so that appropriate measures can be taken to reduce them. Examples of possible side effects include the following:

- risks of the surgery itself such as bleeding, infection, nerve damage
- patients may become aware of other pain elsewhere, e.g. musculoskeletal or back pain, as a result of their primary pain being relieved

- undesirable changes in stimulation can occur with time—these changes can be due to changes in the nerve cells or due to changes in the electrode position
- battery failure and/or battery leakage
- persisting pain at the site of implantation
- movement of the lead causing reduction in pain relief
- allergic response to the implant material
- movement of the implant unit and damage to the overlying skin
- systems may be affected by or adversely affect:
  - pacemakers
  - cardioverter defibrillators
  - external defibrillators
  - MRI
  - diathermy (surgical tissue dissection tool)
  - ultrasonic equipment
  - electrocautery (electrical method of burning tissue)
  - radiation therapy
  - theft detectors
  - security systems
  - aircraft communications systems.

There is a very definite revision rate which has to be factored into costings. It has been variously reported as high as 34% for spinal cord stimulation. There are no figures available for peripheral nerve stimulation alone. The rate of lead migration and the need for revision because of lead migration would be higher as there are more practical problems in anchoring the leads to discourage migration in tissues that are considerably more mobile than the deep fascia of the vertebral erector spinae muscles.

Benefits Peripheral nerve stimulation has the intention of reducing rather than eliminating pain. The benefits of using such a system are as follows:

- improvement in pain relief, providing a 50–70% reduction in pain in 60–70% of patients
- increase in levels of activity
- reduction in the use of narcotic medications
- potentially reduction in the need for hospitalization and surgical procedures
- improvement in overall quality of life for sufferers.

Spinal cord stimulation

Spinal cord stimulation involves the therapeutic use of electricity to produce a specific effect by stimulating the spinal dorsal columns. It is achieved by the insertion of an electrode array into the epidural space at the appropriate level of the spinal cord, *not* at the vertebral level corresponding to the distribution of the pain.

Equipment

Neuromodulation devices consist of three main components: electrodes, an extension cable that connects the electrodes to the impulse generator (IPG) and the impulse generator itself, which may be internal or external to the body.

There are three companies that make neuromodulation electrodes: Advanced Bionics/ Boston Scientific Corporation, St Jude Medical incorporating the old ANS group (Advanced Neuromodulation Systems) and Medtronic Ltd, in both the USA and the UK.

Electrodes

The choice of electrode will be predicated on the size of the target area and the required stimulus density. A discrete nerve plexus may be best stimulated by a quad compact electrode that has four contacts that can be sited very close or, where the contacts are spaced more apart from each other, a quad lead or, where the contacts are broader and spaced more apart, a quad plus. A diffuse subcutaneous area may be best covered by a series of microtens electrodes, which are of the smallest diameter, in parallel. An octrode with eight contacts may suit best when a longer area needs to be covered. Fixation of the electrodes can be problematic in a site that is mobile or subject to stress or strain. Connection to extension cables and their attachment to an IPG can also be problematic.

Extension cable

The electrodes themselves are frequently joined to an extension cable, which is connected in turn the IPG. It consists of a barrel one end, in which the end of the electrode is inserted so that the electrical contacts are in exact opposition to the contacts in the barrel. These are reproduced as contacts at the other end, which is inserted into the IPG. Both electrodes and extension cables are available in different lengths. If the risk of infection is high because of patient factors such as depressed immunity, diabetes or smoking, then the insertion of an extension can sometimes allow one component to be removed alone without the necessity of removal of the entire system. This has obvious economic as well as practical advantages.

Impulse generator

In addition to different electrodes there are two types of electrical activation. The extension cable can be connected directly to an IPG, which contains a battery. This IPG is implanted subcutaneously and has to be replaced at regular intervals. The life of the unit will depend on the length of time in a day the system is turned on, the number of active electrodes and the pulse width and amplitude. With average use, the longevity ranges from three to six years. Thus a direct radiofrequency activation system may be preferred where the patient wears a radiofrequency antenna applied over the skin covering the radio receiver. An example of this is the 'Renew' system made by ANS/St Jude. This is a 'permanent' device and does not have to be replaced.

During a trial it may become apparent that the electrical usage would drain a battery quickly and thus a rechargeable system would be more appropriate. With this system a patient needs to charge the system by placing a radiotransmitter over the skin covering the receiver and charge it in this position for an hour or so once a week. However, it can be rather cumbersome to do this because the recharging radiofrequency unit is quite bulky and it may be difficult in practical terms for the patient to be able to sit still for an hour or so on a regular basis (Fig. 11.4).

Patient selection

The site, speed of development and extent of dissemination of the cancer, and the treatment received or planned all have to be taken into account when planning neuromodulation, to address the *physical* aspects of the pain. However, even significant pain reduction will by no means guarantee a good outcome if the patient's fears, beliefs and avoidance behaviours are left unattended. The eventual outcome will depend on educating the patient about realistic expectations of what can be achieved by the chosen method of neuromodulation. It will also rely on what they, in turn, are able to do as a result of the reduction in the physical sensation of pain, by way of increased activity and resumption of pleasurable activities that had been put on hold or even abandoned once the diagnosis of cancer had been made.

It is therefore imperative that any concomitant depression or other psychiatric disease is treated. Any inappropriate fears and beliefs or psychological co-morbidities that result in fear avoidance behaviours that are harmful to the patient must be rigorously addressed by cognitive behavioural therapy prior to implantation.

Patients with cancer, especially if treatment of the cancer has required prolonged hospitalization, will be physically deconditioned. Restoration of physical functioning will

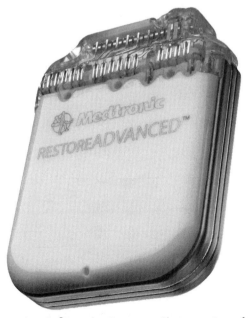

Fig. 11.4 Restore Ultra Medtronic ® Impulse Generator. Photo courtesy of Medtronic, Inc. Also appears in colour in the colour plate section, Plate 46.

require simultaneous and coordinated rehabilitative physiotherapy at the same time as pain reduction by neuromodulation.

Patients with advanced cancer will be treated by several disciplines. It is vital that there is good communication between everyone involved in his or her care so that everybody presents a unified strategy. There should be a clear consensus about the stage of disease, prognosis, expectations of further cancer treatments and a mutual understanding of what can or cannot be achieved by neuromodulation. If the likely prognosis exceeds six months then neurodestructive procedures should be discarded in favour of neuromodulation techniques if medication alone will not suffice in controlling pain.

Appropriate patient selection will rely on a full assessment of the cancer in terms of its site, the tissue involved and spread, treatments received, treatments planned for the future and the likely prognosis (if known). Because cancer patients are likely to have reduced immunological surveillance they will be more susceptible to infection, and screening for any active infection must be rigorous, specifically looking for MRSA. Should the patient be a carrier, this should be treated with vancomycin or teicoplanin, depending on culture sensitivities. There should be three 'clear' swabs before any implant takes place.

It is important to emphasize that neuromodulation should only be considered when other treatment modalities have failed to relieve the pain, and that any direct treatment of the underlying cancer or it's recurrence has been undertaken. In particular, any further surgery should ideally have been undertaken and the patient recovered. Anticoagulants pose specific problems and can be an absolute contraindication to epidurally placed leads in the thoracic and cervical spine because of the danger of cord compression from an epidural haematoma. There is more space in the lumbar spine and the individual clinician must decide if the risks are outweighed by the potential benefits.

Genesis of pain in patients with cancer

Direct tumour spread will create pressure effects when in confined spaces such as bone or a viscera confined within a capsule. It will also cause pain from spreading within lymphatic vessels, causing widespread oedema in patients with breast cancer involving the axillary tail. It can also cause pain from direct infiltration/invasion of a neighbouring nerve plexus such as an apical lung 'Pancoast' tumour invading the brachial plexus. Sudden changes in pain will always signal further spread or recurrence of the cancer in the mind of the patient and should be thoroughly investigated.

Pain will also arise from cancer treatments. Various chemotherapeutic agents, particularly the platins, can cause irreversible nerve damage and, frequently, neuropathic pain. If neuromodulation is to be successful in this situation the system used must be capable of covering the are involved with stimulation—induced paraesthesiae. If it is too big to cover by multiple leads then other forms of pain relief, such as intrathecal pharmacotherapy, need to be considered (see Chapter 6).

Radiotherapy will cause fibrosis, skin atrophy, contracture, telangectasia and lymphoedema, which can cause pain directly by involvement of local neural tissue or by pressure effects.

Surgery will cause pain by direct damage to nerves and via post-operative fibrosis formation as the patient heals. Certain surgical sites are known to cause more post-operative pain than others. For example breast, thoracic, hernia and gallbladder surgery are notorious for causing post-operative pain and several studies have shown that neuropathic pain, thus produced, can last for years if untreated.

However, there is a tendency to under-report pain in cancer patients for fear that treatment may be stopped. Thus the clinician must be aware that considerable pain may be present, which the patient, given the chance, will suffer in silence.

Risks and benefits of spinal cord stimulation
Risks

Side effects are uncommon but do occur, and it is important to be aware of these so that appropriate measures can be taken to reduce them. The list includes all those already cited for peripheral nerve stimulation but also includes specific risks due to the proximity of the devices to the spinal cord. Examples of possible side effects include the following:

- risks of the surgery itself—bleeding, infection, paralysis (very unlikely)
- patients may become aware of other pain elsewhere, e.g. musculoskeletal or back pain, as a result of their primary pain being relieved
- undesirable changes in stimulation can occur with time, these changes being due to changes in the nerve cells or the electrode position
- battery failure and/or battery leakage
- leakage of spinal fluid
- persisting pain at the site of implantation
- movement of the lead, causing reduction in pain relief
- allergic response to the implant material
- movement of the implant unit and damage to the overlying skin
- paralysis, weakness, numbness, clumsiness below the level of the implant
- systems may be affected by or adversely affect:
  - pacemakers
  - cardioverter defibrillators
  - external defibrillators
  - MRI
  - diathermy (surgical tissue dissection tool)
  - ultrasonic equipment
  - electrocautery (electrical method of burning tissue)
  - radiation therapy
  - theft detectors
  - security systems
  - aircraft communications systems.

There is a very definite revision rate which has to be factored into costings. It has been variously reported as high as 34% or as low as 10%. In our unit 15% is a more likely figure. However interpreting the figures is not straightforward because, for example, a renewal of battery while not a complication would be counted as a revision.

Benefits of spinal cord stimulation

Spinal cord stimulation has the intention of reducing rather than eliminating pain. The benefits of using such a system are as follows:

◆ improvement in pain relief, providing a 50–70% reduction in pain in 60–70% of patients
◆ increase in levels of activity
◆ reduction in the use of narcotic medications
◆ potentially reduction in the need for hospitalization and surgical procedures
◆ improvement in overall quality of life for sufferers.

Suggested treatment of refractory cancer pain by region
Head and neck

The cervical extension of the trigeminal nucleus, which includes fibres from the maxillary and the mandibular branches, can be reached by high cervical spinal cord stimulation. To reach the maxillary nerve peripherally is more problematic as the trajectory from the skin surface would put the lead in close contact with the coronoid process of the mandible, which, by virtue of its movement, would make lead migration almost a certainty. However, since the cervical epidural space ends variably at C2 and C3, appropriate paraesthesia coverage of the pain of head and neck cancer by spinal cord stimulation is usually difficult to achieve.

However, there are many discrete peripheral nerves that make appropriate targets for neurostimulation. The greater occipital nerve is easily reached subnuchally with a percutaneously introduced lead. The superficial branches of the trigeminal nerve; the supraorbital and the infraorbital nerves are also easily reached.

If neurmodulation is required following major ENT or maxillofacial surgical resection and reconstruction then deep brain stimulation is likely to be the best option and is outside the scope of this chapter.

Thorax

Thoracotomy for lung resection is notorious for producing neuropathic pain. It tends to be superficial in the chest wall and the painful area is well localized. Spinal cord stimulation is physically feasible and so is peripheral nerve stimulation to the segmental nerves supplying the painful area.

Mesothelioma

The pain from mesothelioma can be very refractory to treatment. Formerly, where life expectancy was rarely longer than a year, percutaneous cordotomy was the treatment of choice.

However, with improving results and thus longer survival times, cordotomy is less ideal because of the development of neuropathic pain on nerve regeneration. This will typically occur after a year to 18 months. The pain of mesothelioma is also mediated by both the autonomic system as well as the somatic system. Thus, depending on level, both the relevant segmental nerves and the sympathetic supply should be stimulated to get complete coverage of the area.

Breast

Breast surgery is fortunately much less radical and resective than formerly. However, it still remains one of the most common causes of post-operative pain. Spinal cord stimulation should provide good paraesthesia coverage to the painful area when it is confined to the thoracic wall and the axilla. Occasionally, direct peripheral nerve stimulation to the affected nerves will provide a more focused area of stimulation. The choice of target will depend on local factors such as scarring, resection and site of pain. As a general rule, peripheral nerve stimulation operates through 'normally' sensitive tissues, so if there is a large area of allodynia, spinal cord stimulation, by avoiding the area, is the better choice.

Upper limb

Satisfactory paraesethesia coverage by spinal cord stimulation can be achieved by cervically placed epidural electrodes. However, because of the mobility of the neck, a surgically placed 'paddle' electrode array is best as this is least likely to migrate. The brachial plexus is an easy target for peripheral nerve stimulation.

Abdomen/viscera

Following resection of abdominal viscera and chemotherapy, occasionally severe visceral hyperalgesia will develop. Spinal cord stimulation of the vertebral levels of the autonomic supply have not, in the main, been very successful. However, there is now evidence that direct stimulation of the splanchnic nerves can be effective in these otherwise refractory cases.

Abdomen/somatic

The abdominal wall can be stimulated by epidurally placed electrodes, which stimulate either the dorsal lemniscal fibres or the segmental dorsal root fibres. The electronic parameters required to achieve satisfactory stimulation are, however, quite different.

Pelvis

Pain arising from intrapelvic organs can, like the abdomen, arise from pain mediated through the autonomic and the somatic system. Electrodes sited at the hypogastric plexus will stimulate both autonomic and somatic sensation. Sacral nerve stimulation has been shown to be effective in reducing the frequency and pain of tenesmus and of micturition in interstitial cystitis that can follow irradiation of cervical neoplasms.

Lower limb

Tumours of the lower limb requiring resection and amputation can result in severe neuropathic pain and phantom pain. A combination of psoas compartment and sciatic nerve peripheral stimulation and/or spinal cord stimulation may be required to control the pain in these circumstances.

The evidence

There are very few published reports on the use of neuromodulation specifically in cancer pain *per se*. There are no randomized controlled trials or meta-analyses for this procedure-based treatment. However, it is a constantly evolving situation; individuals' experiences are necessarily going to involve small numbers. There are several papers in the medical literature on the outcome of peripheral nerve stimulation for neurogenic pain. Most of these studies are retrospective and do not merit comparison. The success rate (defined as greater than 50% pain relief) is reported to be as high as 89% and as low as 32%, with complication rates of 5–27% (19–21). The reader has to extrapolate from reports in cases where the mechanism of the genesis of the pain is similar to that suffered by the patient.

Because of the invasive nature of most forms of neuromodulation, trial designs 'blind-ing' the patient as well as the observer are either unethical or not feasible. Thus we have to rely on less rigid criteria along the Cochrane cascade than would be acceptable for a drug treatment. For example, in one recent report two patients with chemotherapy-induced neuropathic pain were successfully treated with spinal cord stimulation, and pain scores, mobility and medication usage was reduced (22).

Because of the enormous costs involved in randomized trials there is a paucity of 'scientific' evidence of efficacy relying on conventional critical appraisal. We frequently have nothing more than case series to report new uses and are left to evaluate the results individually, hence the need to undertake a trial of stimulation before committing the patient to the full implant.

Neuromodulation is not a panacea and the physician must make an informed choice along with their patient taking into account the risks, benefits and experience of others. The author seeks to emphasize that lack of evidence of efficacy most definitely does not equate with evidence of lack of efficacy.

The future

The applications for neuromodulation continue to broaden. Autonomic stimulation is under evaluation, with promising results for abdominal and pelvic visceral neuropathic pain. Refinements of both technique and equipment will facilitate the provision of effective pain relief in an ever-increasing population of patients who had previously been poorly controlled. One company is promising to produce 'MRI-proof' components, which will be a boon in patients requiring monitoring of tumour progression/regression. Currently, the fear of putting a patient with the existing components (which are non-paramagnetic anyway) in a strong magnet is based on the risk of inducing an electric current, heating the device and wiping the memory of the program in the IPG. In fact, low-field-strength

MRI scanners (<3 Tesla) appear not to adversely affect the presently available systems, but persuading radiological colleagues of this may prove a challenge.

There are different stimulation parameters, e.g. very high stimulation frequencies, with very different neuromodulation effects, currently being explored, or so the makers claim. It is a case of 'watch this space'. There are also new techniques being developed, such as the ability to introduce percutaneously a flat electrode, which then can concentrate the electrical energy in one direction rather than circumferentially, thus producing stimulation of deeper structures within the spinal cord, leading to different stimulation-induced paraesthesiae.

There is an increasing body of evidence attesting to the cost-effectiveness of spinal cord stimulation in previously refractory cases, where life expectancy exceeds three years. Now that we have more and more cancer survivors, there are more and more patients in whom this will make economic sense, irrespective of any ethical issues.

Evidence from spinal cord stimulation fails Cochrane criteria for evidence-based efficacy because of the cost and the problems inherent in the methodology of the trial design required to evaluate neurostimulation. The National Institute of Clinical Excellence (NICE) has approved its employment in a few areas such as neuropathic pain and ischaemic pain (23), but unfortunately not specifically for cancer—as yet. However, there is thus official recognition for neuromodulation as a treatment entity in carefully selected cases. As the body of experience increases so, I am sure, will the spectrum of 'officially' recognized indications.

As cancer survivors are frequently the family breadwinner, we must endeavour to provide the difference between a life of and in pain, and a return to gainful employment having made the 'unbearable' bearable. We have a very potent and useful therapeutic tool in neuromodulation. As physicians we must employ it not only fairly but also wisely. By achieving good outcomes for our patients we will convince our colleagues and our purchasers that there is a viable alternative to strong opioids and neurotropic drugs.

References

1. LoMonaco M, Milone M, Batocchi AP et al. (1992). Cisplatin neuropathy; clinical course and neurophysiological findings. *J Neurol* **239**(4), 199–204.

2. Hilkens PH, Verweij J, Stoter G et al. (1996). Peripheral neurotoxicity induced by docetaxel. *Neurology* **46**(1), 104–108.

3. Aass N, Kaasa S, Lund E et al. (1990). Long-term somatic side-effects and morbidity in testicular cancer patients. *Brit J Cancer* **61**(1), 151–5.

4. Gerl A (1994). Vascular toxicity associated with chemotherapy for testicular cancer. *Anticancer Drugs* **5**(6), 607–14.

5. Jaeckle KA (1989). Nerve plexus metastases. *Neurol Clinics* **9**(4), 857–66.

6. Gybels J, Sweet WH (1989). *Neurosurgical Treatment of Chronic Pain.* Karger, Basel.

7. Shealy CN, Mortimer JT, Reswick JB (1967). Electrical inhibition of pain by stimulation of the dorsal columns: preliminary clinical report. *Anesth Analg* **46**(4), 489–91.

8. Myerson BA, Linderoth B Spinal Cord Stimulation (2000). In: Loeser JD (ed.) *Bonica's Management of Pain*, 3rd edn. Lippincott Williams and Wilkins, Philadelphia.

9. Myerson BA, Linderoth B (2003). Spinal cord stimulation—mechanisms of action in neuropathic and ischaemic pain. In: Simpson BA (ed.) *Electrical Stimulation and Relief of Pain. Pain Research and Clinical Management*, Vol 15. Elsevier, Amsterdam.

10. Urban MO, Gebhart GF (1998). The glutamate synapse: a target in the pharmacological management of hyperalgesic pain states. *Prog Brain Res* **116**, 407–20.

11. Woolf CJ (1983). Evidence for a central component of post-injury pain hypersensitivity. *Nature* **306**(5944), 686–8.

12. Cherny NJ, Catane R (1995). Profesional negligence in the management of cancer pain. A case for urgent reforms (editorial comment). *Cancer* **76**(11), 2181–5.

13. Sapir R, Catane R, Cherny NJ (1997). Cancer pain: knowledge and attitudes of physicians in Israel (Meeting Abstract). *Proceedings of the Annual Meeting of the American Society of Clinical Oncology* **16**.

14. Ikeda H, Stark J, Fischer H *et al.* (2006). Synaptic amplifier of inflammatory pain in the spinal dorsal horn. *Science* **312**(5780), 1659–62.

15. Tsuda M, Shigemoto-Mogami Y, Koizumi S *et al.* (2003). Induction of P2X4 ionotropic ATP receptor in spinal hyperactive microglia gates neuropathic pain. *Nature* **424**(6950), 778–83.

16. Yakhnitsa V, Linderth B, Myerson BA (1998). Modulation of dorsal horn neuronal activity by spinal cord stimulation in a rat model neuropathy: the role of the dorsal funicles. *Neurophysiology* **30**(6), 424–7).

17. Roberts MHT, Rees H (1994). Physiological basis of spinal cord stimulation. *Pain Rev* **1**, 184–98.

18. El-Khoury C, Hawwa M, Baliki SF *et al.* (2002). Attenuation of neuropathic pain by segmental and supraspinal activation of the dorsal column system in awake rats. *Neuroscience* **112**(3), 541–53.

19. Law JD, Sweet J, Kirsch WM (1980). Retrospective analysis of 22 patients with chronic pain treated by peripheral nerve stimulation. *J Neurosurg* **52**(4), 482–5.

20. Long DM, Erickson D, Campbell J *et al.* (1981). Electrical stimulation of the spinal cord and peripheral nerves for pain control: a 10-year experience. *Appl Neurophysiol* **44**(4), 207–17.

21. Nashold BS Jr, Goldner JL, Mullen JB *et al.* (1982). Long term pain control by direct peripheral nerve stimulation. *J Bone Joint Surg Am* **64**(1), 1–10.

22. Cata JP, Cordella JV, Burton AW *et al.* (2004). Spinal cord stimulation relieves chemotherapy-induced pain: a clinical case report. *J Pain Symptom Manage* **27**(1), 72–8.

23. National Institute for Health and Clinical excellence (2008). *Spinal cord stimulation for chronic pain of neuropathic or ischaemic origin. NICE Technology Appraisal Guidance No.159.* Available at: http://guidance.nice.org.uk/nicemedia/live/12082/42369/42369.pdf.

Chapter 12

Transcutaneous electrical nerve stimulation and acupuncture

Mark I. Johnson, Jacqueline Filshie, and
John W. Thompson

Introduction

Interventions that stimulate the body or the nervous system for pain relief have a role in the management of pain in patients with cancer. Transcutaneous electrical nerve stimulation (TENS) and acupuncture are techniques that are used in pain clinics throughout the world. They have a role in oncology and palliative care settings for the management of pain associated with cancer and its treatment and for cancer-related nausea and vomiting, breathlessness, fatigue, xerostomia and vasomotor symptoms. Both techniques are safe and can be used in combination with conventional treatments. However, disease progression needs to be monitored regularly because TENS and acupuncture may mask symptoms (1).

Transcutaneous electrical nerve stimulation

Introduction

TENS is a non-invasive technique that is used for pain of nociceptive, neuropathic and musculoskeletal origin. Factors predicting success with TENS are not yet known, so any patient may respond to TENS. TENS is administered using a portable battery-operated electrical pulse generator, which delivers currents across the intact surface of the skin via self-adhering conducting pads called electrodes (Fig. 12.1). TENS activates endogenous analgesic mechanisms.

TENS is easy to use, with almost no potential for toxicity or overdose, so patients can administer treatment themselves. TENS is inexpensive and available without prescription in the UK, although patients should be assessed for suitability by a medical practitioner and instructed on how to use TENS by a healthcare professional. There should be regular monitoring of progress and a point of contact to troubleshoot any problems.

Electrical stimulation of the skin for pain relief is an age-old technique. The ancient Egyptians (2500 BC), Greeks (400 BC) and Romans (AD 46) treated headache and gout using electrogenic fish (*Malapterurus electricus* and *Torpedo marmorata*). The invention of the electrostatic generator in the eighteenth century led to the development of electrical devices for use in medicine, although these were soon to be superseded by more widespread use of pharmacological agents. Interest in electrical stimulation for pain relief was rekindled

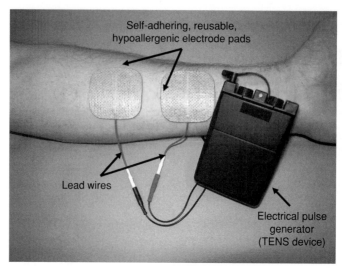

Fig. 12.1 Transcutaneous electrical nerve stimulation. Also appears in colour in the colour plate section, Plate 47.

in 1965 following the publication of the 'Gate Control Theory of Pain'. In 1967, percutaneous electrical stimulation of large-diameter nerve fibres was shown to reduce neuropathic pain, and electrical stimulation of the dorsal columns reduced chronic pain. TENS was used to predict the success of dorsal column stimulation implants until, in the early 1970s it was realized that TENS was effective in its own right.

The use of TENS in oncology and palliative settings date back to the 1970s, although TENS appears to be used only on selected cancer pain patients in the UK. Data on usage in oncology and palliative settings are surprisingly lacking. Only 3% of 2118 patients surveyed over a 10-year period were given TENS in an anaesthesiology-based palliative care programme in Germany. In this setting, TENS was indicated for pains of neuropathic origin (2, 3).

TENS equipment

In health care, the term TENS is used to describe stimulation delivered by a 'standard TENS device' (Fig. 12.2). There are differences in the specifications of standard TENS devices between manufacturers but in general these differences are minor and often cosmetic. TENS-like devices deliver electrical currents across the intact surface of the skin but have output specifications that differ from a standard TENS device. TENS-like devices include interferential current therapy, microcurrent electrical therapy, transcutaneous spinal electroanalgesia (TSE see below) and transcranial electrical stimulation. Claims about the effectiveness of TENS-like devices are often exaggerated (4).

Techniques using a standard TENS device

The intention when using TENS is to selectively activate nerves beneath the electrodes to elicit segmental and/or extrasegmental pain modulatory processes. Large-diameter, non-nociceptive afferents (A-beta) have lower thresholds of activation to electrical stimuli

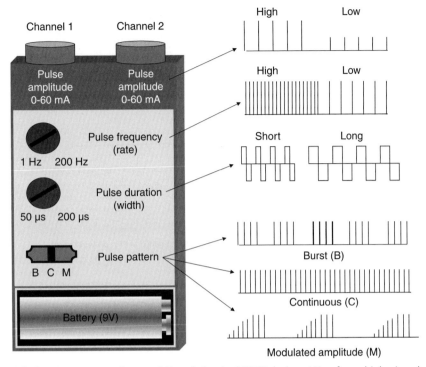

Fig. 12.2 Common output characteristics of standard TENS devices. Waveform, biphasic pulsed electrical currents; pulse amplitudes, 1–60 mA into a 1 kΩ load; pulse frequencies, 1–200 Hz; pulse durations (width), 50–200 μs; pulse patterns, continuous, burst and modulated amplitude, frequencies and/or durations.

than their small-diameter nociceptive counterparts (A-delta and C). Increasing the amplitude of electrical currents will therefore result in non-nociceptive nerve fibres being activated before nociceptive fibres. Good-quality evidence from healthy humans exposed to experimental pain suggests that the parameter combinations are pivotal to optimizing hypoalgesic effects.

Conventional TENS

The International Association for the Study of Pain (IASP) describes conventional TENS as high-frequency (50–100 Hz), short pulse width (50–200 μs), low-intensity (paraesthesia, not painful) TENS covering the painful region. Conventional TENS is used to selectively stimulate large-diameter non-noxious afferents (A-beta fibres) without simultaneously stimulating small-diameter noxious afferents (A-delta and C fibres, Table 12.1). This is akin to 'rubbing skin for pain relief'. In practice, the user increases the pulse amplitude of TENS so that a strong, comfortable, non-painful TENS paraesthesiae is perceived beneath the electrodes. Electrodes are positioned around the site of pain or over nerve bundles arising from the painful area so that large-diameter afferents, segmentally related to the noxious input, are activated. Pain relief is segmental and rapid in onset and offset, so TENS is switched on for prolonged periods to achieve ongoing pain relief.

Table 12.1 Different TENS techniques

	Conventional TENS	AL-TENS	Intense TENS
Physiological intention	Activation of non-noxious afferents	Activation of small-diameter muscle and cutaneous afferents	Activation of small-diameter noxious afferents
Patient experience	Non-noxious TENS paraesthesiae (minimal muscle activity)	Strong TENS generating muscle twitching	Electrical paraesthesiae that is uncomfortable but tolerable with post stimulation hypoaesthesia
Electrode location	Site of pain (dermatomal)	Acupuncture points, trigger points and over motor nerves	Main nerve bundle from origin of pain
TENS characteristics			
◆ Pulse frequency	◆ High (10–200 pps)	◆ Low (<5 pps or <5 bps)	◆ High (>50 pps)
◆ Pulse amplitude	◆ Low (non-painful)	◆ High (non-painful twitching)	◆ High (painful)
◆ Pulse duration	◆ 50–200 µs		◆ >500 µs
◆ Pulse pattern	◆ Continuous in first instance	◆ 100–200 µs	◆ Continuous in first instance
		◆ Burst in first instance	
Analgesic profile	Rapid onset and offset	Rapid onset delayed offset	Rapid onset delayed offset peripheral
	Segmental	Segmental, extrasegmental	Segmental, extrasegmental
Regimen	Apply for long periods of time throughout the day as needed	Apply for ~30 min per session a few times each day	Apply for 15 min per session

bps = bursts of 100 pulses per second

Acupuncture-like TENS (AL-TENS)

AL-TENS was developed to harness the actions of TENS and acupuncture. IASP describes AL-TENS as low-frequency (2–4 Hz), long pulse width (100–400 µs), higher-intensity (to tolerance threshold). Electrodes are usually placed at acupuncture points, trigger points or at the painful region. AL-TENS is a form of hyperstimulation that stimulates small-diameter peripheral afferents (A-delta cutaneous and muscle afferents), which then activate descending pain-inhibitory pathways, so inhibiting central nociceptor cells for up to 2 h (Table 12.1). Strong non-painful muscle twitching is often achieved during AL-TENS. Some patients prefer bursts of high-frequency pulses (~2–5 bursts/s of 100 pps) rather than low-frequency pulses to achieve this. AL-TENS may benefit patients who do not respond to conventional TENS, when it is not possible to position electrodes at the site of pain due to altered skin sensations, and for certain neuropathic pain conditions, e.g. for cancer-related back pain where conventional TENS can be administered in the lumbar region and AL-TENS administered at the same time over the hamstring muscles for radiating pain (5). TENS is occasionally used as a counter-irritant for minor surgical procedures such as wound dressing and suture removal, delivering currents at intensities that are painful but tolerable.

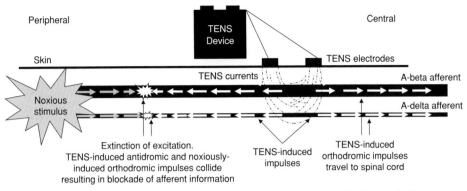

Fig. 12.3 Antidromic activation of nerves by TENS leading to peripheral blockade of afferent information arising from noxious stimuli.

Mechanism of action

TENS activates peripheral nerves both orthodromically and antidromically, and can block incoming afferent impulses arising from natural stimuli (Fig. 12.3). Activity in large- and small-diameter afferents, contributing to a patient's pain experience, may therefore be blocked by different types of TENS. Experiments using anesthetized rats and cats demonstrate that TENS inhibits evoked responses in sensitized wide dynamic range cells. This TENS-induced inhibition of wide dynamic range cells remains after spinal cord transection, which removes the influence of supraspinal structures. This suggests that inhibition is due to a segmental effect (Fig. 12.4). High-intensity TENS (e.g. AL-TENS) generates segmental effects that outlast the period of stimulation for up to 2 h. AL-TENS activates the periaqueductal grey and ventromedial medulla on the descending pain-inhibitory pathways, which project to many levels of the spinal cord producing extrasegmental effects (Fig. 12.4). TENS-induced activity in deep muscle afferents appears to generate larger effects than skin afferents (6).

TENS pharmacology is complex. Gamma-amino butyric acid (GABA) is a key transmitter for conventional TENS and endogenous opioids for AL-TENS. Cholinergic, adrenergic and serotinergic systems also seem to have a role in TENS analgesia. Mu opioid receptors have been implicated in low-frequency TENS and delta opioid receptors in high-frequency TENS.

Indications

TENS is used as a stand alone treatment for mild-to-moderate pain or in combination with analgesic medication for moderate-to-severe pain. Any patient with pain directly or indirectly related to cancer and its treatment may respond to TENS. This can include pains from metastatic cancer, bone metastases, direct infiltration of nerves and nerve compression by a tumour, vertebral collapse or enlarged organs. TENS may also benefit chemotherapy-related pain, post-surgical pain and post-amputation pain. There are reports of success with TENS for neuropathic cancer pain caused by nerve compression by a tumour or infiltration by a tumour, and post-mastectomy and post-thoracotomy

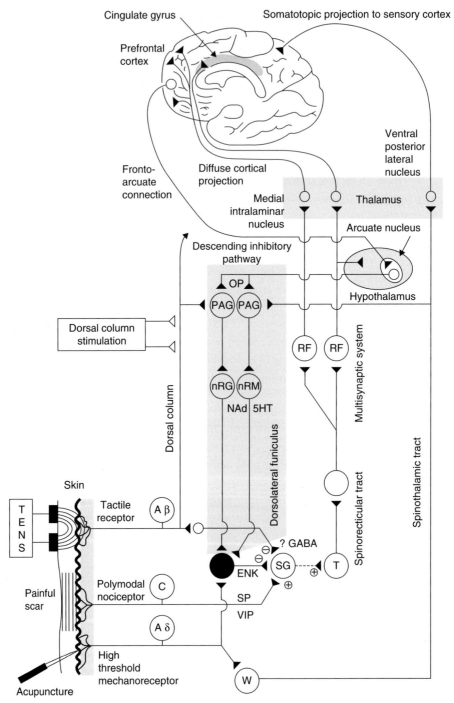

Fig. 12.4 Neurophysiology of TENS and acupuncture. Reproduced from Filshie J, Thompson JW, (2009). Acupuncture. In Hanks G. *et al.* (eds*), Oxford Textbook of Palliative Medicine*, 4th Edn. Oxford University Press, with permission.

pain (7–10). TENS may benefit central neuropathic pain, yet is likely to be more beneficial for peripheral neuropathic pains such as radiculopathies (cervical, thoracic and lumbar), post-herpetic neuralgia, and phantom limb and stump pain.

TENS over the Pericardium 6 (PC6, Neiguan) acupuncture point has been reported to be beneficial for chemotherapy-induced and post-operative nausea and vomiting(11, 12). A TENS-like device worn like a watch to stimulate over PC6 (transcutaneous electrical acupoint stimulation), when combined with ondansetron, has been shown to reduce post-operative nausea and vomiting in post-operative non-cancer patients following laparoscopic surgery. TENS has also been used for the management of lymphoedema by placing electrodes proximal to the lymphoedematous limb.

Practical aspects

In order for TENS to be effective, skin sensation must be intact, so it is important to check skin sensibility prior to application. Conventional TENS should be tried first in most situations, with TENS paraesthesiae directed into the painful area (Fig. 12.5). In the presence of hyperalgesia or mechanical allodynia, electrodes should be positioned over the main nerves proximal to the site of pain in the first instance. Paravertebral electrode placement at the appropriate segments is also useful and stimulation of contralateral and/or ipsilateral dermatomes has been used, especially in post-herpetic neuralgia.

A pragmatic approach is taken in clinical practice: a patient's report of 'strong but comfortable' TENS paraesthesiae beneath the electrodes is the criterion used to ascertain selective large-fibre activation. Patients titrate TENS amplitude to achieve this goal. In theory, high-frequency, low-intensity currents with pulse durations between 50 and 500 μs are most efficient in selective recruitment of large-diameter afferents, although in practice patients are encouraged to experiment with pulse frequency, pulse pattern and pulse duration to achieve what is most comfortable for them at that moment in time. Patients are encouraged to leave electrodes in situ so that TENS can be administered intermittently or constantly throughout the day. It is important to attend to skin care underneath the electrodes.

AL-TENS may be useful for patients who do not respond to conventional TENS or when it is not possible to generate TENS paraesthesiae locally at the site of pain, e.g. neuropathic pain that radiates or patients with hyperaesthesia, hypoaesthesia or dysaesthesia. Because AL-TENS is a form of hyperstimulation, it is usually given intermittently throughout the day, e.g. 20 min, three times per day with electrodes positioned over acupuncture points, trigger points or at the site of pain. AL-TENS can be combined with conventional TENS using a dual-channel TENS device with four electrodes.

Safety

TENS is safe, and serious adverse events appear to be rare, although literature is sparse in this area. TENS worsens pain in some patients and it is difficult to predict when this will occur, although it is more likely when mechanical (tactile) allodynia is present. Patients with a history of autonomic reactions to tactile allodynia may experience nausea and, rarely, syncope. Minor skin irritation (redness and itch) may occur due to contact dermatitis beneath the electrodes.

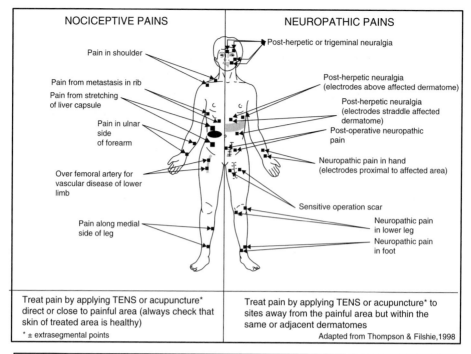

NOCICEPTIVE PAINS	NEUROPATHIC PAINS

Pain in shoulder

Pain from metastasis in rib

Pain from stretching of liver capsule

Pain in ulnar side of forearm

Over femoral artery for vascular disease of lower limb

Pain along medial side of leg

Post-herpetic or trigeminal neuralgia

Post-herpetic neuralgia (electrodes above affected dermatome)

Post-herpetic neuralgia (electrodes straddle affected dermatome)

Post-operative neuropathic pain

Neuropathic pain in hand (electrodes proximal to affected area)

Sensitive operation scar

Neuropathic pain in lower leg

Neuropathic pain in foot

Treat pain by applying TENS or acupuncture* direct or close to painful area (always check that skin of treated area is healthy)
* ± extrasegmental points

Treat pain by applying TENS or acupuncture* to sites away from the painful area but within the same or adjacent dermatomes

Adapted from Thompson & Filshie,1998

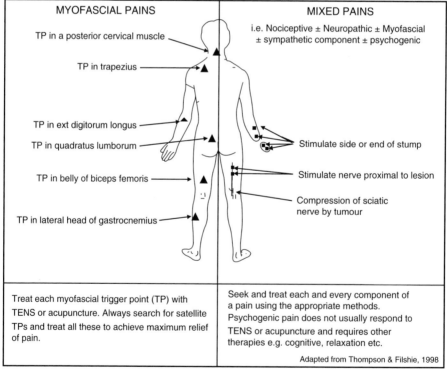

MYOFASCIAL PAINS	MIXED PAINS

TP in a posterior cervical muscle

TP in trapezius

TP in ext digitorum longus

TP in quadratus lumborum

TP in belly of biceps femoris

TP in lateral head of gastrocnemius

i.e. Nociceptive ± Neuropathic ± Myofascial ± sympathetic component ± psychogenic

Stimulate side or end of stump

Stimulate nerve proximal to lesion

Compression of sciatic nerve by tumour

Treat each myofascial trigger point (TP) with TENS or acupuncture. Always search for satellite TPs and treat all these to achieve maximum relief of pain.

Seek and treat each and every component of a pain using the appropriate methods. Psychogenic pain does not usually respond to TENS or acupuncture and requires other therapies e.g. cognitive, relaxation etc.

Adapted from Thompson & Filshie, 1998

Fig. 12.5 Diagram to show examples of the four main types of pain, namely nociceptive, neuropathic, myofascial and mixed, together with an indication of the principles of their treatment using TENS and acupuncture. For the sake of clarity and space, the first two types are depicted on the front of the body, while the second two types are shown on the back of the body. For further details see text. Adapted from Thompson JW, Filshie J (1998). Transcutaneous electrical nerve stimulation (TENS) and acupuncture. In Doyle D, Hanks G, MacDonald N, eds *Oxford Textbook of Palliative Medicine*, pp. 421–437, 2nd Edn. Oxford University Press, Oxford.

It is generally accepted that electrodes should not be positioned directly over a tumour for a patient whose tumour is treatable, although to our knowledge there are no studies that have evaluated the effects of TENS on tumour growth in humans and there are no reports suggesting detrimental effects on tumour growth in case series. However, electrodes can be positioned over areas where there is known disease in the palliative setting, e.g. on skin over a rib metastasis. Electrodes should not be placed on irradiated skin in the immediate weeks after radiotherapy.

The UK Chartered Society of Physiotherapy guidelines list cardiac pacemakers and bleeding disorders as contraindications (13). Patients with certain pacemakers have been given TENS under the careful guidance of cardiologists. TENS should not be used near the site of thrombosis in patients with compromised circulation. TENS should not be administered over or close to the abdomen during pregnancy because, theoretically, currents could inadvertently cause uterine contractions. There have been no reports of TENS affecting foetal development, although TENS can interfere with foetal monitoring equipment. Patients with epilepsy can use TENS, providing electrodes are positioned below the neck and practitioners monitor progress carefully. There are case reports of TENS causing epileptic seizures in patients susceptible to seizures, including a patient with post-stroke pain and a patient with severe psychomotor disorder and epilepsy following viral meningoencephalitis (13a,b). Any risk/benefit decisions are left to the discretion of the medical practitioner.

TENS is used in patients with metal implants, stents, percutaneous central catheters or drainage systems. Practitioners should be alerted to the mechanical stresses on implants due to TENS-induced muscle activity. Electrodes should not be positioned close to transdermal drug-delivery systems as they may cause iontophoresis, leading to drug toxicity. TENS does interfere with monitoring equipment, so medical staff need to be able to identify TENS artefacts. TENS interference can be filtered using interface units under the guidance of the medical physics department.

TENS should not be applied internally (mouth) or over areas of damaged skin such as open wounds. The anterior part of the neck should not be stimulated as this may cause an acute vasovagal reaction. TENS should not be used while operating motor vehicles or any potentially hazardous equipment or while in the shower or bath. Stimulation through the chest using anterior–posterior electrode sites has been reported to compromise respiration. TENS devices with timers that automatically switch off power can be used to reduce pain prior to sleep. Children as young as four can use TENS providing they understand what to expect.

Clinical research

Systematic reviews on acute post-operative pain and labour pain have found no evidence of effects from TENS, although a meta-analysis of 21 randomized controlled trials (RCTs) found that TENS reduced post-operative analgesic consumption providing it was administered using an appropriate technique (14). A Cochrane review found that high- but not low-frequency TENS reduced symptoms of primary dysmenorrhoea, although this was based on only a small number of trials (15). Some systematic reviews of chronic non-cancer pain have been positive for osteoarthritic knee pain, chronic musculoskeletal pain and low back pain, although contradictory review findings exist. In general, Cochrane reviews are inconclusive for rheumatoid arthritis of the hand, low back pain, whiplash and mechanical neck disorders, post-stroke shoulder pain and chronic recurrent headache.

A Cochrane review on TENS for cancer-related pain found two small RCTs, but neither meet the criteria for meta-analysis (16) (Table 12.2).One of the RCTs, using 45 women with chronic pain associated with breast cancer treatment, found that TENS and TSE reduced pain compared to baseline but their effects were no greater than placebo TSE. Interestingly, 15 women preferred to continue TENS treatment compared to five for TSE and six for sham. The other RCT compared AL-TENS, sham AL-TENS and no treatment on 15 patients with various cancers, and suggested that AL-TENS was superior to sham and no treatment.

A systematic review of complementary therapies in patients dying with cancer (17) concluded that TENS may relieve intractable pain, although this finding was based on one RCT and one case series. The non-controlled trial found that 39 out of 60 patients with metastatic cancer, surgery, irradiation and amputation responded to TENS at two weeks. Only 20 patients continued with TENS at three months. Case series report that TENS may be useful in the short term. For example, TENS relieved pain in 50 of 60 patients with painful bony metastases and 35 of 37 cancer patients with pains from compression by large masses over the cervical nerve trunks or neoplastic involvement on maxillofacial tissues. Recently, a feasibility study assessed active and placebo TENS in patients with cancer-related bone pain and found that active TENS had the potential to decrease pain on movement more than pain on rest (18).

A Cochrane review concluded that PC6 acupoint stimulation by a variety of methods, including TENS, was beneficial in non-cancer patients without antiemetic prophylaxis. Interestingly, a subsequent Cochrane review concluded that TENS at acupuncture points was unlikely to benefit chemotherapy-induced nausea and vomiting, although the stimulation parameters chosen may have been suboptimal. Evidence from RCTs suggest that transcutaneous electrical acupoint stimulation of PC6 reduces post-operative nausea and vomiting in non-cancer patients. A phase I–II trial of AL-TENS delivered using a Codetron device found improvements in saliva production and related symptoms in patients with radiation-induced xerostomia.

Acupuncture

Introduction

Acupuncture is a form of stimulation-induced analgesia and is a technique of inserting fine needles in the skin at specific points (from the Latin *acus* 'with a needle' and *punctura*, from *pungere* 'to prick') for symptom control. Acupuncture is used as a first-line treatment for many medical conditions in China and it is gaining popularity in the West for common ailments such as osteoarthritis, back pain, migraine, myofascial pain, and nausea and vomiting. Needles are positioned to stimulate nerve, muscle and sometimes periosteum, and additional (stronger) stimulation can be achieved by manipulating (twirling) the needle or by passing electrical currents through the needles (electroacupuncture). Acupuncture has been integrated into pain management services in many countries and has an increasing role

Table 12.2 TENS for cancer pain—research evidence

Reference	Pain patient sample	Comparison groups and TENS technique	Proportions of patients reporting pain relief
RCTs			
Robb et al. (2007)	45 patients with chronic pain secondary to treatment for breast cancer (41 completed)	Cross-over trial of conventional TENS, TSE, sham TSE	No differences between groups. 15 patients requested to continue to use TENS compared to 5 for TSE and 6 for sham
Gadsby et al. (1997)	15 patients in palliative care setting with various malignancies	Parallel group trial of AL-TENS, sham AL-TENS, no treatment control	Claimed that odds ratio AL-TENS 0.5 times greater than placebo and 0.16 times better than no treatment control but based on 5 patients per group
Pre and post evaluations without control group			
Avellanosa and West (1982)	60 patients with a variety of metastatic carcinomas	Conventional TENS	at 2 weeks = 39/60 patients at 3 months = 20/60 patients
Hasun and Marberger (1988)	45 patients with advanced cancer of prostate, renal cells or urothelial bladder	Uncertain—galvanic current?	'Every other patient responded to TENS'
Ostrowski (1979)	9 patients with various carcinomas	Conventional TENS	At immediate post TENS = 8/9 patients at 6 months = 3/9 patients
Loeser et al. (1975)	7 patients with malignancies in a mixed population of 198 chronic pain patients	Conventional TENS	3/7 patients
Long (1974)	5 patients with malignancies in a mixed population of 197 chronic pain patients	Conventional TENS	3/5 patients
Hardy (1974)	4 patients with malignancies in a mixed population of 53 chronic pain patients	Conventional TENS	2/4 patients
Ventafridda et al. (1979)	37 patients in which cancer was the primary cause	Conventional TENS	In first 10 days = 36/37 patients At 30 days = 4/37 patients
Bates and Nathan (1980)	5 patients with malignancies in a mixed population of 161 chronic pain patients	Conventional TENS	4/5 patients
Rafter, cited in Librach and Rapson (1988)	49 patients with malignancies of musculoskeletal origin	Conventional TENS	37/49 patients

(continued)

Table 12.2 (Cont'd)

Reference	Pain patient sample	Comparison groups and TENS technique	Proportions of patients reporting pain relief
Dil'din et al. (1985) Abstract only	84 patients with malignancies and post-operative procedures	Conventional TENS using a Soviet device	84/84 patients
Reuss and Meyer (1985)	60 patients with bony metastasis	Conventional TENS	50/60 patients
Hidderley and Weinel (1997)	4 patients undergoing radiotherapy for head and neck cancer	TENS on acupuncture points away from the site of pain (TENS intensity very low)	4/4 patients

TSE, transcutaneous spinal electroanalgesia. See reference (16) for list of references of original articles.

in the treatment of cancer pain and symptom management. Patients consider acupuncture as 'very important' when integrated into cancer clinics. The increasing use of acupuncture in veterinary medicine lends some credence to the view that acupuncture is more than merely a placebo.

The Yellow Emperor's *'Classic of Internal Medicine* is one of the earliest texts referencing acupuncture, although acupuncture may have been practiced as early as the twenty-first century BC in China. Traditional Eastern-style acupuncture was based on the principles of traditional Chinese medicine, which involved diagnosis and treatment based on normalization of vital 'energy flow' or 'Qi' round the body. The Qi is said to flow along invisible energy channels (meridians), which are joined by a series of acupuncture points on the surface of the body. Herbal treatment is often administered as well.

Types of acupuncture

Acupuncturists select their techniques according to disease and treatment approach, which depends on training and background. There are two main approaches: traditional Chinese acupuncture using Eastern-style acupuncture or Western medical acupuncture using orthodox medical principles and practice (Table 12.3).

Western medical acupuncture

Western medical practitioners make a diagnosis following orthodox history, examination and investigation (19). In clinical practice, Western medical practitioners tend to use a mix of traditional points that have an appreciable evidence base, trigger points and segmental points appropriate to the symptom and region affected. A vast amount of neurophysiological evidence supports the view that acupuncture modulates multiple endogenous homeostatic mechanisms, including endogenous endorphins, serotonin and oxytocin (see Mechanism of action section below). Acupuncture can be blocked by prior injection with local anaesthesic and thus relies on nerves for transmission and to initiate a cascade of endogenous molecular changes. Western medical acupuncturists no longer subscribe to the view that acupuncture balances 'vital energy'.

Table 12.3 Acupuncture techniques

Technique	Description
Manual acupuncture	Western approach medical acupuncture
	◆ Diagnosis following orthodox history, examination and investigation
	◆ Use a mix of segmental points, trigger points and traditional points
	◆ Stimulation usually 10–20 min
	◆ Embraces neurophysiological mechanisms
	Traditional Chinese acupuncture
	◆ Elaborate diagnosis uses 'laws', tongue and pulse diagnosis
	◆ Points selected to achieve 'De Qi' and to balance Yin and Yang, forces of opposite polarities
	◆ Vigorous stimulation and/or moxibustion
	◆ Embraces abstract concepts of Qi and Yin and Yang
Electroacupunture	Electrical currents passed through pairs of needles using a portable electrical stimulator
	◆ Low frequency = 2–4 Hz
	◆ High frequency = 50–200 Hz
	◆ Modulated frequency 2–100 Hz
Laser acupuncture	No needles—not strictly acupuncture
	Use low-level laser device and principles of laser therapy to administer to acupuncture points
Acupressure	No needles—weaker stimulus than acupuncture
	Massage at acupuncture points
	Can be self-administered
Auricular acupuncture	Needling points on the ear
	Based on claims that there are somatotopic representations of the body on ear
	Point specificity has been challenged
Moxibustion	Thermal stimulus applied to needle or held above acupuncture points
Ryodoraku	Uses electrodermal testing to identify reduced skin impedance prior to electroacupuncture-like treatment

Traditional Chinese acupuncture

The traditional Chinese view utilized 'laws' to guide a complex tongue and pulse diagnosis, although the authenticity of pulse diagnosis has been seriously challenged. The traditional Chinese acupuncturist uses needles to manually stimulate acupuncture points in order to balance Yin and Yang forces of opposite polarities. Points are selected to achieve 'De Qi' (needling sensation), which the patient reports as sensations of aching, numbness, tingling, heaviness and 'fullness'. Abstract concepts such as Qi, Yin and Yang have contributed to scepticism about the merits of acupuncture in some quarters of the medical fraternity. If Yin and Yang are taken to represent homeostatic mechanisms such as autonomic balance, and circulation of Qi taken as the circulation of blood containing oxygen and endogenous chemical substances such as hormones, then parallels to modern medical knowledge are more understandable.

Electroacupuncture

Electroacupuncture is a treatment using weak electric currents that pass through pairs of needles using a portable electrical stimulator. Low-frequency electroacupuncture (2–4 Hz) has been shown to increase circulating levels of enkephalins and cortisol, while high-frequency electroacupuncture (50–200 Hz) increases serotonin (5-HT) and dynorphin. Electroacupuncture was developed to generate additional stimulation similar to the vigorous manual stimulation used during peri-operative acupuncture analgesia. It is used when stronger stimulation is required for complex pain problems such as chronic back pain, and for acute pain. Ryodoraku is a Japanese form of electroacupuncture where measurement of skin impedance is used to aid diagnosis and a form of electroacupuncture is used to modify abnormalities.

Laser acupuncture/therapy

Laser treatment is not strictly acupuncture as it does not involve the use of needles, yet the term 'laser acupuncture' is widely used. Laser therapy consists of stimulating acupuncture points using a low-level laser. Laser therapy is non-invasive and is more acceptable for children or patients with needle phobias. When administered at the site of a painful soft-tissue injury, low-level laser therapy has been shown to modulate biochemical markers of inflammation and to reduce acute pain in a dose-dependent manner. Systematic reviews conclude that low-level laser therapy provides short-term relief in a range of chronic pain conditions but is equivocal for post-mastectomy lymphoedema. RCTs suggest that low-level laser therapy is effective for mucositis induced by chemotherapy in cancer patients (20–22) and that laser acupuncture reduces peri-articular swelling (23), chronic tension-type headache (24) and radicular pain (25).

Acupressure

Acupressure involves massage rather than needles to stimulate acupuncture points. Acupressure is non-invasive and can be self-administered but is a weaker stimulus than acupuncture. A Cochrane review shows that acupressure at PC6 is effective for early nausea and vomiting post chemotherapy (PONV) (26), and RCTs have shown that acupressure at PC6 is effective for chemotherapy-induced PONV. Acupressure is also used for chronic obstructive pulmonary disease.

Auricular acupuncture

Auricular acupuncture involves needling points on the ear. The pinna has rich innervation, including the vagus nerve. It has been claimed that there is a somatotopic representation of the body on the ear, although the precise importance of point specificity has been challenged. Auricular acupuncture is used for habitual drug abuse, especially narcotic and alcohol addiction using the National Acupuncture Detoxification Association (NADA) treatment, although a Cochrane review found no evidence to support effectiveness for the treatment of cocaine dependence (27). It is widely used for smoking cessation, yet a Cochrane review found no clear evidence that acupuncture, acupressure, laser therapy or electrostimulation was effective for smoking cessation. A randomized placebo-controlled trial reported that auricular acupuncture was effective in reducing chronic peripheral or central neuropathic pain after treatment of a cancer (28). Pilot studies also show significant improvements in pain following auricular acupuncture in cancer patients.

Related techniques

Moxibustion consists of a thermal stimulus applied to the needle or held above acupuncture points. Moxibustion has been reported to help breech babies turn in the last trimester, although a Cochrane review was inconclusive. Other microsystems have been used, such as scalp and hand acupuncture.

Acupuncture equipment

In general, acupuncture needles are fine disposable needles (0.2–0.3 mm) made of surgical stainless steel. Needles are available in a variety of sizes, lengths and gauges, and are chosen according to practitioner preferences. Plastic introducing guide tubes can facilitate needle insertion. Semi-permanent needles are used extensively to prolong the effects of acupuncture for treatment of cancer-related pain, dyspnoea, anxiety and hot flushes. Wall charts and models are available to aid accurate point localization. Manufacturers provide a wide range of electrical and laser equipment.

Mechanism of action

Neurophysiological evidence provides a sound scientific basis for acupuncture analgesia (29). Acupuncture analgesia is mediated through polymodal receptors and high-threshold small-diameter A-delta and C fibres, although needling will also activate lower-threshold A-beta afferents and autonomic efferents. It has been shown that in humans acupuncture points are excitable skin–nerve–muscle complexes with a high density of nerve endings and that acupuncture actions are blocked by local anaesthetic. The afferent input resulting from acupuncture stimulation leads to inhibition of second-order nociceptive transmission cells through segmental and extrasegmental mechanisms.

The segmental effects of acupuncture result from activity in high-threshold mechanoreceptors stimulating A-delta afferents that terminate in inhibitory enkephalinergic interneurons in the substantia gelantinosa (Fig. 12.4). This leads to post-synaptic inhibition of nociceptive transmission cells in the substantia gelatinosa of the spinal cord, preventing onward transmission of noxiously-generated information.

Acupuncture-induced activity in small-diameter peripheral afferents also activates second-order cells in lamina I of the spinal gray matter, which form the ascending pathways of the spinothalamic tract. The spinothalamic tract is a fast-transmitting noxious pathway, which relays information such as pin-prick to the somatosensory cortex. Collaterals of this fast-transmitting ascending system activate midbrain and brain-stem structures, which switch on descending pain-inhibitory pathways throughout all levels of the spinal cord and inhibit onward transmission of noxious information. This supraspinal feedback loop explains the extrasegmental actions of acupuncture. Research demonstrates that acupuncture activates descending pain-inhibitory structures, including the ventromedial medulla and periaqueductal grey.

Acupuncture activates multiple endogenous neural systems, leading to the release of a complex array of neurochemicals, including opioids, serotonin, noradrenaline, adrenocorticotrophic hormone, cholecystokinin, nerve growth factor and oxytocin, to name but a few. There is a wealth of research evidence that suggests that beta-endorphin, met-enkephalin and dynorphins acting on mu, delta and kappa (OP3, OP1 and OP2) opioid receptors mediate acupuncture analgesia. Opioid gene production is up-regulated by acupuncture and may be frequency dependent with low-frequency electroacupuncture causing preproenkephalin mRNA expression and high-frequency electroacupuncture causing preprodynorphin mRNA expression. Such up-regulation may explain the role of acupuncture 'top-ups', which may maintain gene expression in a 'switched-on' mode.

Brain-imaging studies suggest that acupuncture influences structures extending from the brainstem and cerebellum to the cerebrum, although studies often suffer from significant within subject variability (30). Evidence supports a somatotopic representation of acupuncture points in the primary somatosensory cortex, and a critical role for limbic system structures such as the anterior cingulate, hippocampus, insula, amygdala and nucleus accumbens. These structures are likely to have a role in positive affect and in the pleasurable feelings associated with acupuncture. This may account for reports that pain remains but is less unpleasant. Brain activation patterns suggest differences between patients in pain and healthy volunteers when exposed to experimental pain, suggesting that acupuncture differs in its actions in normal versus abnormal pathological states. Specific brain activation patterns are produced during acupuncture when compared with sham and electroacupuncture, and when acupuncture is given at different points and for different durations. Post-stimulation analgesia may result from activation of a positive feedback loop in the mesolimbic system, causing continuous outflow from descending pain-inhibitory pathways (31). Acupuncture may be acting in part by activating diffuse noxious inhibitory controls.

No convincing theory to support the existence of meridians has emerged. Physiological correlates of meridians have been suggested, including electrical conductive properties and intermuscular or intramuscular connective tissue planes. Associations between acupuncture points and trigger points, and tendino-muscular and tendino-fascial structures have been reported. Acupuncture may produce immunomodulating effects akin to moderate exercise, although evidence is limited and mainly from studies in experimental animals. Further details of recent developments can be found elsewhere (32).

Practical aspects

Acupuncture treatment is individualized for each patient and requires a trained specialist practitioner (see www.medical-acupuncture.co.uk). Approaches to treatment can vary considerably in point selection, type of acupuncture, length of stimulation and frequency of follow-up treatments. Treatment is modified on a trial-and-error basis, according to patient responses.

Needles need to be inserted in areas where there are normally functioning nerves in order to stimulate subcutaneous, intramuscular and/or periosteal tissue. Western medical practitioners adopt a segmental approach to point selection by locating needles at dermatomes, myotomes and sclerotomes related to the affected structure (19). They often combine these with trigger points, tender points and 'strong' traditional extrasegmental points (e.g. L14) for maximum benefit. Trigger points are needled in patients with myofascial pain and musculoskeletal problems. Trigger points are hyperirritable spots in taut bands of muscle, which are painful on compression and give a classical referral pattern accompanied by a twitch response in many cases. These are common in cancer patients, for example those with breast cancer (33), and are exacerbated by stress, which is a common symptom in cancer patients. Interestingly, some acupuncture points are tender to palpation in health and worsen in disease. These points often appear in acupuncture 'recipes' for various conditions.

A typical initial course of acupuncture may consist of one or two treatments each week for up to six treatments. Acupuncture effects can be slow in onset and tend to be cumulative over time. Sometimes there is a lengthy induction time or inadequate analgesia, which requires initial analgesic supplementation. It is best not to start reducing current analgesic intake until any benefit kicks in. During each treatment, needles may be inserted for 10–30 minutes, although this depends on both acupuncturist and the individual response. Cancer patients tend to be sensitive to acupuncture so it is important to assess whether a patient is a 'strong reactor' at the initial visit. Cancer patients may rarely become sleepy during acupuncture, so nursing assistance is advised, especially during the first treatment. Treatment is then tailored according to need, with strong reactors given shorter, gentle treatments. Some practitioners attempt to elicit the needling sensation—'De Qi'—because they believe it is important for outcome.

Practice guidelines for the use of acupuncture for cancer patients have been published (34). These include the provision of clear instructions on how to use the needles for patients administering acupuncture to themselves, for example for hot flushes. Practitioners should give patients realistic expectations about the likely benefits of acupuncture for symptom control and coincidental improvement of other conditions such as migraine and hay fever.

Cancer patients with both early and advanced disease often need continuing intermittent 'top-ups' of acupuncture to maintain analgesia. Some cancer patients report a reduced response to acupuncture over time, and there seems to be an inverse relationship between tumour size and longevity of response to acupuncture, with larger tumours and more active disease having shorter analgesic benefits from acupuncture. Semi-permanent needles can also be used to prolong analgesia, and patients can massage them on an as-needed basis to increase pain relief.

Tolerance to acupuncture can develop over time and has been observed experimentally in animal models during prolonged electroacupuncture. Increasing the frequency of treatments has been used in late-stage disease to overcome acupuncture tolerance, although this is labour intensive. If sudden tolerance to acupuncture analgesia appears, the patient should be referred to the oncologist for further investigation as this may be a sign of the development of further metastases. Such patients may become acupuncture-responsive again following successful treatment of the metastases.

Indications

Acupuncture is increasingly being used for patients with cancer to manage a range of symptoms, which may or may not be related to cancer and its treatment. These include pain, nausea and vomiting, dyspnoea, xerostomia, radiation-induced intestinal hurry, ulcers that fail to heal, intractable fatigue, insomnia and vasomotor symptoms such as hot flushes (32, 34).

Cancer-related pain

Like TENS, acupuncture is useful as a stand alone treatment for a wide variety of pains that are acute or chronic in nature, with nociceptive and neuropathic components. Factors predicting success are not known and many patients with pain related to cancer and/or its treatment may respond to acupuncture. It can be used alone if patients present early, but more often it is used as an adjunct to analgesics or coanalgesics for cases that fail to respond to conventional approaches. Acupuncture is particularly useful for patients who are sensitive to medication and who experience unacceptable side effects. It can reduce peripheral neuropathic pain.

Acupuncture has been used alongside anaesthesia for cancer patients having major gastrointestinal surgery and has improved post-operative recovery with decreased analgesic requirement post surgery (35). Acupuncture is seldom used as a sole anaesthetic because it provides only a minority of patients with sufficient analgesia during surgery and it does not give adequate muscle relaxation for abdominal surgery and mechanical ventilation. Acupuncture can also be useful for phantom pain, possibly by sympathetic blockade via needling the paravertebral upper lumbar sympathetic blocking points to warm up cold leg stumps. Also, paravertebral upper thoracic sympathetic blocking points are used for phantom limb pain and pain in the upper limb or quadrant (Jacqueline Filshie, personal communication). There is emerging evidence to support the use of acupuncture and electroacupuncture for joint pains resulting from treatment with adjuvant aromatase inhibitors.

Acupuncture for non-pain symptoms

Stimulation of PC6 and/or ST36 with acupuncture, electroacupuncture or acupressure reduces nausea and vomiting associated with surgery and chemotherapy. Nausea and vomiting in late-stage palliative care is often due to a combination of factors, including medication, metabolic and electrolyte imbalance, anorexia, dehydration and gastrointestinal obstruction. If feasible, treatment should include targeting the cause.

RCTs for breathlessness in non-cancer patients with chronic obstructive cardiopulmonary disease have been positive. A case series found cancer-related breathlessness at rest was reduced using sternal and LI4 acupuncture in 14 of 20 patients, but a subsequent pilot RCT was inconclusive.

Anxiety, sickness and dyspnoea upper sternal points are used to control anxiety, sickness and dyspnoea using semiperminant needles in the form of indwelling studs. To maintain relief, patients self-administer on an as-needed basis by gently massaging the studs for one to two minutes. These studs can remain in place for up to four weeks at a time, covered with a clear plastic dressing.

A number of RCTs show acupuncture to be beneficial for xerostomia, including radiation-induced xerostomia, but not for Sjögren's syndrome. It is noteworthy that acupuncture relieved post-radiotherapy xerostomia (refractory to pilocarpine) in patients with head and neck cancer (36) and also in those with advanced cancer (37). Stimulation of parasympathetic outflow, which increases salivary volume and release of calcitonin gene-related peptide may contribute to success. Local facial points appear to be best.

Acupuncture can help control troublesome vasomotor symptoms associated with cancer treatment in both women as well as men. Prolonged relief can be maintained by weekly self-needling, although RCTs need to be performed to confirm these findings.

Acupuncture has also been shown to help heal radionecrotic ulcers, which classically never heal, and vascular problems, including ischaemic skin flaps. One clinical report showed that acupuncture improved radiation-induced intestinal hurry following radiotherapy for carcinoma of the cervix. Acupuncture is widely used by HIV-infected patients and can reduce HIV/AIDS-related diarrhoea and sleep disturbance. Acupuncture failed to produce any benefit for peripheral neuropathy, although a subsequent study was positive.

Safety

Contraindications to acupuncture include patients with needle phobia, intracardiac defibrillators (electroacupuncture) and severe clotting dysfunction. Acupuncture should not be administered locally to patients over an unstable spine due to metastatic disease because it is theoretically possible that the acupuncture may remove any protective muscle spasm around the unstable area, which would lead to cord compression or even transection. This is especially important in patients with good neurological function below that level. Acupuncture should not be given to limbs with or prone to lymphoedema, arms following axillary dissection or to tumour nodules or areas of ulceration. Semipermanent needles should not be used for patients with valvular heart disease, significant neutropenia or post splenectomy (34).

Acupuncture is relatively safe with a low incidence of serious adverse events when compared with conventional drug treatment (38). The incidence of significant minor adverse events arising from acupuncture has been estimated as 13–14 per 10,000 treatments, including a forgotten needle, fainting, bleeding and bruising, pain, and aggravation of symptoms (39). Other adverse effects include delayed or missed diagnosis of the condition treated, negative reactions such as vertigo, sweating, bacterial and viral infections (hepatitis B, C and HIV), and trauma of tissues and organs. Very rarely, serious damage to organs from needling has been reported, including unilateral and bilateral pneumothorax, and damage to the heart, liver, spleen, kidney, vessels and nerves. A working knowledge of basic anatomy and avoidance of deep-needling techniques suggested in some traditional textbooks should prevent such events. Cachectic patients should be needled superficially with particular care. All needles should be single use and disposable because bacterial infection has been described, including bacterial endocarditis, hepatitis B and hepatitis C.

A review of safety aspects of acupuncture in cancer patients emphasizes the need to continuously monitor disease progression because acupuncture can mask, for example, the pain of bone metastases (34). Hence, acupuncture should ideally be delivered by a physician/healthcare professional who has full knowledge about the stage and clinical condition of the patient, or by a practitioner who works alongside the oncologist. Artefacts have been reported on bone scintigraphy, where a patient with thyroid carcinoma had abnormal accumulation of iodine-131 on whole-body scan, which appeared similar to metastases. However, the cause appeared to be related to the presence of small gold needles used for acupuncture treatment. Practitioners should be aware of the possibilities of burns from faulty electrical apparatus for electroacupuncture and moxibustion. Needles which 'fall out' are a hazard and should be disposed of in a sharps box. Kits given to patients for self-needling should include a sharps box, which should be returned to the hospital for disposal.

Clinical research

A systematic review of acupuncture for cancer-related pain concluded that evidence was insufficient to determine effectiveness (40). Three RCTs were included in the review but only one was of good quality. It included 90 patients with neuropathic pain resulting from cancer treatment and found that auricular acupuncture was superior at reducing pain when compared with auricular acupuncture at non-acupuncture points and non-penetrating auricular acupuncture at non-acupuncture points (28). A further low-quality RCT of 76 patients with chest pain related to upper-body malignancies showed that acupuncture reduced pain when added to radiotherapy and chemotherapy when compared with radiotherapy and chemotherapy alone. A number of case series were included in the review and all reported benefits from acupuncture. Sample populations were cancer-related neuropathic pain, abdominal pain, nerve compression pain and breathlessness when pain was included as a secondary outcome measure. One study compared massage/acupuncture together with usual care and showed alleviation of pain and depressive mood in 138 post-operative cancer patients, although it was not possible to directly attribute the effects to acupuncture as it was combined with massage.

Clinical research is needed to establish whether acupuncture at specific points on the body can generate clinically meaningful effects. There are many challenges to acupuncture research. One approach has been to compare acupuncture point stimulation with non-acupuncture point stimulation. Western medical acupuncturists argue that stimulation of any point on the skin will produce neurophysiological effects as both treatments work on nerves and will have neurophysiological effects. This means that any needling sham treatment is an active control, even minimal needling. Another approach is to compare acupuncture with a sham intervention, although inappropriate sham controls are often used, e.g. dummy TENS and dummy laser. These controversies have led Dincer *et al.* (41) to conclude that it was scientifically unacceptable to summarize the variety of approaches used in acupuncture trials as 'sham or placebo controls' when assessing outcome in systematic reviews. Some investigators have invented sham acupuncture needles which telescope inside the handle instead of penetrating the skin, e.g. the Streitberger and Park needle, although they are also not completely inert because they cause some degree of acupressure. The Streitberger needle also engendered less activity on PET scanning, but less than a real needle, but more activity than a pin prick, described as an inert stimulus (42).

In 2001 the Centre for Reviews and Dissemination in the UK concluded that acupuncture was superior to no treatment or waiting list controls in most studies, but studies were evenly balanced between acupuncture and sham techniques (43). There are so many RCTs on acupuncture that investigators have started to systematically review the systematic reviews on the topic. Recently, one systematic review of the systematic reviews concluded that acupuncture improved nausea and vomiting (post-operative and chemotherapy-related), insomnia, fibromyalgia, osteoarthritis of the knee, non-specific back pain, dental pain, epicondylitis and idiopathic headache (44). Since then, two meta-analyses of acupuncture for osteoarthritis of the knee published within six months of each other seemed to have contradictory conclusions, with both showing clinical benefit when compared with waiting list or no treatment groups (45, 46). The widespread use of 'sham' control treatments, which are physiologically active, is widely responsible for conflicting reviews about the efficacy of acupuncture.

There remain great methodological inadequacies that bias trial outcomes in both directions. For example, the use of controls with active therapeutic effects and insufficient doses of acupuncture may bias outcome against acupuncture, whereas lack of blinding and inappropriate randomization may bias outcome in favour of acupuncture. This leads to conflicts in interpretation of RCTs and tremendous challenges for future investigators [47].

Summary

In summary, TENS and acupuncture have potential benefit for pain experienced by patients with cancer. There is considerable low-level evidence that TENS and acupuncture are effective, and limited high-level evidence to support their use to date. Both techniques are useful as an adjunct to pharmacological treatment and also for patients who have failed to respond to pharmacological treatment. Both techniques deserve further clinical scrutiny in well-designed RCTs. The methodological issues that hamper acupuncture research in particular might be best addressed by direct comparison with best standard treatment.

Case study–Pain in a cancer survivor

P is a 70-year-old lady whose endometrial cancer was treated by surgery and radiotherapy six years previous to her referral. She was well for two years post treatment but then developed long-term side effects of radiation with perineal neuropathic pain and bowel movements up to ten times per day. Since retirement, she had enjoyed a very active social life, which included walking up to ten miles a day.

She was otherwise in good general health, although was taking carbimazole latterly for thyrotoxicosis. She initially developed pain on sitting, which was exacerbated by walking, and the pain was so intense she was unable to sit down long enough to eat a meal or write a letter. When referred she needed to sit on two chairs with the perineum unsupported in the gap between the chairs to avoid overwhelming pain. Her pain scores varied between 3–4/10 and 8/10. Pain was exacerbated by bowel movements, necessitating a lie down for 30 min to recover. She had tried amitryptyline, which kept her awake at night, and co-dydramol, which reduced the pain by 50%. She was offered tramadol and gabapentin or acupuncture by another pain consultant. Her quality of life was greatly compromised and she became socially quite isolated by her symptoms. She was referred for a trial of acupuncture.

When referred, the plan was to give six weekly treatments using paravertebral and abdominal points predominantly for gastrointestinal symptoms and pain control.

After her first treatment her pain was slightly modified.

After her second treatment she was more mobile and felt much better generally.

After her third treatment there was significant improvement in perineal pain.

After her fourth treatment she could sit on a chair and recommence driving, also a decrease in nocturia and gastrointestinal symptoms was noted.

After her fifth treatment she could walk four miles again.

After her sixth treatment she was pain free.

After a six-week gap there was good symptom control.

She was subsequently given 'top-ups' at increasing intervals and is now pain free at her most recent six-month appointment.

Learning point

The benifits of acupuncture can sometimes build up over a number of weeks.

Acknowledgement

The authors would like to thank Mrs Jane Brooks at the Royal Marsden Hospital for her secretarial help. We wish to thank Oxford University Press for allowing reproduction of Figure 12.4.

References

1. Filshie J (2001). Safety aspects of acupuncture in palliative care. *Acupunct Med* **19**(2), 117–22.
2. Zech DF, Grond S, Lynch J *et al.* (1995). Validation of World Health Organization Guidelines for cancer pain relief: a 10-year prospective study. *Pain* **63**(1), 65–76.
3. Grond S, Radbruch L, Meuser T *et al.* (1999). Assessment and treatment of neuropathic cancer pain following WHO guidelines. *Pain* **79**(1), 15–20.
4. Johnson MI (2001). Transcutaneous electrical nerve stimulation (TENS) and TENS-like devices. Do they provide pain relief? *Pain Rev* **8**(3–4), 121–58.
5. Johnson MI (1998). The analgesic effects and clinical use of acupuncture-like TENS (AL-TENS). *Phys Ther Rev* **3**, 73–93.
6. DeSantana JM, Walsh DM, Vance C *et al.* (2008). Effectiveness of transcutaneous electrical nerve stimulation for treatment of hyperalgesia and pain. *Curr Rheumatol Rep* **10**(6), 492–99.
7. Avellanosa AM, West CR (1982). Experience with transcutaneous electrical nerve stimulation for relief of intractable pain in cancer patients. *J Med* **13**(3), 203–13.
8. Ventafridda V, Saganzerla EP, Fochi C *et al.* (1979). Transcutaneous nerve stimulation in cancer pain. In: Bonica J, Ventafridda V (eds). *Advances in Pain Research and Therapy* Raven Press, New York.

9. Librach S (1988). The use of transcutaneous electrical nerve stimulation (TENS) for the relief of pain in palliative care. *Palliat Med* **2**(1), 15–20.

10. Reuss R, Meyer SC (1985). The use of TENS in the management of cancer pain. *Clin Manage* **5**(5), 26–8.

11. Dundee J, Yang J, McMillan C (1991). Non-invasive stimulation of the P6 (Neiguan) antiemetic acupuncture point in cancer chemotherapy. *J Roy Soc Med* **84**(4), 210–2.

12. Pearl ML, Fischer M, McCauley DL *et al.* (1999). Transcutaneous electrical nerve stimulation as an adjunct for controlling chemotherapy-induced nausea and vomiting in gynecologic oncology patients. *Cancer Nurs* **22**(4), 307–11.

13. Chartered Society of Physiotherapy (2006). *Guidance for the clinical use of Electrophysical agents.* Chartered Society of Physiotherapy, London.

13a. Rosted P (2001). Repetitive epileptic fits—a possible adverse effect after transcutaneous electrical nerve stimulation (TENS) in a post-stroke patient. *Acupuncture Med* **19**, 46–9.

13b. Scherder E, Van Someren E, Swaab D (1999). Epilepsy: a possible contraindication for transcutaneous electrical nerve stimulation. *J Pain Symptom Manage* **17**, 152–3.

14. Bjordal JM, Johnson MI, Ljunggreen AE (2003). Transcutaneous electrical nerve stimulation (TENS) can reduce postoperative analgesic consumption. A meta-analysis with assessment of optimal treatment parameters for postoperative pain. *Eur J Pain* **7**(2), 181–88.

15. Proctor ML, Smith CA, Farquhar CM *et al.* (2003). Transcutaneous electrical nerve stimulation and acupuncture for primary dysmenorrhoea (Cochrane review). *Cochrane Database of Systematic Reviews* **1**, CD002123.

16. Robb KA, Newham DJ, Williams JE (2007). Transcutaneous electrical nerve stimulation vs. transcutaneous spinal electroanalgesia for chronic pain associated with breast cancer treatments. *J Pain Symptom Manage* **33**(4), 410–419.

17. Pan CX, Morrison RS, Ness J *et al.* (2000). Complementary and alternative medicine in the management of pain, dyspnea, and nausea and vomiting near the end of life. A systematic review. *J Pain Symptom Manage* **20**(5), 374–87.

18. Bennett MI, Johnson MI, Brown SR *et al.* (2010). Feasibility study of transcutaneous electrical nerve stimulation (TENS) for cancer bone pain. *J Pain* **11**(4), 351–59.

19. White A, Cummings M, Filshie J (2008). *An Introduction to Western Medical Acupuncture.* 1st Edn. Churchill Livingstone Elsevier Philadelphia.

20. Arun Maiya G, Sagar MS, Fernandes D (2006). Effect of low level helium-neon (He-Ne) laser therapy in the prevention & treatment of radiation induced mucositis in head & neck cancer patients. *Indian J Med Res* **124**(4), 399–402.

21. Cowen D, Tardieu C, Schubert M *et al.* (1997). Low energy helium-neon laser in the prevention of oral mucositis in patients undergoing bone marrow transplant: results of a double blind randomized trial. *Int J Radiat Oncol Biol Phys* **38**(4), 697–703.

22. Bensadoun RJ, Franquin JC, Ciais G *et al.* (1999). Low-energy He/Ne laser in the prevention of radiation-induced mucositis. A multicenter phase III randomized study in patients with head and neck cancer. *Support Care Cancer* **7**(4), 244–52.

23. Yurtkuran M, Alp A, Konur S *et al.* (2007). Laser acupuncture in knee osteoarthritis: a double-blind, randomized controlled study. *Photomed Laser Surg* **25**(1), 14–20.

24. Ebneshahidi NS, Heshmatipour M, Moghaddami A, Eghtesadi-Araghi P (2005). The effects of laser acupuncture on chronic tension headache—a randomised controlled trial. *Acupunct Med* **23**(1), 13–8.

25. Kreczi T, Klingler D (1886). A comparison of laser acupuncture versus placebo in radicular and pseudoradicular pain syndromes as recorded by subjective responses of patients. *Acupunct Electrother Res* **11**(3–4), 207–216.

26. Ezzo J, Streitberger K, Schneider A (2006). Cochrane systematic reviews examine P6 acupuncture-point stimulation for nausea and vomiting. *J Altern Complement Med.* **12**(5), 489–95.

27. Gates S, Smith LA, Foxcroft DR (2006). Auricular acupuncture for cocaine dependence. *Cochrane Database Syst Rev* **1**, CD005192.

28. Alimi D, Rubino C, Pichard-Leandri E *et al.* (2003). Analgesic effect of auricular acupuncture for cancer pain: a randomized, blinded, controlled trial. *J Clin Oncol* **21**(22), 4120–26.

29. Zhao ZQ (2008). Neural mechanism underlying acupuncture analgesia. *Prog Neurobiol* **85**(4), 355–75. PM:18582529

30. Lewith GT, White PJ, Pariente J (2005). Investigating acupuncture using brain imaging techniques: the current state of play. *Evid Based Complement Alternat Med* **2**(3), 315–319.

31. Han JS, Yu LC, Shi TS (1986). A mesolimbic loop of analgesia. III A neuronal pathway from nucleus accumbens to periaqueductal grey. *Asia Pac J Pharmacol* **1**, 7–22.

32. O'Regan D, Filshie J (2010). Acupuncture and Cancer. *Autonomic Neuroscience: Basic and Clinical,* **157**(1–2), 96–100.

33. Torres Lacomba M, Mayoral del Moral O, Coperias Zazo JL, Gerwin RD, Goñí AZ (2010). Incidence of myofascial pain syndrome in breast cancer surgery: a prospective study. *Clin J Pain* **26**(4), 320–5.

34. Filshie J, Hester J (2006). Guidelines for providing acupuncture treatment for cancer patients—a peer-reviewed sample policy document. *Acupunct Med* **24**(4), 172–82.

35. Kotani N, Hashimoto H, Sato Y *et al.* (2001). Preoperative intradermal acupuncture reduces postoperative pain, nausea and vomiting, analgesic requirement, and sympathoadrenal responses. *Anesthesiology* **95**(2), 349–56.

36. Johnstone PA, Peng YP, May BC *et al.* (2001). Acupuncture for pilocarpine-resistant xerostomia following radiotherapy for head and neck malignancies. *Int J Radiat Oncol Biol Phys* **50**(2), 353–7.

37. Rydholm M, Strang P (1999). Acupuncture for patients in hospital-based home care suffering from xerostomia. *J Palliat Care* **15**(4), 20–3.

38. White A (2004). A cumulative review of the range and incidence of significant adverse events associated with acupuncture. *Acupunct Med* **22**(3), 122–33.

39. MacPherson H, Thomas K, Walters S, Fitter M (2001). The York acupuncture safety study: prospective survey of 34 000 treatments by traditional acupuncturists. *BMJ* **323**(7311), 486–7.

40. Lee H, Schmidt K, Ernst E (2005). Acupuncture for the relief of cancer-related pain-a systematic review. *Eur J Pain* **9**(4), 437–44.

41. Dincer F, Linde K (2003). Sham interventions in randomized clinical trials of acupuncture—a review. *Complement Ther Med* **11**(4), 235–42.

42. Pariente J, White P, Frackowiak RS, Lewith G (2005). Expectancy and belief modulate the neuronal substrates of pain treated by acupuncture. *Neuroimage* **25**(4), 161–7.

43. Vickers A (2001). Acupuncture. *Effective Health Care Bulletin* **7**(2), 1–12.

44. Ernst E. (2006). Acupuncture—a critical analysis. *J Intern Med* **259**(2), 125–37.

45. White A, Foster NE, Cummings M, Barlas P (2007). Acupuncture treatment for chronic knee pain: a systematic review. *Rheumatology (Oxford)* **46**(3), 384–90.

46. Manheimer E, Linde K, Lao L *et al.* (2007). Meta-analysis: acupuncture for osteoarthritis of the knee. *Ann Intern Med* **146**(12), 868–77.

47. Thompson JW, Filshie J (1998). Transcutaneous electrical nerve stimulation (TENS) and acupuncture. In: Doyle D, Hanks G, MacDonald N (eds). *Oxford Textbook of Palliative Medicine,* 2nd edn. Oxford University Press, Oxford.

Chapter 13

The patient's perspective

Rosanna Heal

'If there's pain, it must be somebody or something's pain; somebody or something must be in it.' (Jerry Fodor, 'Headaches have themselves', a review of 'Consciousness and its place in nature: does physicalism entail panpsychism?' by Galen Strawson and others in *The London Review of Books* 24 May 2007)

The aim of this chapter is to highlight the relevance of the patient's perspective to the management of cancer pain, and to help clinicians appreciate the value of incorporating this perspective into their assessment and management plans. Although it would be helpful to focus in particular on the experiences of cancer patients undergoing interventional procedures for pain control, in practice the literature does not yield much in relation to this question: studies on interventional pain control concentrate above all on effectiveness defined mainly in terms of pain relief and avoidance of adverse physical consequences, with limited reference to the patient's view of the experience (1–5). This chapter therefore reviews some of the literature on pain assessment and management to see what can be said about the impact of both on the patient. How far has their viewpoint been explicitly considered, and does it tell us anything that can be applied to the context of particular pain control procedures? Does what we learn about pain and quality of life (QOL) help us look at aspects of cancer pain management from a different angle?

What *is* the value of listening to what patients have to say about their pain? Ever since Cicely Saunders coined the term 'total pain' (6), it has been recognized that pain is a multidimensional experience (7) and one that varies in expression and meaning from one individual to another. However, it has also been suggested that despite this holistic definition, a narrower biomedical model of care continues to dominate, even in palliative care, prioritizing symptom control over other aspects of care and regarding pain and other symptoms as, for example, 'the predominant cause of suffering in the dying'(8). Indeed, definitions of pain have sometimes reflected these differing emphases, being patient-centred or professionally defined to a greater or lesser degree. Paying attention to what patients say helps clinicians understand both the nature of the pain and what it signifies for the patient. If pain has a different significance for each of us, then so will its management. So while assessment alone is not enough ('asking patients about pain, without action, is a needless activity' (9)), a full and multidimensional assessment of pain is likely to lead to a better management plan (10). The patient's views need to be included in the management plan too, not only because their consent and cooperation are required, but because once the physical sensation of pain has been dealt with, other dimensions of pain, which may hitherto have been hidden, may be exposed. It is in these circumstances that the involvement of the multiprofessional team may be beneficial, and the chapter identifies some of the advantages of a multiprofessional interpretation of pain and how this can be balanced with the patient's voice.

In recent years a shift has taken place towards greater involvement in health care by users. A by-product of this environment in which patients are consulted, or at least asked, about their response to the care they receive may be stronger partnerships between patients and clinicians. Such partnerships are built on being able to look at treatment from the patient's point of view, seeing the patient in the context of their social environment and on clear communication about the purpose and possible outcomes of treatment; in other words, on clinicians being able to imagine themselves in the patient's shoes (Box 13.1).

Finding out what patients think: the context

Clinicians, in the UK at least, operate in an environment where the expectation is that patient views will be heard. In part this has come about because the growth of consumerism has made both providers and users of health care more aware of patients' rights, and patients better at voicing their increased expectations of good care. The last decade has seen a burgeoning of efforts to improve the quality of health care through different kinds of user feedback, consultation or advice, sometimes initiated by government (13, 14) and at other times through campaigns by individuals or organizations representing specific interest groups. Small and Rhodes give a comprehensive account of user involvement in health care, its many contradictory elements and the mixed motives for many initiatives ostensibly designed to maximize patient choice (15). They point out how choice may be an illusion when patients are in crisis and want a rapid response. Nonetheless, structures to facilitate patient and public involvement have been established, and evidence for building strategies to strengthen patient engagement is growing (16).

Box 13.1 Seeing the world through the eyes of the patient

The key question is what does the world look like through the eyes of my patient? The problem is that we only have access to our own perspective. We are not wired to our patient. We will never know what it is like to be him or her. The question has to be put over and over again without getting a final answer. In Zen buddhism there is a saying that when you have not seen someone for more than two minutes, you no longer know him (11).

'. . . you must have your antennae out as well for the unspoken things that people don't, can't quite voice because they don't think it's legitimate to voice it, but you must somehow hear those things as well if you can.' (12)

Initiatives designed to 'empower' patients in order to encourage genuine partnerships with clinicians have gone beyond regarding patients simply as consumers (17). Empowerment and genuine consultation are a tall order. But even on a more modest scale, attempts to obtain feedback on various aspects of care have proliferated. Surveys (18), focus groups and patient interviews (19) have begun to give healthcare providers better information about which aspects of care are experienced as satisfactory or unsatisfactory. Healthcare organizations in both the public and independent sectors have for some time been expected to demonstrate that they have undertaken surveys of patient care (20), even though it has been acknowledged that knowing just how much weight to give to patient perceptions is not a straightforward task (21).

As mechanisms for consulting and obtaining feedback from patients develop, so does patient access to alternative sources of knowledge, especially via the internet. Provision of clear patient information is regarded as an important quality measure and is included as a healthcare standard in the UK (22). Information has some potential to rebalance the power relationship between patient and clinician, and this may be one of the reasons that patient access to information and patient education are also emphasized in the pain management literature (23).

However, despite a social and political climate in which user consultation and feedback are encouraged and facilitated, and one where there is better access to information on disease and treatment, good communication between patients and healthcare professionals is still a challenging area of practice. While patients may now be more assertive and expect clinicians to justify their treatment decisions, it does not follow that they will be able to show such assertiveness when they are in pain or afraid.

Assessing cancer pain: the patient's perspective?

At the heart of what we know about pain lies the belief that pain is what the patient says it is (24). But patients do not or cannot always tell us all there is to say about their pain, nor do clinicians always know how to 'hear' what is behind the patient's expressions of suffering. By the time patients are being considered for procedures such as epidurals or blocks, they may have already experienced long periods of pain. How has their attitude been affected by previous pain control measures and with what expectations do they come to this 'new' pain treatment? Patient narratives reveal some of the complexities behind pain and its meaning (25, 26). Pain may mean different things to different people at different points in their illness (27). Larsson and Wijk carried out unstructured interviews aimed at exploring patient experiences of pain at the end of life (28). Some of the themes that emerged were the way in which pain became bound up with a preoccupation with the disease, uncertainty about the future and patients' contradictory need both to reveal and conceal their pain. Improved understanding of such factors has influenced the development of programmes designed to help people manage chronic pain of different kinds, such as the INPUT Programme at St Thomas's Hospital, London, a residential pain management programme, which recognizes, for example, the importance for patients of unshackling fear from pain before they can cooperate with pain management strategies (29).

Although pain assessment tools may appear to offer clinicians a clear route to the most appropriate form of pain management, assessment itself is not straightforward. Twenty years ago Walker *et al.* (30) remarked that 'pain charts in the printed literature are mainly concerned with assessment of acute pain whereas patients with cancer usually have chronic pain'. They go on to say that their research indicates that the assessor's view often carries more weight than that of the patient. More recently, Holen *et al.* highlighted the unsuitability of many pain assessment tools for palliative care patients either because they are too burdensome and therefore poorly completed or because they contain 'dimensions of limited relevance' (31). Caraceni *et al.,* while noting that clinicians do not always clearly define the outcomes they are seeking to achieve from pain control, they also identify problems in the use of pain measurement instruments, and observe that five of the studies into cancer pain assessment in clinical trials between 1999 and 2002 did not include any subjective pain assessment scale or questionnaire (32). The use of particular tools may arouse suspicion in some patients (33), who see them as only for the benefit of healthcare professionals. The importance of *simply asking people about their pain* has been stressed again and again, and while the signs are that this aspect of care is getting better, there is still room for improvement (34). The literature cites many examples of discrepancies between clinician measures of pain and those of the patient. There does not therefore seem to be any justification for not involving patients, even if patients do not or cannot communicate the full extent of their pain (35, 36) or have difficulty understanding the pain assessment tools used (37).

Pain management: the patient's perspective?

Barriers to pain management have been categorized as clinician-related, healthcare system-related and patient and family-related (38), and research has shown the many obstacles that stand in the way of patient cooperation with pain management plans (39). Other research has shown how culturally influenced beliefs about pain and cancer may be overlooked or misunderstood by pain clinicians, who as a consequence miss important opportunities not only to understand better the patient's view of the pain but also to treat it effectively (40).

What are the patient's and family's attitude to the use of opioids (41)? How does their culture or ethnicity affect their beliefs about pain? Do they regard pain with cancer as inevitable or think that it is impossible to control the pain any better (42)? It has been shown that stoicism and fatalism influence attitudes to pain and pain relief, as do other factors (43), all of which can create an unfortunate symbiosis with clinician-related barriers such as fear of patient tolerance of opioids or routine under-assessment of pain (44, 45). While elderly hospice patients may understand basic concepts of pain management, some nonetheless express the view that older people cope better with pain and observe that they are not taken seriously when they complain about their pain (46). Elderly people may be inclined to believe that they have no choice but to put up with pain (47). More specific fears can also interfere with patients' willingness to talk to clinicians about their pain, for example, the belief that 'good' patients do not complain, or that (cancer) pain means that the disease has progressed. Fear of injections is another factor that may make patients reluctant to be open about pain (48).

Patient 'satisfaction' and pain management

A common way of judging the success or otherwise of pain management is the admittedly ill-defined concept of 'patient satisfaction' (49, 50). Wilkinson has helpfully set out some considerations for establishing patient views on palliative care services, some of which could apply to other settings (51). For example, care must be taken when selecting the wording of satisfaction questionnaires as the same question differently expressed can provide very different answers. There can be problems with ceiling effects and response acquiescence (where respondents give the answers they believe the questioner wants to hear), and this is likely to be a bigger problem the greater the power imbalance between patient and questioner. Demographic determinants of satisfaction must also be taken into account (52). McKracken *et al.* in their study of satisfaction with treatment for chronic pain, review earlier studies on the topic and find that their applicability cannot easily be extended to patients who have different characteristics or who receive different treatments (53). They observe that 'commonly used satisfaction inventories reveal contamination with items related to the treatment context' and therefore do not actually measure patient satisfaction. The instrument they developed (the pain service satisfaction test) includes what the authors refer to as the behavioural, emotional and verbal components of satisfaction and their findings (based on less than half their sample of 114 patients attending a university pain clinic) suggested that 60% of satisfaction with treatment for chronic pain was accounted for by trust and confidence with the service provider, pain reduction and length of time waiting in the clinic. Significantly, the greatest influence on patient satisfaction derived from the nature of the patient's relationship with the pain physician. The authors claim that the findings can be extended to other chronic pain treatment contexts.

Indeed, other research has shown that patients may paradoxically express satisfaction with pain management even while they continue to experience pain. The investigation by Dawson *et al.* (54) into this phenomenon involved a study of a sample of 316 cancer patients in a primary care setting, of whom more than 75% were satisfied or very satisfied with their overall pain management, despite almost half of all patients reporting recent moderate-to-severe pain within the previous three days. The authors attempted to identify independent predictors of patient satisfaction with pain management by examining the multivariate relationship of satisfaction to patient demographics, the pattern of pain and pain treatment, patient beliefs and expectations about pain and pain relief, their behaviours such as willingness to report pain or take pain medication, and care from the provider. They identified two factors as being significantly predictive of higher levels of patient satisfaction: a primary care doctor or nurse expressing commitment to treating their pain, and long-term changes in pain. The results indicated, amongst other things, that low expectations were predictive of lower rather than higher satisfaction, and the authors suggest that 'if patients' initial expectations for pain relief are not fulfilled, they might adjust expectations downward, yet still remain dissatisfied with their pain management'.

In fact, the patient comments quoted in the study highlight the influence exerted by the patient's relationship with the healthcare professional: in the context of a good relationship, poor pain management could be regarded as satisfactory, confirming earlier research findings that patients express greater satisfaction if clinicians communicate that they want to provide pain treatment, even if the treatment is subsequently unsuccessful (55). Other studies, however, indicate that patients' trust in the clinician increases their willingness to participate in pain management, but that this is more problematic if patients have experienced earlier failures (56), an aspect that may be relevant to cancer patients contemplating interventional pain control measures. Efforts that concentrate on other aspects of the pain control system may bring all kinds of improvements, but not necessarily ones that are recognized by the patient. For example, a recent project designed to improve paediatric oncology pain control in Germany resulted in 'improvement in the structure, process and outcomes quality' of pain control services, but did not succeed in improving pain control 'to a magnitude significant to the patient' (57).

Research on patient-controlled analgesia (PCA) suggests ways of helping patients gain a different perspective on pain (58). Interestingly, Lehmann claims that one of the most important benefits of PCA has been the acceptance by clinicians of the principle of WYNIWYG (what you need is what you get), thus conveying the importance of assessing individual analgesic needs *and* of trusting the patient (59).

As indicated earlier, provision of information is often seen as a way of empowering patients to collaborate with clinicians rather than being passive recipients of clinicians' pain management strategies, but information has to be balanced with sensitivity to how much information the patient can manage before feeling overwhelmed (60). Patient expectations, the pain relief achieved, the intensity of their current pain experience and the information they have received about pain management are not necessarily factors in predicting satisfaction (61). A study of unmet analgesic needs in cancer patients concluded that patients who were dissatisfied with their pain control were also less likely than satisfied patients to have found that the pain information their doctor had given them was adequate (62). They were more likely to believe that their doctor was not as concerned about their pain as they were. Patients' understandable anxiety about whether or not they are believed is one that punctuates the literature on pain (63), with some justification perhaps, as health professionals do sometimes harbour doubts about the nature of patients' pain (64).

In situations where pain has not been effectively controlled, patients may be reluctant to consider an invasive procedure or, equally, be so desperate to achieve pain relief that they barely listen to the clinician's explanations of what the procedure involves. Patients who want to feel in control of events may find the risks that attend epidural or intrathecal procedures particularly difficult. These findings reinforce the importance of a trusting relationship between patient and clinician as the basis of good pain management. Without trust it seems doubtful that attempts to elicit patient views will meet with much success. The box below (box 13.2) offers some suggestions for establishing the patient's views on pain management.

Box 13.2 Establishing the patient's views

1. Communicate your commitment to tackling the patient's pain.

2. Make time to listen to what the patient has to say about the pain. Take account of cultural and individual perspectives.

3. Establish the patient's fears, hopes and expectations in relation to the pain control measure that you are considering.

4. Consider, together with the patient, different possible outcomes, their consequences and how this would fit with their priorities in life.

5. Establish what the carer's views are in relation to care that might be required once the procedure has been carried out.

6. After the procedure, seek feedback, either directly from the patient/carer or from other members of the multidisciplinary team.

7. Be prepared to find that improved pain control uncovers other issues the patient or carer may need help with.

Communication challenges in pain management

The value of good communication, encompassing listening and conveying understanding, has already been noted. Communication that takes account of patients' experiences and knowledge, and that of their families and carers is vital when describing the intended outcomes of procedures, the possible complications, how long the treatment is likely to be effective and how the procedure fits into the overall plan of treatment (65), as is conveying these matters honestly. Gilbert comments on the 'subtle forms of paternalism' that sometimes lurk behind the way in which clinicians describe the benefits of treatment options in order to avoid facing potentially distressing discussions with patients (66). Establishing the patient's, the carer's and the family's expectations of treatment (which may differ) is essential as it may uncover some of the deeply held beliefs mentioned earlier. Documenting the patient's goals for pain relief may also be helpful (67). Frames of reference may well differ between generations (68) and with different cultures (69, 70), but the same principles of careful listening and pacing of information apply. The encouragement given to healthcare professionals to develop better communications skills and to find out what patients' wishes are in relation to care at the end of their lives (71) may help them elicit patient preferences sensitively. Whatever difficulties may need to be overcome in order to communicate with patients about their pain can be magnified in patients for whom communication presents particular challenges, including the cognitively impaired, people with learning difficulties, and the very ill and frail.

Cognitively impaired patients are known to be at risk of under-treated pain (72). Communication of discomfort by cognitively impaired care home residents can be misunderstood: it may be perceived as confusion or agitation (73). Scherder *et al.*, reviewing recent developments in pain in dementia, argue therefore that more work is needed on differentiating between subtypes of dementia and different aspects of pain as well as suggesting that observation scales are useful in assessing motivational-affective aspects of pain for all patients, irrespective of cognitive status (74). Family members or carers may be in a position to interpret pain expressions, although the evidence indicates that use of proxies can be problematic (75–77).

Similar issues have emerged with people with learning difficulties. If difficult behaviour is treated at face value rather than as an expression of pain or fear, how well can the pain management strategy for a patient with learning difficulties be evaluated (78)? How much effort is put into establishing how much the patient understands and how far they are able to consent to a procedure? Fortunately, strategies and tools for communicating with cancer patients with learning difficulties are being developed (79, 80).

Cancer patients approaching the end of their lives have been the subject of separate study, but some of the same factors emerge about the challenges of seeking feedback from a patient group who may be unable always to speak for themselves (81). There is less time, and their priorities may have changed, reflecting a preoccupation with quality of life rather than treatment. What we are learning about quality of life may help clinicians think more widely about the context in which pain treatment services are provided.

Pain management and quality of life

The assessment of patients' QOL has become a recognized way of measuring patient-based outcomes of palliative care, where active treatment may have ceased and the aim is to support the patient, family and carers in the period up to the patient's death (82, 83). Multidimensional tools for assessing QOL have been developed by asking patients what concerns and factors they think contribute most to their QOL (84). Carr and Higginson (85) have argued that since QOL is by definition subjective and individual, any tools used to measure it should be patient-centred, sufficiently sensitive to the changes that occur at the end of life, yet not burdensome. This is a complex area where the relationship between pain and QOL is not straightforward (86), and pain may not always be the main concern for patients at the end of life (87). Mean QOL levels of a sample of patients with advanced cancer improved significantly during symptom control admission to a palliative care unit, but many patients who on admission had said that relationships with others were a more significant factor in their QOL than symptoms subsequently found that symptoms became important when they interfered with relationships (88). So, while symptoms may not always be the most important aspect in patients' lives, 'adequate symptom control may be a condition for the attainment of patients' most important life goals'. The QOL of patients with a short time to live may be affected by the side effects of analgesic techniques, once pain has been relieved (89). Yan and Myers' recent systematic review of the efficacy and safety of neurolytic plexus blockade compared with standard treatment in randomized controlled trials was unable to reach any conclusions about patients' QOL (90), and Kawamata *et al.* recommended further study into the relationship between pain management and QOL in patients at the end of life, their research having shown that QOL did not improve significantly after pain was controlled by coeliac plexus block (although they suggest that coeliac plexus block may have prevented further deterioration of QOL) (91). All these findings highlight the importance of exploring the relationships between pain and other aspects of patients' lives. However, in practice the pain clinician will not always have the time to do this, and this is where the benefits of a multiprofessional team can be appreciated.

Multiprofessional work and its contribution to pain management

The goal of integrating different aspects of cancer care in order to provide a seamless service for patients was a recurring theme in the Calman Hine report, which led to the reconfiguration of cancer services in the UK (92). The importance of a multiprofessional approach with what has been called an 'extremely complicated patient population' has been recognized before as a way of providing smoothly coordinated and appropriate care (93). However, a survey carried out in the UK suggests that 'few anaesthetists are involved in delivery of an integrated palliative care service and (that) only a small proportion of patients who could benefit from advanced pain management techniques do so' (94). Yet early multiprofessional assessment of pain and a coordinated response could mean less suffering and a swifter decision to offer interventional pain relief in appropriate cases. Of course, not all members of a multiprofessional team necessarily require face-to-face contact with the patient (indeed, some multiprofessional teams may be virtual rather than actual), but each will have a different body of knowledge upon which to draw (95), which can contribute to an effective pain management strategy. If it is true that 'a primary factor in the patient's experience of pain rests on the multi-factorial nature of cancer pain and suffering' (96), then a multiprofessional response would seem to be the right one. Sheldon has pointed out that patients will say different things to different people (97), so by bringing together the various accounts the patient has given of his or her pain, a deeper understanding can be reached, and even small improvements in the intensity of interprofessional collaboration seems to have benefits in terms of cancer patient pain management (98).

We know that pain affects not just the patient but also those around him or her (99), and that carers can spend a significant part of the day on pain management and worrying about the future (100). Nursing staff and social workers may be able to provide a fuller picture of the patient's needs and how they interact with those of the family or carer. This information is particularly vital if the patient is returning home with an indwelling epidural, for example, where the burden of managing the epidural and the fear of breakdown is likely to fall on the carer, and where normalizing experiences such as taking a bath are no longer possible for the patient. On the other hand, the pain of *not* being able to die at home may be such that professional and carer anxieties about effective support systems may have to take second place.

Many patients and families will be aware that interventional procedures are a final attempt to manage pain, and that they have run out of other options. This situation can magnify feelings of loss and fear of further deterioration and death. Awareness of the spiritual dimensions of pain, and of the fact that some people describe their spiritual pain in physical terms (101, 102), may be more quickly perceived and understood by some members of the team than others (Box 13.3).

Box 13.3 A person or a patient?

Our patients don't only want to be free of pain—they long to be useful, to be wanted, and to be needed. Yet our care system so easily makes people into patients. From being givers they become receivers. From doers they become passive recipients (*Doyle*, 103).

Conclusion

While research into patient perspectives on cancer pain assessment and management has enhanced understanding in this field, there remains more to be done, particularly in relation to patient views on interventional pain techniques. What contribution do such techniques make to the patient's overall disease journey, and do the timeliness of pain assessment and the pattern and nature of the previous pain management strategy affect how patients view them? The relationship between such techniques and the patient's quality of life is still largely unknown. What are the particular dilemmas created for patients and families by such interventions? Discharge of terminally ill patients with indwelling epidurals, for example, remains rare in the UK because of reluctance on the part of clinicians to shift the burden of responsibility onto patients and carers against a backdrop of minimal professional expertise in the community. This might mean that a patient who wants to die at home is prevented from doing so.

These questions are likely to remain relevant in the changing landscape of pain control and cancer services, while the patient's experience continues to play a crucial role in determining best practice for the future.

References

1. Williams JE, Louw G, Towlerton G (2000). Intrathecal pumps for giving opioids in chronic pain: a systematic review. *Health Technology Assessments* **4**(32) iii–iv, 1–65.
2. Perello A, Ashford NS (1999). Coeliac plexus block using computed tomography guidance. *Palliat Med* **13**(5), 419–25.
3. De Leon-Casasola OA, Kent E, Lema MJ (1993). Neurolytic superior hypogastric plexus block for chronic pelvic pain associated with cancer. *Pain* **54**(2), 145–51.
4. Kairalouma PM, Bachmann MS, Rosenberg PH, Pere PJ (2006). Preincisional paravertebral block reduces the prevalence of chronic pain after breast surgery. *Anaesth Analg* **103**(3), 703–708.
5. Wong GY, Carns PE Neurolytic celiac plexus block. In: de Leon-Casasola OA (ed.) (2006). *Cancer Pain: Pharmacological, Interventional and Palliative Care Approaches.* Saunders, Elsevier, Philadelphia.
6. Saunders C (2003). A voice for the voiceless. In: Monroe B, Oliviere D (eds). *Patient Participation in Palliative Care: a Voice for the Voiceless.* Oxford University Press, New York.
7. McGuire DB (1992). Comprehensive and multidimensional assessment and measurement of pain. *J Pain Symptom Manage* **7**(5), 312–19.
8. Corner J, Dunlop D (1997). New approaches to care. In: Clark D, Hockley J, Ahmedzai A (eds). *New themes in palliative care.* Oxford University Press, Buckingham, Philadelphia.

9. Maiaskowski C (2000). Two double-edged swords. *Pain Manag Nurs* 1, 27–8.

10. Frost M (2000). The role of systematic overviews of the research literature in identifying clinical evidence for pain management. In: Hilier R, Finlay I, Welsh J, Miles A (eds). *The Effective Management of Cancer Pain.* Aesculapius Medical Press, London.

11. Maex E, De Valck C (2006). Key elements of communication in cancer care. In: Stiefel F (ed.) *Communication in Cancer Care.* Springer, Berlin. 1–5.

12. Sheldon, F. quoted in Clark D, Small N, Wright M, Winslow M, Hughes N. (2005). *A bit of heaven for the few? An oral history of the modern hospice movement in the United Kingdom.* Observatory Publications, Lancaster. p186.

13. Department of Health (2007). Patient Advice and Liaison Services. Available from: http://www. dh.gov.uk/en/Policyandguidance/Organisationpolicy/PatientAndPublicinvolvement/ Patientadviceandliaisonservices/DH_4081305. Accessed 10 January 2010.

14. National Health Service Act (2006). *Section 242.* HMSO, London.

15. Small N, Rhodes P (2000). User involvement: selected review of the literature. In: Small N, Rhodes P. *Too Ill to Talk? User Involvement and Palliative Care.* Routledge, London.

16. Coulter A, Ellins J (2007). Effectiveness of strategies for informing, educating, and involving patients. *BMJ* 335, 24–7.

17. Department of Health (2006). Expert Patients Programme, and various websites such as www.cancer-pain.org.

18. Picker Institute website. http://www.pickereurope.org/page.php?id=1. Accessed 10 January 2010.

19. Wiles R (1996). Quality questions. *Nursing Times* 92(44), 38–40.

20. Department of Health (2002). *National Standards for Independent Healthcare,* C6.1–C6.4 pp 9–10. Available at: http://www.dh.gov.uk/prod_consum_dh/groups/dh_digitalassets/@dh/@en/documents/ digitalasset/dh_4078367.pdf. Accessed 15 February 2011.

21. Sofaer S, Firminger K (2005). Patient perceptions of the quality of health services. *Ann Rev Pub Health* 26, 513–59.

22. Care Quality Commission (2009). Essential standards of quality and safety. *Outcome 1: Respecting and involving people who use services,* p. 42. Care Quality Commission, London.

23. Lebovits A (2006). Psychological interventions In: de Leon-Casasola OA (ed.) *Cancer Pain: Pharmacological, Interventional and Palliative Care Approaches.* Saunders Elsevier, Philadelphia.

24. SIGN Publication no.44 (2008). *Control of pain in adults with cancer.* Section 1, Introduction, p 2. Available at: http://www.sign.ac.uk/pdf/SIGN106.pdf. Accessed 10 January 2011.

25. Kleinman A (1988). *The Illness Narrative: Suffering, Healing and the Human Condition.* Basic Books, New York.

26. Carr DB, Loeser JD, Morris DB (eds) (2005). *Narrative, Pain and Suffering.* IASP Press, Seattle.

27. Nekolaichuk CC, Bruera E, Spachynski K *et al.* (1999). A comparison of patient and proxy symptom assessment in advanced cancer patients. *Palliat Med* 13, 311–24.

28. Larsson A, Wijk H (2007). Patient experience of pain and pain management at the end of life: a pilot study. *Pain Manag Nurs* 8(1), 12–16.

29. Guy's and St Thomas' NHS Foundation Trust (2004). INPUT Pain Management. Available at: http://www.inputpainunit.net/. Accessed 10 January 2010.

30. Walker VA, Dicks B, Webb P (1987). Pain assessment charts in the management of chronic cancer pain. *Palliat Med* 1(2), 111–16.

31. Holen JC, Hjermstad MJ, Loge JH, *et al.* (2006). Pain assessment tools: is the content appropriate for use in palliative care? *J Pain Symptom Manage,* 32(6), 567–80.

32. Caraceni A, Brunelli C, Martini C *et al.* (2005). Cancer pain assessment in clinical trials: a review of the literature 1999–2002. *J Pain Symptom Manage* 29(5), 507–15.

33. Eun-Ok I (2006). White cancer patients'perception of gender and ethnic differences in pain experience. *Cancer Nurs* **29**(6), 441–52.

34. National Audit Office (2005). *Tackling Cancer: Improving the Patient's Journey.* The Stationary Office. London.

35. Breitbart W (1987). Suicide in cancer patients. *Oncology* **1**, 49–53.

36. Chan A, Woodruff RK (1997). Communicating with patients with advanced cancer. *J Palliat Care* **13**(3), 29–33.

37. Loftus LA, McIntosh J, Pearce E, Tolson D (2007). Implementation of SIGN 44 guidelines for managing cancer pain in a community setting. *Int J Palliat Nurs* **13**(7), 315–24.

38. Pargeon KL, Hailey B J (1998). Barriers to effective cancer pain management: a review of the literature. *J Pain Symptom Manage* **18**(5), 358–68.

39. Thomason TE, McCune JS, Bernard SA *et al.* (1998). Cancer pain survey: patient-centred issues in control. *J Pain Symptom Manage* **15**(5), 275–84.

40. Núñez Olarte JM (2003). Cultural differences and palliative care. In: Monroe B, Oliviere D (eds). *Patient Participation in Palliative Care: a Voice for the Voiceless.* Oxford University Press, New York.

41. Reid CM, Gooberman-Hill R, Hanks GW.(2008). Opioid analgesics for cancer pain: symptom control for the living or comfort for the dying? A qualitative study to investigate the factors influencing the decision to accept morphine for pain caused by cancer. *Ann Oncol* **19**, 44–8.

42. Koffman J, Higginson IJ (2003). Symptom severity in advanced cancer, assessed in two ethnic groups by interviews with bereaved family members and friends. *J Roy Soc Med* **96**, 10–16.

43. Ward SE, Goldberg N, Miller-McCauley V *et al.* (1993). Patient-related barriers to management of cancer pain. *Pain* **52**(3), 319–24.

44. Cleeland CS (1984). The impact of pain on the patient with cancer. *Cancer* 54/11 Suppl 2635–41.

45. Taye GA (2006). Pain issues from the palliative perspective: a survey of doctors in Hospital Melaka. *Med J Malaysia* **61**(4), 405–9.

46. Brockopp DY, Warden S, Colclough G, Brockopp G (1996). Elderly hospice patients' perspective on pain management, *Hosp J* **11**(3), 41–53.

47. Yates P, Dewar A, Fentiman B (1995). Pain: the views of elderly people living in long-term residential care settings. *J Adv Nurs* **21**(4), 667–74.

48. Ward SE, Goldberg N, Miller-McCauley V *et al.* (1993). Patient-related barriers to management of cancer pain. *Pain* **52**(3), 319–24.

49. Hall JA, Dornan MC, (1988). What patients like about their medical care and how often they are asked: a meta- analysis of the satisfaction literature. *Soc Sci Med* **27**, 935–9.

50. Scott A, Smith RD (1994). Keeping the customer satisfied: issues in the interpretation and use of patient satisfaction surveys. *Int J Qual Health Care* **6**(4), 353–9.

51. Wilkinson EK (1999). Patient and carer satisfaction. In: Bosanquet N, Salisbury C (eds). *Providing a Palliative Care Service.* Oxford University Press, New York.

52. Ipsos MORI (2008). *Frontiers of performance in the NHS II.* Available at: http://www.ipsosmori.com/DownloadPublication/1221_sri_health_frontiers_of_performance_in_the_NHS_II.pdf. Accessed 11 January 2010.

53. McKraken LM., Klock PA., Mingay DJ *et al.* (1997). Assessment of satisfaction with treatment for chronic pain *J Pain Symptom Manage* **14**(5), 292–9.

54. Dawson R, Spross JA, Hoyer DR *et al.* (2002). Probing the paradox of patients' satisfaction with inadequate pain management. *J Pain Symptom Manage* **23**(3), 211–20.

55. Ward SE, Gordon DB (1996). Patient satisfaction and pain severity as outcomes in pain management: a longitudinal view of one setting's experience. *J Pain Symptom Manage* **11**(4), 242–51.

56. Boström B, Sandh M, Lundberg D, Fridlund B (2004). Cancer-related pain in palliative care: patients' experience of pain management. *J Adv Nurs* **45**(4), 410–9.

57. Zernikow B, Hasan C, Hechler T *et al.* (2008). Stop the pain! A nation-wide quality improvement programme in pediatric oncology pain control. *Eur J Pain* **12**(7), 819–33.

58. Larsson A, Wijk H (2007). Patient experience of pain and pain management at the end of life: a pilot study. *Pain Manag Nurs* **8**(1), 12–6.

59. Lehmann KA (2005). Recent developments in patient-controlled analgesia. *J Pain Symptom Manage* **29**(5S), S72–89.

60. Hilier R, Wee B (2000). Decision making at the bedside: what constitutes 'best medical practice' in the management of cancer pain? In: Hillier K, Finlay I, Welsh J, Miles A (eds). *The Effective Management of Cancer Pain*. Aesculapius Medical Press, London. 25–30.

61. Corizzo CC, Baker MC, Henkelmann GC (2000). Assessment of patient satisfaction with pain management in small community inpatient and outpatient setting. *Oncol Nurs Forum* **27**(8), 1279–86.

62. Zhukovsky DS, Gorowski E (1995). Unmet analgesic needs in cancer patients. *J Pain Symptom Manage* **10**(2), 113–99.

63. McHugh G, Thomas G (2001). Patient satisfaction with chronic pain management. *Nurs Stand* **15**(51), 33–8.

64. Pasero C, McCaffery M (2001). The patient's report of pain: believing vs accepting. *There's a big difference. Am J Nurs* **101**(12), 73–4.

65. Phan CP, Madhuri A, Hassenbusch III J *et al.* (2006). Epidural intracheal analgesia and neurosurgical techniques in the palliative setting. In: Bruera E, Higginson IJ, Ripamonti C, Von Gunten C (eds) *Textbook of Palliative Medicine*. Oxford University Press, Oxford. 431–49.

66. Gilbert J. (2003). Palliative medicine. In: Monroe B, Oliviere D (eds). *Patient Participation in Palliative Care: a Voice for the Voiceless*. Oxford University Press, New York.

67. Ward SE, Gordon DB (1996). Patient satisfaction and pain severity as outcomes in pain management: a longitudinal view of one setting's experience. *J Pain Symptom Manage* **11**(4), 242–51.

68. Bird J (2005). Assessing pain in older people. *Nurs Stand* **19**(19), 45–52.

69. Surbone A (2006). Cultural aspects of communication in cancer care. In: Stiefel F (ed.) *Communication in Cancer Care,* Vol **168**: Recent results in cancer research. Springer, Berlin. 91–104.

70. Lister AN (1997). The influence of culture in pain assessment. In: De Conno F (ed.) *Proceedings of the IV Congress of the European Association for Palliative Care*. EAPC, Milan. 22–5.

71. NHS (2009). *National End of Life Care Programme*. Available at: http://www.endoflifecareforadults.nhs.uk/eolc/acp.htm. Accessed 10 January 2010.

72. Morrison RS, Siu AL, (2000). A comparison of pain and its treatment in advanced dementia and cognitively intact patients with hip fracture. *J Pain Symptom Manage* **19**(4), 240–8.

73. Cohen-Mansfield J (2004). The adequacy of the MDS assessment of pain in cognitively impaired nursing home residents. *J Pain Symptom Manage* **27**(4), 343–51.

74. Scherder E, Oosterman, Swaab D *et al.* (2005). Recent developments in pain in dementia. *BMJ* **330**/7489, 461–4.

75. Nekolaichuk CL, Bruera E, Spachynski K *et al.* (1999). A comparison of patient and proxy symptom assessment in advanced cancer patients. *Palliat Med* **13**, 311–23.

76. Hinton J (1996). How reliable are relatives' retrospective reports of terminal illness? Patients' and relatives' accounts compared. *Soc Sci Med* **43**(8), 1229–36.

77. Field D, Douglas C, Jagger C *et al.* (1995). Terminal illness: views of patients and their lay carers. *Palliat Med* **9**(1), 45–54.

78. Kerr D, Cunningham C, Wilkinson H (2006). *Responding to the Pain Experiences of Older People with a Learning Difficulty and Dementia*. Joseph Rowntree Foundation, York.

79. Royal College of Psychiatrists (2009). Books beyond words. Available at: http://www.rcpsych.ac.uk/publications/booksbeyondwords.aspx. Accessed 11 January 2010.

80. Donaghey V, Bernal J, Tuffrey-Wijne I, Hollins S (2002). *It's not all bad news*. Gaskell/St George's, University of London, London.

81. Fowler FJ Jr, Coppola KM, Teno JM (1999). Methodological challenges for measuring quality of care at the end of life. *J Pain Symptom Manage* **17**(2), 114–19.

82. Massaro T, McMillan SC. (2000). Instruments for assessing quality of life in palliative care settings. *Int J Palliat Nurs* **6**(9), 429–33.

83. Morgan G (2000). Assessment of quality of life in palliative care. *Int J Palliat Care* **6**(8), 406–10.

84. Bart HP, Osse MD, Vernooij MJFJ *et al.* (2004). Towards a new clinical tool for needs assessment in the palliative care of cancer patients: the PNPC instrument. *J Pain Symptom Manage* **28**(4), 329–41.

85. Carr AJ, Higginson IJ (2001). Measuring quality of life: are quality of life measures patient-centred? *BMJ* **322**, 1357–60.

86. Hwang SS, Chang VT, Kasimis B (2002). Dynamic cancer pain management outcomes: the relationship between pain severity, pain relief, functional interference, satisfaction and global quality of life over time. *J Pain Symptom Manage* **23**(3), 190–200.

87. Powis J, Etchells E, Martin DK *et al.* (2004). *Can a 'good death' be made better?: a preliminary evaluation of a patient-centred quality improvement strategy for severely ill in-patients*. Available at: http://www.biomedcentral.com/1472-684X/3/2. Accessed 13 September 2007.

88. Echteld MA, Van Zuylen L, Bannink M *et al.* (2007). Changes in and correlates of individual quality of life in advanced cancer patients admitted to an academic unit for palliative care. *Palliat Med* **21**, 199–205.

89. Kawamata M, Ishitami K, Ishikawa K *et al.* (1996). Comparison between celiac plexus block and morphine treatment on quality of life in patients with pancreatic cancer pain. *Pain* **64**, 597–602.

90. Yan BM, Myers RP (2007). Neurolytic plexus block for pain control in unresectable pancreatic cancer. *Am J Gastroenterol* **102**(2), 430–8.

91. Kawamata M, Ishitami K, Ishikawa K *et al.* (1996). Comparison between celiac plexus block and morphine treatment on quality of life in patients with pancreatic cancer pain. *Pain* **64**, 597–602.

92. Department of Health (1995). A policy framework for commissioning cancer services: a report by the expert advisory group on cancer to the chief medical officers of England and Wales. Department of Health, London.

93. Coyne PJ (2003). When the World Health Organisation analgesic therapies ladder fails: the role of invasive analgesic therapies. *Oncol Nurs Forum* **30**(5), 777–86.

94. Kay S, Husbands E, Antrobus JH, Munday D (2007). Provision for advanced pain management techniques in adult palliative care: a national survey of anaesthetic pain specialists. *Palliat Med* **21**(4), 279–85.

95. Payne M. (2000). *Teamwork in Multi-professional Care*. Palgrave, Basingstoke.

96. Chapman E, Hughes D, Landy A *et al.* (2005). Challenging the representations of cancer pain: experiences of multidisciplinary pain management in a palliative care unit. *Palliat Support Care* **3**(1), 64–9.

97. Frances Sheldon, cited in Clark D, Small N, Wright M, Winslow M, Hughes N (2005). *A Bit of Heaven for the Few? An Oral History of the Modern Hospice Movement in the United Kingdom*. Observatory Publications, Lancaster.

98. San Martin-Rodriguez L, D'Amour D, Leduc N (2008). Outcomes of interprofessional collaboration for hospitalized cancer patients. *Cancer Nursing* **31**(2), E18–27.

99. Ferrell B R, Grant M, Borneman T *et al.* (1999). Family caregiving in cancer pain management. *J Palliat Med* **2**(2), 185–95.

100. Ferrell BR, Ferrell BA, Rhiner M, Grant M (1991). Family factors influencing cancer pain management. *Postgrad Med J* **67**(Suppl 2), s64–9.

101. Mako C, Galek K, Poppito SR (2006). Spiritual pain among patients with advanced cancer in palliative care. *J Palliat Med* **9**(5), 1106–13.

102. Mystakidou K, Tsilika E, Parpa E *et al.* (2006). Psychological distress of patients with advanced cancer: influence and contribution of pain severity and pain interference. *Cancer Nurs* **29**(5), 400–405.

103. Doyle D (1992). Have we looked beyond the physical and psychosocial? *J Pain Symptom Manage* **7**(5), 302–11.

Appendix

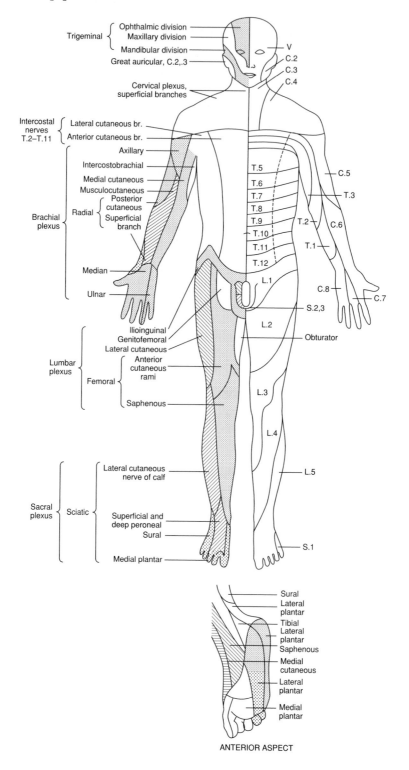

Trigeminal { Ophthalmic division
Maxillary division
Mandibular division
Great auricular, C.2,.3

V
C.2
C.3
C.4

Cervical plexus,
superficial branches

Intercostal nerves T.2–T.11 { Lateral cutaneous br.
Anterior cutaneous br.

Axillary
Intercostobrachial
Medial cutaneous
Musculocutaneous
Posterior cutaneous
Radial { Superficial branch

Brachial plexus

Median

Ulnar

T.5
T.6
T.7
T.8
T.9
T.10
T.11
T.12
L.1

C.5
T.3
T.2
C.6
T.1
C.8
C.7
S.2,3

Ilioinguinal
Genitofemoral
Lateral cutaneous
Femoral { Anterior cutaneous rami
Saphenous

Lumbar plexus

Obturator

L.2
L.3
L.4

Lateral cutaneous nerve of calf

Sacral plexus Sciatic { Superficial and deep peroneal
Sural
Medial plantar

L.5
S.1

Sural
Lateral plantar
Tibial
Lateral plantar
Saphenous
Medial cutaneous
Lateral plantar
Medial plantar

ANTERIOR ASPECT

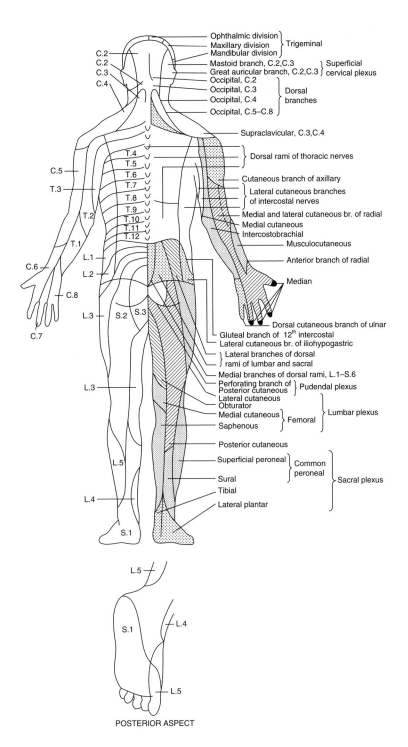

Ophthalmic division ⎫
Maxillary division ⎬ Trigeminal
Mandibular division ⎭

C.2
C.2 — Mastoid branch, C.2,C.3 ⎫ Superficial
C.3 — Great auricular branch, C.2,C.3 ⎭ cervical plexus
C.4 — Occipital, C.2 ⎫
— Occipital, C.3 ⎬ Dorsal
— Occipital, C.4 ⎭ branches
— Occipital, C.5–C.8

Supraclavicular, C.3,C.4

T.4
T.5 ⎫ Dorsal rami of thoracic nerves
T.6 ⎭
C.5
T.7 — Cutaneous branch of axillary
T.3
T.8 — Lateral cutaneous branches
T.9 — of intercostal nerves
T.2
T.10 — Medial and lateral cutaneous br. of radial
T.11 — Medial cutaneous
T.12 — Intercostobrachial
T.1 — Musculocutaneous
L.1
C.6 — Anterior branch of radial
L.2
C.8 — Median

L.3 S.2 S.3
— Dorsal cutaneous branch of ulnar
C.7 — Gluteal branch of 12ᵗʰ intercostal
— Lateral cutaneous br. of iliohypogastric
— Lateral branches of dorsal
— rami of lumbar and sacral
— Medial branches of dorsal rami, L.1–S.6
L.3 — Perforating branch of ⎫ Pudendal plexus
— Posterior cutaneous ⎭
— Lateral cutaneous
— Obturator
— Medial cutaneous ⎫ Femoral ⎫ Lumbar plexus
— Saphenous ⎭ ⎭

— Posterior cutaneous
L.5 — Superficial peroneal ⎫ Common
— Sural ⎭ peroneal ⎫ Sacral plexus
— Tibial
L.4 — Lateral plantar

S.1

L.5

S.1   L.4

L.5

POSTERIOR ASPECT

Dermatomes and sensory innervation.

Reproduced with permission from Longmore *et al.* (2010), *Oxford Handbook of Clinical Medicine*, 8th edn, Oxford University Press, Oxford.

Index

The index entries appear in letter-by-letter alphabetical order.